# DIABETE

**How to improve patient education**

# DIABETES EDUCATION
## How to improve patient education

Proceedings of the 2nd European Symposium of the
Diabetes Education Study Group (Geneva, 3–6 June 1982)
and selected topics held at workshops of the DESG

*Edited by*
**J.-Ph. Assal, M. Berger,
N. Gay, J. Canivet**

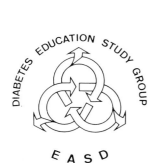

**1983**

**EXCERPTA MEDICA, Amsterdam-Oxford-Princeton**

International Congress Series No. 624

ISBN 0 444 90338 0

*Publisher:*
Excerpta Medica
305 Keizersgracht
P.O. Box 1126
1000 BC Amsterdam

*Sole Distributors for the USA and Canada:*
Elsevier Science Publishing Co. Inc.
52 Vanderbilt Avenue
New York, NY 10017

Printed in The Netherlands by Casparie - Amsterdam

# List of Contributors

John G. ALIVISATOS, M.D.
Director, Department of Endocrinology and Metabolism, Athens Polyclinic,
3 Piraeus Street, ATHENS, Greece

Jean-Philippe ASSAL, M.D.
Chief, Diabetes Treatment and Teaching Unit, Medical Polyclinic, WHO
Collaborating Center for Diabetes Education, University Cantonal Hospital,
1211 GENEVA 4, Switzerland

Michel BARTHOLOME, Eng.
Department of Applied Mathematics and Information Processing, University
of Liège au Sart-Tilman, 4000 LIEGE, Belgium

Michael BERGER, M.D.
Professor of Medicine, Medizinische Klinik E, University of Düsseldorf,
Moorenstrasse 5, 4000 DÜSSELDORF, Federal Republic of Germany

Charlotte BOENINGER, M.D.
Diabetesklinik, Wielandstrasse 23, 4970 BAD OEYNHAUSEN, Federal
Republic of Germany

Jean CANIVET, M.D.
Professor of Medicine, Hôpital St. Louis, 40, rue Bichat, 75010 PARIS,
France

M. Gyuala R. CEY-BERT
Sociologist, Research Director, Institut de Recherches de Communication et
de Motivation, 3 rue de la Cité, 1204 GENEVE, Switzerland

Ernst CHANTELAU, M.D.
Medizinische Klinik E, University of Düsseldorf, Moorenstrasse 5, 4000
DÜSSELDORF, Federal Republic of Germany

André CRUCHAUD, M.D.
Professor of Medicine, Dean, Faculty of Medicine (1978–1982), Geneva
Medical School, and Head of the Division of Immunology and Allergology,
University Cantonal Hospital, 1211 GENEVA 4, Switzerland

Christian DANTHE, M.D.
General Practitioner, 61 rue de l'Ancienne Poste, 1337 VALLORBE,
Switzerland

John K. DAVIDSON, M.D., Ph.D.
Professor of Medicine, Emory University School of Medicine, Director,
Diabetes Unit, Grady Memorial Hospital, 69 Butler St. SE, ATLANTA, GA.
30303, U.S.A.

John DAY, M.D.
Consultant Physician, Ipswich Hospital, Heath Road, IPSWICH, Suffolk,
United Kingdom

Françoise DOURVER, R.D.
Registered Dietician, Diabetes Treatment and Teaching Unit, University Cantonal Hospital, 1211 GENEVA 4, Switzerland

Donnell D. ETZWILER, M.D.
Pediatrician, St. Louis Park Medical Center, Director, Diabetes Education Center, 4959 Excelsior Boulevard, MINNEAPOLIS, MN 55416, U.S.A.

Nancy GAY, Ed.D.
Educational Consultant, Seyfferstrasse 18, 7000 STUTTGART 1, Federal Republic of Germany

Willy GEPTS, M.D.
Professor of Medicine, President, European Association for the Study of Diabetes, Department of Pathology, Akademisch Ziekenhuis, Laarbeeklaan 101, 1091 BRUSSELS, Belgium

Rolf GFELLER, M.D.
Assistant Head, Unité de Psychiatrie et de Psychologie Médicale, University Cantonal Hospital, 1211 GENEVA 4, Switzerland

Torbjørn GJEMDAL, M.D.
Assistant Head, Medical Department, Østfold County Hospital, Medisinsk Avdeling, Sentralsykehuset, 1601 FREDRIKSTAD, Norway

Colette GODART, R.N.
Division of Diabetes, Institute of Medicine, University of Liège, Bd. de la Constitution 66, 4020 LIÈGE, Belgium

Anne GÖRANSSON, B.A.
Department of Education, University of Linköping, LINKÖPING, Sweden

Vilius GRABAUSKAS, M.D.
Medical Officer, Office of the Director, Division of Noncommunicable Diseases, World Health Organization, 1211 GENEVA 27, Switzerland

Winfried GRANINGER, M.D.
II. Medizinische Universitäts Klinik, University of Vienna, Garnisongasse 13, 1090 VIENNA, Austria

Johannes J. GROEN, M.D.
Emeritus Professor of Internal Medicine (University of Jerusalem, Israel) and of Psychobiological Research (University of Leiden, Holland), c/o Department KNO, Academisch Ziekenhuis, LEIDEN, The Netherlands

André HAYNAL, M.D.
Professor of Psychiatry, Institutions Universitaires de Psychiatrie, P.O. Box 165, 1211 GENEVA 4, Switzerland

Mutien-Omer HOUZIAUX, D.Phil.
Department of Applied Mathematics and Information Processing, University of Liège au Sart-Tilman, 4000 LIEGE, Belgium

Lutz HORNKE, Ph.D.
Professor of Educational Science, University Institute, Kreuzenbergstrasse 45,
4000 DÜSSELDORF, Federal Republic of Germany

Michael O.C. JANUARY, Ed.D.
Educational Consultant, Seyfferstrasse 18, 7000 STUTTGART 1, Federal
Republic of Germany

Viktor JORGENS, M.D.
Medizinische Klinik E, University of Düsseldorf, Moorenstrasse 5, 4000
DÜSSELDORF, Federal Republic of Germany

Sven-Gunnar KARLANDER, M.D.
Department of Medicine, St. Erik's Hospital, 112 82 STOCKHOLM, Sweden

Alessandra KUNZ, R.N.
II. Medizinische Universitäts Klinik, University of Vienna, Garnisongasse 13,
1090 VIENNA, Austria

Anne LACROIX, M.S., Psych.
Educational Consultant, Diabetes Treatment and Teaching Unit, University
Cantonal Hospital, 1211 GENEVA 4, Switzerland

Pierre J. LEFEBVRE, M.D., Ph.D.
Professor of Medicine, Head, Division of Diabetes, Institute of Medicine,
University of Liège, Bd. de la Constitution 66, 4020 LIEGE, Belgium

Sylvia LION, Pharm.
Diabetes Treatment and Teaching Unit, University Cantonal Hospital, 1211
GENEVA 4, Switzerland

Johnny LUDVIGSSON, M.D.
Department of Pediatrics, University of Linköping, LINKÖPING, Sweden

Alfred S. LUYCKX, M.D., Ph.D.
Associate Professor of Internal Medicine, Head, Division of Clinical
Pharmacology, Institute of Medicine, University of Liège, Bd. de la
Constitution 66, 4020 LIEGE, Belgium

Ingrid MÜHLHAUSER, M.D.
Medizinische Klinik E, University of Düsseldorf, Moorenstrasse 5,
4000 DÜSSELDORF, Federal Republic of Germany

Henk PELSER, M.D.
Endocrinologist, Velazquezstraat 13, 1077 NG AMSTERDAM, The
Netherlands

Jean PIRART, M.D.
234 avenue Winston Churchill, 1180 BRUSSELS, Belgium

Albert E. RENOLD, M.D.
Professor of Medicine, President (1979–1982), International Diabetes
Federation, Director, Institut de Biochimie Clinique, Sentier de la Roseraie,
1211 GENEVA 4, Switzerland

Ulla RIIS, Ph.D.
Department of Education, University of Linköping, LINKÖPING, Sweden

Guido RUFFINO, M.A., Phil.
Professor, Collège Rousseau, 43 rt. de Frontenex, 1207 GENEVA, Switzerland

Myriam SCHEEN-LAVIGNE, R.N.
Division of Diabetes, Institute of Medicine, University of Liège, Bd. de la Constitution 66, 4020 LIEGE, Belgium

Wolfgang SCHNELLE
Expert for Group Communication, Managing Director, Institute METAPLAN, Goethestrasse 16, 2085 QUICKBORN, Federal Republic of Germany

Pierre SCHULZ, M.D.
Unité de Psychopharmacologie Clinique Extrahospitalière, Department of Psychiatry, University of Geneva, 1211 GENEVA 4, Switzerland

Gabriele SONNENBERG, M.D.
Medizinische Klinik E, University of Düsseldorf, Moorenstrasse 5, 4000 DÜSSELDORF, Federal Republic of Germany

Kerstin SPARRE, R.N.
Department of Endocrinology, Karolinska Hospital, Radmansgatan 1, 104 01 STOCKHOLM, Sweden

Katherine WASSER-HEININGER, R.N.
Medizinische Klinik E, University of Düsseldorf, Moorenstrasse 5, 4000 DÜSSELDORF, Federal Republic of Germany

# Table of Contents

# 1.  Foreword

J.-Ph. ASSAL, M. BERGER, J. CANIVET AND N. GAY

The idea of patient education and self-management as an integral part of treatment is now generally accepted for many chronic diseases. However, reality shows that patient education is far from being understood by medical teams in their daily routine. Our general concern is how we can better teach the diabetic patient for the improvement of metabolic control and prevention of acute and late complications of diabetes, but the principles described in this volume could be applied to the treatment of any other chronic disease.

The improvement of the educational process requires a systematic analysis of the various factors involved in the transmission of the message from the 'emitter' (the physician, the nurse, and the dietician who teach) all the way to the 'receptor' (the individual with diabetes). The teaching procedure should be analyzed just as systematically as if we were to examine the blood-glucose-lowering effect of a given insulin dose or analyze the insulin receptor site to better understand the biological effect of the hormone. Since we are deeply convinced that teaching patients is an essential part of treatment, we have to examine the teaching process as systematically as biochemical pathways or the pharmacology of a drug.

The chapters of this book include lectures given at the annual meeting of the European Association for the Study of Diabetes (EASD) in Amsterdam in 1981 and at the Second European Symposium on Diabetes Education in Geneva in 1982. Other articles deal with subjects which were discussed during the workshops of the Diabetes Education Study Group (DESG).

It was the editor's wish to include some personal experiences of physicians who have attempted to begin patient education programs on their own. Physicians, nurses and dieticians were also asked to write articles related to the psychological and pedagogical aspects of their work. This was a challenge and a calculated risk. The results may not be the typical medical papers which are found in professional journals. However, the readers within the medical community may find the educational and psychological aspects of patient education more understandable and relevant when discussed by their colleagues.

In addition, there are 3 articles from professionals in education, communications and audio-visual technology. These authors provide an objective, outside viewpoint on the application of their speciality area in diabetic patient education.

A global approach to the patient implies that the person who treats the patient is able to understand not only metabolic problems, but also other medical dimensions such as patient education and the reciprocal doctor/patient relationship. To delegate these dimensions to specialists would signify an unacceptable limitation of the physician's role in the delivery of diabetic care.

The editors are of the opinion that each chapter should be introduced by a small editorial note which will try to present the paper in a wider global context.

The editors are greatly indebted to Les Laboratoires Servier, France, which have been financially supportive since the beginning of the DESG in 1979, donating grants to cover the first 5 years of the DESG's activities. Without their support the numerous workshops, as well as this book, would not have been possible. The Second Symposium on Diabetes Education was made possible through the financial assistance of Becton and Dickinson, Boehringer Mannheim, Novo Industry and Les Laboratoires Servier, that the editors also wish to thank.

We also acknowledge the invaluable secretarial help of Mrs. J. Mange, Miss J. Meynet, Miss A.M. Niquille (all of Geneva) and Mrs. J. Garrett (Stuttgart).

# 2. History and aims of the Diabetes Education Study Group

J.-Ph. ASSAL, M. BERGER AND J. CANIVET

## EDITORIAL

*The following article is written by 3 officers of the Diabetes Education Study Group (DESG): J.-Ph. Assal, President; J. Canivet, Vice-President, and M. Berger, Secretary. They trace the history of the DESG since its beginning in 1977, relating both its accomplishments and its conflicts. The objectives of the organization, and the ways in which these could be reached, are outlined with indications of what has been completed as well as what is yet to be done. (The editors.)*

The Diabetes Education Study Group (DESG) is a section of the European Association for the Study of Diabetes (EASD). Its aim is to help the medical profession to realize the importance of patient education as a therapeutic measure and to analyze the needs and difficulties experienced by medical teams when they have to teach diabetics. The large and varied membership participation in the different medical fields concerned with diabetic education and care from all European areas, North, South, East, and West, provides the unique opportunity for multidimensional studies and approaches to the many facets involved in the successful education of diabetic individuals. This is well illustrated in the article *Difficulties encountered with patient education in European diabetic centers* (Chapter 13), which outlines the results of 6 workshops conducted by the DESG.

The starting point of the DESG was the annual meeting of the EASD in Geneva in 1977, when a day devoted to patient education was attended surprisingly by over 400 physicians. However, from that beginning in 1977, it took over 2 years before the actual creation of the DESG took place at the First European Symposium on Diabetes Education in Geneva in 1979.

The initial meeting in 1977 made us painfully aware of how mistaken we had been to believe that it would be easy to encompass the whole problem of patient education. As doctors, we had severe problems even to define our objectives for teaching patients. Furthermore, our academic training based on the physiological approach to diseases and our method of thinking (which is often binary, true or false) were of little help for analyzing the educational, sociological and psychological needs of the patients.

3

*J.-Ph. Assal, M. Berger and J. Canivet*

## THE NAME 'DESG'

The denomination of 'Diabetes Education Study Group' was not our first choice, but was selected after the process of rejecting 3 other names. Each of the first 3 names contained aspects which were not satisfactory to one or another of the medical interests within the DESG. Our developmental passage through a total of 4 names represents elements of almost all the problems involved in patient education.

We first thought of the name 'Study Group of Teaching Aids for Diabetic Patients'. This name did not last long. After the first DESG meeting, held as an adjunct to the annual EASD meeting in Geneva in 1977, it was evident that teaching aids are only a small part of the general process of learning. Teaching aids alone could not solve the many problems that patients encountered.

'Study Group on Patient Education' was the second proposal. This name seemed more appropriate than the first. However, only 'the receiver' (the patient) was included in the title without mention of the teacher (doctor/nurse/dietician) who provides the message. So the name was changed to the 'Study Group on Doctor-Patient Education'.

The third name represented the 2 poles of the educational process, the teacher and the student, who are linked by the information and feedback which flows between them. Nevertheless, this name also was replaced because several physicians said that teaching patients was not their duty. They viewed problems of inefficiency in patient education as almost always being caused by the patient. To prevent negative reactions from these physicians, the words 'doctor' and 'patient' were deleted from the Group's name, leaving the official title 'The Diabetes Education Study Group'.

The story of the development of the Group's name is not just an anecdote. It reflects a deep, almost unspoken problem in patient education. Doctors, nurses or dieticians who are knowledgeable in the field of diabetes and can express themselves easily among colleagues can be unaware of their own difficulties in a new role as teacher.

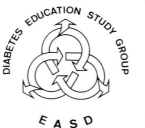

Fig. 1

## THE EMBLEM

The DESG needed an emblem which would symbolize its activities. We first thought of the famous symbol from Russian history, the 'Troika', which depicts a chariot being pulled by a team of 3 horses abreast. The 3 horses would represent diet, insulin, and exercise, equally pulling the wheels of diabetes. However, the horses did not symbolize clearly enough the *inter-dependence* among the 3 elements of diet, medicine, and exercise.

The emblem which we chose expresses the interdependence and interaction among 3 areas of *equal* importance (Fig. 1). A comprehensive treatment of individuals with the chronic illness of diabetes requires of the physician not only sound knowledge and skill in the medical field, but also in the psychosocial and educational domains.

The annual meetings of the EASD provide a remarkable stimulus for investigations into the causes of diabetes and its biochemical abnormalities. However, clinicians who experience the daily frustrations in treating the 10 million diabetics under their care in Europe need more than this yearly stimulus. Diabetic patients present these medical care providers with the psychosocial as well as the medical consequences of the disease. Self-care information and techniques need to be taught so that they are understood and used by these patients. It is in these psychosocial and educational realms that the Diabetes Education Study Group can make great contributions.

All of these biological, psychosocial, and educational aspects of diabetes are interdependent. A patient who is better controlled biochemically feels better psychologically. With a feeling of well-being, the patient is usually more ready and able to learn about the disease. It then follows that the patient who knows his or her diabetes and feels better psychologically is far easier to treat metabolically (Fig. 2).

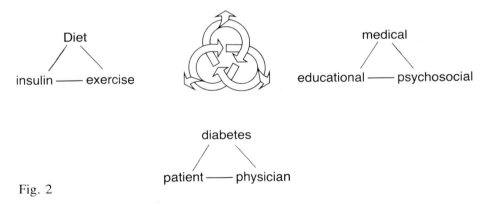

Fig. 2

## THE AIMS OF THE DESG

1. To increase effectiveness and efficiency in the treatment of diabetes.
2. To improve the quality of control in the non-acute phase of diabetes in which patient education and a meaningful doctor/patient relationship oriented to patient needs are crucial.

3. To foster diabetic research in the fields of diabetic treatment and patient education, and to develop means of evaluating patient education.

## SHORT-TERM OBJECTIVES

### I. Establishment of a list of members and centers

1. *Members:* The DESG is open to all persons who are actively involved in the treatment and education of diabetic patients, particularly physicians, nurses, dieticians and other health care personnel. Patients are also welcome. After 3 years of DESG activity, there are about 550 members, mostly physicians.

2. *Centers for patient education:* These are centers which have patient education organized into their daily routine; after 3 years there are approximately 240 centers registered in the DESG throughout Europe. About 80 of them run a patient education program daily.

3. *Centers for training doctors, nurses and dieticians for patient education:* Training of doctors, nurses and dieticians has to be organized at a post-graduate level. Some diabetic centers should be able to accept health care personnel for training sessions in patient education. A list of training centers throughout Europe is in the process of being compiled.

### II. Organization of workshops

To improve interaction and in order to share experiences among participants, small workshops with 20 to 40 people are organized with the following objectives:

1. To create inventories of the problems, needs, and ideas coming from the daily practice of the various medical professionals with diabetic patients. The results will help to plan training programs which will really meet the medical personnel's needs.

2. To create training workshops which would operate at national, regional and European levels. During the first 3 years of DESG activities, there were 10 workshops at the European level and 17 national workshops held in 11 different European countries.

## CONCLUSIONS

The complexity of the educational and psychological approach to patient education requires a wide range of knowledge and skill. The help of specialists in education and psychology is fundamental for understanding the effects of our actions and words on patients in educational programs. Such understanding will help in more effective future planning of training programs for patients and medical teams. This might help not only diabetic therapy but also the therapy of other chronic diseases, such as obesity, arterial hypertension, pulmonary and cardio-vascular diseases, etc.

Studies in the field of patient education are mandatory. The DESG should promote such studies, which should contribute to the improvement of the level of health care of the diabetic patient.

# 3. Patient education – the viewpoint of the World Health Organization

V. GRABAUSKAS

## EDITORIAL

*The opening remarks of Vilius Grabauskas, MD, representing the World Health Organization (WHO) at the Second European Symposium on Diabetes Education held in Geneva, Switzerland, stress the growing importance of controlling the world threat of diabetes mellitus. He outlines how both the WHO and the Diabetes Education Study Group (DESG) of the European Association for the Study of Diabetes (EASD) believe that effective patient and public health education is an absolute necessity to slow the increasing spread of chronic degenerating diseases such as diabetes. Dr. Grabauskas hopes that the results of this symposium will help to create the innovative ideas which can make diabetes education successful. The articles which follow his speech represent some of the thoughts presented at the symposium. (The editors.)*

It is a great pleasure and honor to address you on behalf of the Director-General of the World Health Organization (WHO), and to welcome all the participants who have found the time and possibility to attend the Second European Symposium On Diabetes Education convened in Geneva, June 4-6, 1982, to organize our knowledge in the combat against diabetes mellitus through education.

Amongst non-communicable diseases, diabetes mellitus has always been recognized by WHO as a problem of public health importance. The data available on morbidity and mortality, the expected population increase and the expected age group changes in terms of a higher proportion of older people make diabetes likely to become a worsening problem with an increased frequency of its complications. Becoming an increasing problem in both developed and developing countries, diabetes requires, in the framework of its management in the community, the organization of an adequate infrastructure of health services at the national level to cope with the problems.

It must be mentioned that despite tremendously expended research over the last 2 decades, which has resulted in impressive advances in knowledge with regard to diabetes mellitus, our ability to prevent or control the disease is unsatisfactory. On the other hand, even by implementing the knowledge we have at present, diabetes mellitus might be used as one of the model diseases to develop a community-oriented, chronic, degenerative disease control program because, in this particular case, the disease control depends very much on how the patient himself, his family, the medical personnel and the community understand the problem. As a matter of fact, the routine long-term management of diabetes mellitus (and this is also true of other chronic diseases!) rarely requires continual specialist experience provided that expert guidance is available when it is needed. This suggests that the most efficient way of using specialist skills is on a consultative basis combined with a greater effort to disseminate understanding of the problem to all health workers involved in the care process.

For specialists to act more as consultants would call for corresponding developments in primary health care, so that workers at this level would be better fitted to carry out control measures and to undertake routine long-term management. Redeployment of certain other services would be necessary since full exploitation of primary health care would be possible only if many diagnostic and therapeutic procedures were generally available at this level.

With the possible exception of the control of obesity, primary preventive programs for diabetes mellitus are difficult to conceive at the present time (further research is needed). On the other hand, secondary preventive measures must be stressed through mass education programs for the patients and their families as well as the public and health professionals, through early detection of high risk groups, case reporting and follow-up, and through the provision of comprehensive medical care.

At the present time it is difficult to correlate therapeutic measures for the control of diabetes with the prevention of its complications. However, special emphasis should be placed on the necessity of instituting the best possible course of treatment for each individual case.

One of the essential components in combating chronic diseases in general and diabetes in particular, is the intensive education of health personnel since each part of the public health service, preventive or curative, requires health personnel. Technical cooperation between countries in health manpower planning and education, especially for those in need, with first priority being given to developing countries, remains an important consideration in the program of the WHO.

The system to combat diabetes (and not only diabetes) at the population level among other important components includes health education, which must be considered as an integral part of intervention and as an activity aimed at assisting people to participate actively in health matters relevant to their personal and community interest on a sustained basis. Like general education, the goal of health education is a change in the knowledge, feelings and behavior of people. Usually health education concentrates on developing the health practices which will bring about the best possible state of well-being. In order to be effective, the planning, methods and procedures must take into account the process by which people acquire knowledge and change their feelings and behavior, as well as the factors that influence such changes.

In the case of patient/health-team-member communication, the effectiveness of the educational process will depend on the closeness between the teacher and the patient, and how successfully the teacher evaluates the motivation of the patient's behavior and can adapt to its changes. Patient instruction alone does not guarantee improved control of the disease. Patients must be willing to use that increased knowledge in a cooperative program of health care. Sustained behavioral changes require continuing communication and support.

My feeling is that the International Diabetes Federation, the Diabetes Education Study Group and the WHO certainly need special studies on individuals' attitudes toward their own health, motivation, etc. in order to improve our knowledge for creating more efficient educational programs incorporated into a community-oriented disease control program. As a matter of fact, the action to be taken to combat unhealthy behaviors on a large scale at the community level goes much further than the scope of diabetology. Such factors as poor nutrition, obesity, lack of physical activity, smoking, etc., contribute very much to the increased risk of the development of a group of chronic degenerating diseases, and their management is equally important for the primary as well as for the secondary prevention of these diseases. The WHO policy in this respect is to develop a community oriented, comprehensive approach in which health, social services and the community itself are to play equally important roles.

The First European Symposium on Diabetes Education, which was also held here in Geneva, was one of the starting points in combining the efforts of WHO and Non Governmental Organizations (NGO's), such as the IDF, EASD and DESG in the field of educational activities. And it happened, not by chance, that 1 of the 4 officially designated WHO Collaborating Centres for Diabetes was and is here in Geneva with Dr. J.-Ph. Assal as principal director. This WHO Collaborating Centre for Diabetes Education assists WHO in developing diabetes education programs as well as disseminating international experience in this important field. I think that this particular symposium will also contribute considerably to this task.

In conclusion I should like to return once again to the point indicating WHO's interest and concern in developing and implementing community-based national diabetes prevention and control programs. Within the context of these programs, educational aspects are among those of utmost importance. Surprisingly enough this field has been given appropriate attention on an international scale only relatively recently. Looking at the first report of the WHO Expert Committee on Diabetes you will not find education mentioned. The second report contains a whole section on this important subject dealing with the patient, the family, health care personnel, the community and policy planners in education and includes a list of resources needed and the role of various organizations involved. This shift reflects the progress made between the time of the first and the second report.

This particular meeting again is a demonstration of a great need for further developments in diabetes education, and I sincerely hope that it will contribute considerably to defining the most efficient strategy in achieving our mutual goal, Health for All, in which diabetes has an important role to play. I wish you great success in your deliberations.

# 4. World dimension of patient education

A.E. RENOLD

The present session on the activities of the Diabetes Education Study Group (DESG) of the European Association for the Study of Diabetes is the first formal and extensive opportunity for this Study Group to report on its activities.

It is not by chance that the President of the IDF has been asked to speak right after the President of the EASD. It was, and is, the natural consequence of the fact that my predecessor, Professor Rolf Luft, was one of the godfathers present at the official baptism of the Group interested in creating the DESG during the EASD Annual Meeting in 1977. Following the first large coordinating symposium in Geneva in 1979, the Group then undertook an exceptionally full and active programme under the energetic leadership of Drs. Jean-Philippe Assal in Geneva, Jean Canivet in Paris, and Michael Berger in Düsseldorf. Since then I have had personal experience of several 3-day Workshops organised during the past 12 months. I can report that these workshops have been enriched and made more profitable by the participation of all who were present – diabetologists, educators and paramedical personnel. The degree of interaction during these Workshops has both surprised and convinced me yet again that the concept of teaching patients and of teaching their teachers how to teach is a much more complex medical and social activity than generally acknowledged.

When I was assigned the topic: 'World dimension of patient education', what was probably intended was my reaffirmation of the universal urgency to provide all human beings, diabetic or not, and whatever their status of socio-economic development, with all the information available and needed to help them achieve the best quality of life. Patient education is of particular importance in chronic disease states, of which diabetes is a good example.

Prevention and treatment of most diseases involves some degree of modification of behavior. These modifications are based on the current understanding of the various disease processes involved. The modification of behavior required may be a simple one – such as the regular intake of vitamin C-containing foods in scurvy; the daily intake of thyroid hormones in hypothyroidism or the observance of straightforward rules of hygiene in avoiding many orally transmitted diseases. The behavioral modifications required may be more complex – such as giving up the belief that the wisdom and courage of ancestors and/or enemies may be acquired by eating their brains (thereby favoring slow-virus lethal disorders, for example); avoiding vitamin D intoxication as a result of repeated ingestion of highly prized morsels of shark liver by most Maori and Polynesian fishermen, or delaying coronary vascular accidents by modification of diet, of physical exercise, and of emotional adaptation to the stresses of daily life.

Transmission of behavior from one generation to the next or its occasional modification, has always been most successful when based on mystic, ancestral, religious or traditional authority. This is true even when no fact or evidence demonstrating the advantages of traditional behavior is known or remembered. Thus, the avoidance of pork in many parts of the world may well have originated from frequent observation of signs and symptoms associated with trichinosis, for example, but the great majority of strict adherents to pork avoidance accept this behavior on the basis of interdiction by sacred texts or the wise old men of their own population group. In general, strict and detailed rules of behavior are the hallmark of all tribal or otherwise closely-linked population units. Such rules serve many purposes, including the preservation of the identity of these groups and recognition of any foreign individual as a potential competitor or enemy.

In contrast to previous generations, people in a large part of the world are now often less closely bound in family or other traditional groups. As a consequence, factors other than ancestral tradition may become more influential in behavioral modifications. It would be ideal if such modifications could be directly related to new understanding of the disease process. The medical team can suggest such behavioral changes with the greatest authority only when they themselves are convinced of the validity of the basis for the change. On the patient's side there are additional factors which may well be linked with the ultimate success or failure of attempts at behavioral modifications. These factors are related to the patient's understanding of what he is being asked to do, the difficulty of what is being asked of him and to much more complex phenomena associated with the patient's perception of the cause/effect relationship as witnessed by the patient's own symptomatology. For example, it is much easier for a patient to understand the reason for treatment which immediately relieves symptoms, e.g. pain, than to understand the necessity for chronic treatment of an illness such as hypertension, which is presently symptomless but which may give rise to severe complications in the future. Thus, even the almost universally accepted negative relationship between good health and smoking or chronic alcohol abuse, exerts remarkably little influence upon the worldwide use of tobacco or liquor. Yet it is very likely that this influence would become greater if clear clinical or laboratory evidence of an *early* stage of evolution toward pulmonary cancer or hepatic cirrhosis occurred within weeks or months of beginning the abuse, and if the effectiveness of withdrawal could similarly be checked.

As far as diabetes is concerned, the behavioral modifications required of the patient are multiple, often perceived as indirect and inconvenient. In addition, the medical team has often considered the suggested modifications to be of largely unproven effectiveness. However, on a more positive note, there have recently been major advances in our knowledge of the scientific fields surrounding diabetes. These have given rise to a greater understanding of the heterogeneity of diabetes, to the hope of increased therapeutic efficiency through new insulin delivery systems and/or transplantation, and to the means for home blood glucose monitoring. These and other advances must be assimilated and rigorously tested by the medical team. More and more cross-information should then become available about the detailed nature and general effectiveness of the principal measures used to prevent the crippling complications of diabetes, and eventually those that might even prevent the disease. One of the results will be that the medical team will approach the patient with increasing conviction of the validity of their propositions. Surely this is an opportunity which must be explored in close collaboration with all interested and willing participants, in the hope of achieving sufficient motivation and participation of all patients and their families in the difficult and repetitive process of absorbing and applying the necessary educational input. Only this will permit each diabetic patient optimal participation in the increasingly effective prolongation of his life while striving for continued amelioration of its quality.

These are some of the reasons – of worldwide significance – that have brought us all together here today, and to which the Diabetes Education Study Group is seeking the best available responses.

# 5.   Patient education — the viewpoint of the European Association for the Study of Diabetes

WILLY GEPTS

The aims of the European Association for the Study of Diabetes are to encourage and support research in the field of diabetes and to facilitate the application of newly acquired knowledge to the care of diabetic patients. The organization by the Association of only one annual scientific meeting clearly does not represent an effective means to achieve this goal. Therefore the EASD has fostered the creation of Study Groups which provide adequate forums where specific problems related to particular aspects of diabetes are dealt with in more depth.

The Diabetes Education Study Group started in 1979 and, thanks to the activities of several physicians of this Group, soon proved to be one of the most active and effective. In the past 3 years, it has organized a large series of workshops which have helped to concentrate attention on what is well recognized as being the keystone of good treatment: education.

The aim of education is to motivate the patient to a proper understanding of his disease and thus improve the quality of his life. Diabetes is one of the most prevalent disorders affecting mankind. The improvement of its care should represent the ultimate goal of all those who are involved in its study. Maintaining lines of information about recent discoveries is only one of the goals of the EASD. Providing a scientific approach to the teaching of doctors, health care workers and patients is, in my opinion, an even more important duty.

It is well recognized that education, the transfer of knowledge, is a complicated process. This is especially so in the case of diabetes, a disease that affects individuals of all ages with different educational, social and environmental backgrounds. The principal aim of the Diabetes Education Study Group is to tackle the problems of patient education with scientific methods. These include a proper analysis of the problems and of the techniques available to solve them, the development of new, more appropriate techniques and a continuous re-evaluation of the achievements.

My presence at this European Symposium is intended to emphasize the recognition by the Association of the fundamental importance of the scientific study of patient education. It gives me great pleasure, as the President, to express the appreciation of the Association to the active members of this Study Group, for their admirable efforts to improve diabetes education as the most effective means of improving diabetes care.

15

# 6.   Patient education — the viewpoint of the Dean of the University of Geneva Medical School

A. CRUCHAUD

I feel certain that there is general agreement that at least some forms of diabetes may now be classified as autoimmune disease. The concept of autoimmunity was established about 25 years ago when it appeared that some people and experimental animals would raise reactions against self-components and develop autoantibodies. At that time we did not know what the pathogenetic mechanisms were and how autoantibodies would react against self-antigens. Later, we learned that on some occasions, autoantibodies may cause direct damage to cell membranes, as is the case, for instance, in autoimmune hemolytic anemia and thrombocytopenia. Also it appeared that autoantibodies may cause indirect damage to tissues by combining either locally or in the circulation with their corresponding antigens. When the resulting immune complexes deposited in the tissues are engulfed by phagocytic cells those release lysosomal enzymes or neutral protease which damage the neighbouring tissues. Finally, we learned that some autoantibodies may act on receptors present on cell membrane as is the case in thyroid diseases. In Graves' Disease, for instance, autoantibodies bind to TSH-receptors. This binding may activate the cells which then produce more thyroid hormones. In myasthenia gravis, autoantibodies are directed to the acetylcholine receptors at the neuromuscular junction; they compete with the binding of acetylcholine and therefore inhibit the process of muscle fibre activation. Finally, in diabetes there may be autoantibodies to insulin receptor(s) on the membrane of some cells and these antibodies may prevent the effect of insulin on these cells.

Now there are other receptors which have been alluded to in the foreword to the programme of this meeting. These receptors are the patients themselves. And these receptors, according to the talent of the teacher — that is to say, the physician, the nurse or the dietician — may be either activated or deactivated. This may result in a great deal of change in the control of their disease. I am sure that all participants at this meeting are not going to behave as inhibiting autoantibodies, but rather as activating mediators who turn on the receptors and make patients profit more from what they know and from what they have been taught.

# 7. From the diabetic to the medical world

NANCY GAY

## EDITORIAL

*This hard-hitting article from a diabetic reflecting on 32 years of living with the disease and the professionals in the medical field who have treated her, is based on the opening remarks to the Second European Symposium of Diabetes Education, June 1982, in Geneva. Based on the real life experiences of this diabetic, who is also an experienced educator, the article makes a strong case for patient education to be an integral part of the medical treatment for all diabetics and for a highly interactive relationship to be developed between patient and physician.*

*Prefaced by the author's personal history, thought-provoking examples of both negative and positive patient-physician interactions and attempts at diabetic education are discussed. A series of recommendations of successful educational techniques with patients challenges prevalent medical thinking.*

*If the views of the author are taken to be representative of the treatment and interactions experienced by a majority, or even a significant number of diabetics, then physicians face tremendous, but not impossible, tasks. A feasible, realistic approach to diabetic education based on a sound medical, educational, and psychological viewpoint needs to be developed with the ideas of the diabetics themselves integrated into the planning and formation of the programs. (The editors.)*

For 32 years of my 40 year life span I have been on the receiving end of insulin needles. Of those 32 years, I have lived 24 years in the USA, 4 years in Belgium, 2 years in England, 1 year in Switzerland, and I have just finished my first year in Germany. And by the medical community, to whom I am usually quite grateful, I have been:

| | | |
|---|---|---|
| treated | guided and | the lucky recipient of correct |
| well-treated | misguided | medical judgement and the |
| ill-treated | | unlucky recipient of both short- |
| untreated | trusted and | and long-term incorrect medical |
| mistreated | mistrusted | judgement |

17

If we can take some time in a relaxed mood, as if over a coffee in a comfortable restaurant, to consider some of my impressions and reactions to the medical professionals with whom I have been in contact, can I assume to speak to you as a typical, representative, long-term, insulin-dependent diabetic? You will have to decide.

A summary of my credentials to represent living with the real world of diabetes includes the following:

1. *The type of blood glucose (bG) control which I have maintained over the years has varied according to what was popular in the medical community at a given time:* From 1950 onward I began with 3 injections of regular insulin per day with a transition to 1 morning injection daily in 1954. During the first half of my diabetic life I was told to relax and not to be overly concerned with tight sugar control. Then, increasingly, I met the physicians who warned me that only tight control would slow the ever approaching diabetic complications. At age 34 another physician suddenly announced to me, 'You don't have to take only 1 injection a day'. It was like a very sacred, limiting rule had been erased for me. I was free to try 2, 3, or 4 injections daily of both long-term and short-term insulin in my constant efforts to understand the mysteries of blood glucose control.

2. *Luckily I had a good beginning:* A kind and wise pediatrician started Mother and Father well on the diabetic road with me. He spent the necessary time to educate them, and later me, so that we were not so afraid of diabetes and the family could have fun together.

3. *Early diabetic education was helpful, but not good enough:* Intensive diabetic education began for me around 12 years of age when I attended a diabetic summer camp. I appreciated the positive approaches to me as a child trying to learn selfcare and regretted the negative ones at this camp, although in 1954 I would not have put my feelings into those educational words.

4. *The stress of adolescence:* Later, as a teenager, I rebelled against my mother who then represented to me all of the diabetic schedules and restrictions. But then, near 18 years of age, I wanted to assume complete control of the diabetic balancing act so that I could leave home to attend a university. One of my greatest fears was that I would never be completely independent.

5. *A decade of unawareness:* In my 20's I didn't know whether I had good blood glucose control or not – sometimes I would seemingly forget that I was diabetic, except for that 1 injection daily. Thinking back over these years, the only real problems I encountered with my diabetes were during the long periods of frustration with either difficulties in one of my teaching positions or in my marriage. This was the beginning of my all too slow realization that months of anxiety and discontent could always, slowly, destroy my diabetic balance.

6. *Stress, conflict, and lack of good medical help:* The period of age 30 to 39 included agonizing too long over a divorce to end an unfortunate

marriage and finishing the many exams and long dissertation for the Doctor of Education degree. It was also a time when I lived in a small town and had difficulty finding a physician who understood my health problems.

I was ignorant that I had the subtle beginnings of diabetic complications and that the 3 medical doctors with whom I had consulted in this small town did not recognize the diabetic influences either. These 2 unfortunate conditions gave the complications time to develop. I am now aware that at all times I must know myself whether the medical doctor, on whose advice I am depending, is current on the care and treatment of diabetes. If she or he is not at least as current as I am in diabetic information, I must quickly find another doctor.

7. *The complications:* These began appearing during my mid-to-late 30's and included retinopathy; neuropathy of the feet, legs, intestines, and sixth nerve palsy; nephropathy; and hypertension. I discovered what a state of misery autonomic neuropathy can cause with endless nocturnal diarrhea followed by nausea with dry heaves.

I have had multiple laser photocoagulation therapy both with Argon and Xenon techniques since 1975. In the summer of 1978 I became legally blind from several major hemorrhages. Complete blindness lasted 5 to 6 months. During this time I was greatly helped both physically and psychologically by living for 5 weeks in a state institution to learn the basic living skills for the blind.

8. *Blood glucose testing:* Since 1977, I have traded urine testing techniques for a blood glucose reflector meter and Dextrostixs. This seemed necessary when I became aware (thanks to a good diabetic specialist) of my high renal threshold. With 4 bG tests per day, I can vary my dosage of regular and/or slow-acting insulin according to my actual needs.

9. *Diabetic Associations' help:* In the last 20 years of my diabetes the Diabetic Associations of both the USA and Europe have been an important source of information and support. I have worked for these associations as a volunteer counsellor to parents of young diabetics, an educator to adult diabetics, a speaker for clubs and schools, and a member of the Board of Directors for the American Diabetes Association in the very large city of Houston, Texas.

10. *Self-education:* Interviewing truly knowledgeable doctors from all the medical fields as well as teaching nurses and dieticians has helped me to keep up with the newer ideas and practical applications of same in the treatment of my own diabetes. Information and tips from fellow diabetics, who have already experienced complications which may occur for me in the future, have helped to increase my resolve to stay in good blood glucose control and to know the first signs of a new complication, so that I can seek medical assistance early rather than waiting until the problem is severe.

In addition I have needed to read as much as possible in the layperson's diabetic journals and information books which are helpful, as they summarize the latest research in language which is understandable to me without having to constantly refer to a medical dictionary. Lately, I have found it necessary to do research into various drugs and their interaction and side effects on diabetes when different medical specialists prescribe drugs for me without taking into account what another specialist has prescribed for me to take at the same time.

*11. Lifetime diabetic considerations:* Several major decisions in my life such as the selection of full time job positions, physical locations for living, and the choice of a husband have been made with diabetic considerations always present. According to several recent medical opinions, I may be headed toward possible renal failure, and probably a whole new phase of my diabetic life.

There you have an outline of the diabetic events which I think have helped to shape my thoughts on the interaction between medical professionals and the individuals with diabetes. These impressions and my own professional training and work have led me to the recommendations I wish to make to you – the medical people concerned with diabetes – while knowing full well that diabetics like myself are only alive because of people in your professions. Can there be an adequate 'thank you' from me to you for your work?

My university background includes a Bachelor Degree in English literature and history followed some 10 years later by 2 graduate degrees in Special Education. The 2 graduate degrees prepared me to work with the physical and psychological problems of handicapped students of any age as well as the highly intelligent, gifted student who often finds himself bored and unchallenged in the normal classroom situation.

The reason I stopped teaching in public schools to return to the university for graduate study in special education, was to attempt to help the students I found in my classes year after year who were emotionally disturbed, learning disabled, or exhibited severe behavioral problems which made academic learning impossible. Much of my recent work includes educational, legal, and psychological consulting with parents, teachers, and entire school systems.

After completing the Doctoral Degree in 1976, I received a scholarship for 12 months to work and study in the Departments of Education and Psychology at the University of Geneva. This was an outstanding opportunity because I had long been a supporter of the theories and application to education of developmental intelligence concepts as described in the many writings of Jean Piaget. Those of you who are familiar with the writings by Piaget and about his theories will, no doubt, recognize his influence in many of my references to the successes and failures I have witnessed in the attempts to educate diabetics.

## SUBTOPICS OF REFLECTIONS

An inner examination of the many reactions I've had towards the medical world leads me to suggest the following as important considerations for the medical professional who often works with diabetics: (1) respect for the individual with diabetes – LISTEN; (2) build the diabetic individual's self-confidence through a trustful partnership with yourself; and (3) create a total support system EARLY through personal, practical, concrete education with the sweet smell of success and the best learning often achieved through mistakes.

*1. Respect for the individual with diabetes – LISTEN:* Unfortunately several times I have met doctors either in a routine, first medical visit or in some sort of semi-emergency situation where the setting is something like this:

It is the first time you have met.

The doctor has no medical records on you.

The doctor views you with knowing sarcasm and says within the first 5 minutes, with a slight jeer, 'How many times have you been in ketoacidosis in the last year?' or 'How often do you eat something you shouldn't?'

Feeling strongly the distrust of the doctor and, therefore, pulling away psychologically and often physically, I was always put on the defensive as a young person. As I became older and more knowledgeable in diabetes, I simply felt disappointment in the physician for I knew we could never work together. So I would seek out a doctor who didn't prejudge me, but it saddens me to think of the many diabetics who are less experienced with both diabetes and the medical world and have to accept this type of attitude.

In talking with diabetics from teenagers through adulthood, the majority of them tell me observations about their diabetes that I know the doctor who is treating them needs to know in order to make a complete evaluation, but when I ask them if they have told their doctor the same information they are telling me, over half of them say, 'No, I can't tell him. He doesn't have time. (or) He won't listen'. Then I become frustrated because I know serious conditions exist which easily could be corrected if only the doctor knew about them.

Recently I had a rather violent reaction to the drug Reglan, which had been prescribed for me to help with the gastrointestinal disturbances related to autonomic neuropathy. After 5 doses I seemed to be unable to stop pacing the floor, my tongue swelled up and my neck went rigid with pain. I tried to remain calm as I realized the conditions were getting worse. Upon calling the local hospital where I normally go, I had to say that I had an emergency to be able to speak to a doctor. The physician who normally treated me was absent so a young doctor, who had spoken to me several times previously, answered. He had not heard of the drug, so he said he doubted that I had an emergency and that I shouldn't have telephoned to say I had an emergency when it was not so.

Later in the Emergency Room of the hospital, this same young doctor came to apologize for his statements on the telephone. He said he had been tired at the end of a long day, but how often can he afford to prejudge the patient without a fair hearing before a serious mistake is made?

In my own profession I would hate to think of the damage I could do if, when required to formally assess the intelligence and emotional stability of a student, I simply wrote, 'emotionally disturbed' or 'mentally retarded' on the student's permanent records because I'm too tired to do the job correctly and want to finish quickly.

2. *Build the diabetic individual's self-confidence through a trustful partnership with yourself, the medical person:* If I feel that doctor, nurse, or dietician trusts that I'm truly trying to do my best to control blood glucose, then I'm encouraged to keep and give correct and accurate information to that person. When I feel distrust, I think, 'What's the use of trying? He or she won't believe me anyway.' The atmosphere is set early for success or failure by the amount of trust I feel from the medical professional, for trust leads to a working partnership between the health care provider and the diabetic while distrust leads to isolation of each from the other.

The feeling that I do have the power, myself, to control my life – and for me that means to control my diabetes – grew through the efforts of every doctor, nurse, and dietician who made me feel that we were working together in a spirit of mutual trust to achieve the best possible health for me. If the trust was missing in my relationship with the medical professional, my self-confidence had to exist on its own, despite their attitude, until I could find a medical person who did send out a feeling of trust and cooperative teamwork between the two of us.

Without self-confidence about my diabetes everything else in my life becomes secondary. For me, an insulin-dependent diabetic whom many doctors quickly label as 'brittle', the very core of my existence is to be at peace with my diabetes. Many adults who have had diabetes for at least 5 years tell me the same thing. Of course, an individual's acceptance of and coping with diabetes is dependent on that person's degree of intellectual and emotional maturity, and how much accurate information he or she has received from the medical world.

Medical distrust, with an attitude of dictating what to do without any explanations as to the 'why's and wherefore's', leaves me with a dependency on the doctor that is dangerous. Diabetes is with me all the time; the doctor is not. So if the doctor is the only one in command of the necessary information to do all the reasoning, what happens when a problem occurs on Sunday afternoon and the doctor's nowhere to be found (as always seems to happen)?

I did not know the relationship of fever, vomiting, and diabetes for the first 15 years of being a diabetic. Somewhere in my mid-twenties I developed a violent case of the flu while traveling and a strange doctor, whom I had never seen before or since, treated me for emergency ketoacidosis in a hospital and took the time to explain what the diabetic should do during periods of flu and fever. Often it has simply been a matter of good or bad luck as to whether I find the needed information to understand the various problems in the management of diabetes.

Do the doctors and nurses really want to produce nonthinking diabetics who don't know how to handle an infection so that they always end up in an emergency situation in the hospital? Reason would say 'no', but that's what happens when the doctor seems not to have the time to explain or actually expects the diabetic to make no decisions without speaking with the doctor first (as all the early books on diabetes used to state so smuggly).

When I am in a lucky time period in which I have found a knowledgeable doctor who wants to think and work as a team to reach maximum blood glucose control, I become spoiled and start believing that the general treatment of diabetes is improving throughout the medical world. However, I only have to move to a new location and have to begin searching again for a new doctor, to become painfully aware how few up-to-date, knowledgeable, general medical doctors there are, who are not threatened by a diabetic who knows something about the disease. The doctors with no time to educate or explain as they work along, either have too many patients already or want to have more, for increased numbers represent more money.

Other doctors who do not share information with the diabetic patients themselves usually tell me of past negative experiences with patients who either didn't understand the explanations or used the information incorrectly. Then these doctors generalize the failures to the entire diabetic population when the failure initially may have been that the doctor explained in medical language far beyond the understanding of the patient. This is a common occurrence through which I have lived often, but I have gotten older and self-assured enough to say, 'Wait, I don't understand what that means'.

Many diabetics have told me that it's all too difficult to even try to understand medical explanations and yet when I explain the diabetic reactions in very simple, everyday language with examples from the diabetic's life, they often say, 'Oh, that's what the doctor meant'. Personally, I finally got so frustrated with medical jargon, that I bought a big, expensive dictionary of medical terms in self-defense.

Unfortunately, I have met several doctors who don't provide explanations for they seem insecure of their own self-image. They appear to want a vast difference created between what they perceive as their social and professional status and the patient's. Keeping the patients ignorant insures a relationship of very high to low (god-like to peasant). The relationship precludes team work and may be simply an insecure personality or one who has accepted, consciously or unconsciously, the cultural norm which dictates a god-like status for doctors. Or this may be a medical person who is just disgusted with the work altogether.

This point reminds me of a diabetologist to whom I was referred about age 16 or 17 when my pediatrician finally decided that I might be too old for him. I visited this diabetologist once with my mother. The doctor immediately told us that everything we were doing was wrong and that we should change it all beginning the next morning with the type of long acting insulin I was taking. His entire approach was to lecture and dismiss questions at the end of the session because he said we would see how much better things would be later. We were dismissed quickly and efficiently.

I don't remember which type of insulin this diabetologist recommended, but I remember how glad I was to get out of his office. Even as a teenager I wanted to be able to ask questions. On the second day of taking the insulin he prescribed, I almost passed out from low blood glucose while singing in the church choir on Sunday. I immediately returned to the same pediatrician who would talk with me. Maybe some of the diabetologist's ideas were good, but for me the thoughts were lost in his attitude.

3.   *Create a total support system* EARLY *through personal, practical, and concrete education with the sweet smell of success for the patient:* For me the ultimate goal of educating diabetics is to provide the possibility for each person's development into an 'active' (thinking) diabetic who is trying to understand his or her disease rather than passively following the last orders of the doctor with little or no understanding of what is happening or why. 'Active' diabetics can deal with emergencies or changes in time schedules that come with normal living. They are aware of what information to record for sharing with medical professionals and what types of questions they need to ask the doctor, nurse, or dietician when the opportunity arises. 'Active' diabetics do not wait until a minor problem has become a major one before going to see a doctor, because they are mentally involved in following each event to its possible conclusion.

'Active diabetics' are created through education that is matched to their level of intelligence, experience, and emotional development. This individualized approach to diabetic education may sound too difficult and time consuming considering all the uneducated diabetics, but actually it can be achieved by introducing all concepts with concrete examples and objects rather than by simply talking about them. After the diabetic begins to grasp the ideas being presented through concrete, actual objects, the education can move to the semi-concrete presentation of films, slides, and pictures. When the patient can ask intelligent questions and demonstrates understanding of the concepts presented concretely and semi-concretely, then the educator can use lecture alone and/or discussion groups to enlarge the concepts already presented.

The support which I have been lucky enough to receive as a young person was a mixture of correctly and incorrectly presented information. One summer at the age of 12 years, I attended a diabetic camp complete with horses, swimming, and camping out. The concrete aspects of this camp, like meeting teenagers who admittedly had not been taking care of their diabetes and already had serious complications or learning how to give an injection by watching other 12 year olds giving their own injections, left strong impressions on me that are with me still. Unfortunately, the concepts like the diet, the effects of exercise, or the action of various types of insulin were only introduced with lectures and pictures. These teachings did not even last long enough to go home with me after camp.

All the teachings could have had a lasting effect if the counselors (residents from the nearest medical school hospital) at the summer camp had introduced the concepts in the context of our daily lives rather than in abstract lectures. Mealtime would have been a good time to select one's own food from a buffet to be checked and discussed with other diabetics and finally approved by the dietician. The dietician could have asked questions of the diabetics sitting at each table to lead them into reasoning out the answers for themselves with the help of peer interaction rather than simply being told the answers, as is most often the case. The final decisions on food selection could have been approved by the dietician. Anything I 'discovered' by myself was always better remembered than anything which was only explained to me.

One of the greatest aids to my concrete diabetic learning has been the blood glucose machine. Never had the doctor's comments that I had 250 mg/dl or 320 mg/dl of glucose in my blood meant as much to me as when I was taking my own blood glucose at home, while thinking and charting insulin dosages daily by the blood glucose readings. Everything I had read and what various doctors had said to me about the changes in blood glucose began to make sense. It was like a whole new world and I was so glad to finally arrive there.

Blood glucose readings are a very strong reinforcer to continue good glucose control because they provide me with immediate, concrete evidence of success and, if not success, I have the necessary information to improve control. Blood glucose has always been an abstract concept for me which only became real when I started to have a hypoglycemic reaction or a 'cotton-mouth' with too high blood glucose. Now with blood glucose readings I know much more about my own diabetes. For example, I know how my body responds to 1 unit of regular insulin at a blood glucose range under 200 mg/dl as compared to a range over 200 mg/dl. I know exactly how much grape or orange juice to drink when the blood glucose is too low and that information keeps me from swinging up too high after the hypoglycemic state. What an improvement from the cave-man days of urine testing! I can avoid going into the high blood glucose ranges during flu and other illnesses for I can keep a constant, accurate check on blood glucose while using the readings to take the necessary regular insulin to combat the infection.

However, all this learning about my own body and reactions means that I have had to go through many periods of learning by my mistakes and, of course, those lessons so learned are well remembered. It was a great pleasure for me when I found doctors (and they are in the minority) who would use my mistakes, not to lecture or punish, but to ask questions that led me to 'discover' the reasons for my mistakes. These were the doctors who asked me why I thought a blood glucose of 300 to 400 mg/dl or a hypoglycemic reaction had taken place at a certain time and, after I had explained my thoughts on the question, this type of doctor would share information and/ or suggestions which would enable me to reach a more feasible conclusion. The medical professionals who do not take the time to help diabetics reach any of their own conclusions through their mistakes, rob the diabetics of one of their greatest learning tools.

If all information given to diabetics at any age was first introduced on the concrete level, there would be a good chance that everyone, except those with true mental defects, could assimilate and use the information. So why do medical professionals spend most of their time trying to teach only through talking? If current educational and psychological research is correct that 50% to 75% of the population – diabetic or not – must be physically involved in the action of doing something to understand a completely new concept well enough to actually use it in their own lives, then lectures and films alone are a waste of time. Most of the people who face diabetic education have the same need for the concrete, but I find it in very few diabetic educational programs. The best concrete approaches I have discovered so far have been in Geneva, Switzerland.

I have prepared a list of books which provide ideas and examples for converting any educational program into a developmental, concrete approach. This approach begins on the Concrete Operational Level and only progresses to the Semi-Concrete and Formal Operations (Abstract) Levels as the students exhibit that they understand and are using in their own lives the material which has been presented. This list is not in alphabetical order, but proceeds from the easiest to comprehend, most practical treatments of the subject to the more difficult theoretical writings. The list, which includes the prices and sources of the books, can be found at the end of this article.

The theory of keeping a concrete technique in teaching can also be enhanced by introducing material in accordance with students' interests rather than the planned agenda of a teacher. When the concepts under discussion relate directly to the thoughts of the student, the concepts become much more concrete for that student. The best example of this approach in operation that I have seen is holding a well organized and monitored discussion group. This is a chance for the psychological and medical world to cooperate to create a total approach to the problem of living with diabetes. Also, nothing will better help you, the medical professional, in gaining a more complete understanding of the personal, social, and medical concerns of your patients' diabetic lives (without having to live it) than to attend some of these meetings, but without saying one word in judgement about the behavior or feelings expressed by the participants.

26

RECOMMENDATIONS

**General recommendations to professionals in all the various medical fields involved with diabetes**

1.  Please use any approach which works – personal contacts, workshops, seminars, pressure on the medical schools for doctors, nurses, and dieticians – to spread knowledge of *current* diabetic education and treatment techniques to the front line general practitioners and medical people because they are frequently out-of-date. Many prescribe treatments from years ago. Educating the diabetic is still regarded as an extra frill if one has plenty of time and money. As a result, newly diagnosed diabetics and those with minor problems end up being referred to specialists because of poor early treatment.

2.  Try to create an atmosphere of trust and respect with any diabetic from your first meeting by listening carefully. You may be the first medical professional who has ever done so with this particular patient. The diabetic will feel more at ease to give you the necessary information to do your job well if he or she feels you are really interested in listening.

3.  Educate diabetics to become 'active' participants in the control of their disease by presenting all new concepts first with concrete, physical examples before any semi-concrete or abstract approach is used. Let the interests of the students influence the timing of the information given and use the patients' mistakes to lead them into 'discovering' the cause and effect of their actions rather than delivering a 'Don't do that again' lecture.

4.  Include the psychological and social as well as the medical aspects of living with diabetes to produce a total person approach for helping the diabetic during the difficult times. Well organized groupings of diabetics and also groups including those people most important in each diabetic's life can provide the needed interaction for concept formation.

5.  There is a desperate need for coordinating all of the various medical specialists who work with the diabetic. I have seriously considered writing a survival guide for diabetics on how to get your endocrinologist or internist together with your retinologist, neurologist, nephrologist, dietician, teaching nurse, etc. As the medical world becomes more and more specialized, the diabetic can be killed off by cross-medication as I have recently learned with antibiotics. I spend much time trying to make certain one specialist knows what the other is doing.

**Recommendations especially for medical doctors**

1.  Strive to maintain a trustful partnership with each diabetic as together you work to reach maximum control of blood glucose. A feeling of teamwork with the medical doctor leads the diabetic into a feeling of teamwork with his or her disease and isn't this attitude the key to success?

2.    Present the realities of all complications truthfully, concretely and early in the person's diabetic life. Do not paint too rosy a picture of life with diabetes, but make it very clear that the best hope to retard or stop the terrible complications is to maintain good blood glucose control. Of course, the approach must be adjusted to fit the age and maturity of the diabetic, but we all need the truth, EARLY!

3.    All the various specializing doctors must become part of the effort to educate so that the complications can be reduced or retarded. I have my eyesight now for 2 reasons: (a) laser and xenon treatments were done well and early (because of my own reading and research) and (equally important), (b) an internal medicine doctor had compiled a list of physical actions which can lead to bleeding in the eyes. He shared this list with me in the early stages of my retinopathy. Thank goodness!

Without this education I would never have regained my sight. Instead, I would have been like all the diabetics I met in the state institution for the blind who, never having been informed about the precautions, continued to bleed. They had received many laser treatments, but laser treatments without an adequate education program were a waste of time and money. Now I have compiled my own list including all the 'don'ts' given to me by the physicians who tried to warn me about dangerous physical actions, plus a few of my own discoveries. I pass the list out to retinologists and to diabetics with retinopathy.

The continuing frustration for me is that when I am now examined by retinologists they all make statements like, 'Amazing that you have such good vision. I can hardly believe it'. And when I try to mention the importance of good blood pressure control and avoidance of physical conditions that cause bleeding, it's as if I've said nothing. All they can say is, 'Look at that beautiful laser work. Who did the last treatment?'

4.    There are still medical doctors telling diabetics that it is not so important that they try to maintain good blood glucose control all the time (and I only mean under 200 mg/dl)! In speaking to several such doctors, I get the feeling that some of them don't want to put out the necessary effort and time to work for good control with each diabetic.

**Recommendations especially for teaching dieticians and teaching nurses**

Where are you? There just are not enough of you!! You can be found in rare numbers in the hospitals, but 95% of the doctors working mainly with diabetics have neither a teaching dietician or nurse on their team.

The diabetic cannot succeed without a complete understanding of the food he or she eats and I have met few doctors who give good instruction in diet. Unless the diabetic is a hospital inpatient, it is almost impossible to have a private or group session with a dietician.

The teaching nurses are crucial to the success of educating the diabetic! Teaching nurses, who are with the diabetics daily, have the most opportunities to teach through the concrete approach. These nurses can also be the link between the medical world and the diabetic's real world.

Doctors, why aren't you pushing for more of these people and letting them know how important they are?

## SUMMARY

This article presents recommendations for improving the effectiveness of medical personnel working with the treatment of diabetics. I combine my experience as an insulin-dependent diabetic with my professional background as a Doctor of Education specializing in the psychological and educational problems of handicapped students to present a pointed critique of the interactions between diabetics and the medical community as outlined from my own experiences. My overriding aim is to stress that a positive human relationship between the medical professional and the diabetic is basic for attaining a high quality of lifestyle for the patient.

## ACKNOWLEDGEMENTS

I am deeply grateful for the strong emotional support of Michael O.C. January and the midnight help of Shannon M.M. January.

## BOOKLIST FOR ADAPTING ANY EDUCATION PROGRAM TO THE DEVELOPMENTAL APPROACH ACCORDING TO PIAGET

This list is arranged to begin with the easiest to understand, most practical treatments of Piaget's theories in practice to the more difficult, theoretical writing. All books are in English with prices in dollars ($) unless otherwise indicated. Usually the fastest way to get books is to write directly to the publisher. All Piaget's original works are in French, but are somewhat difficult to understand for the beginner. The total library of his writings are at the Université de Genève.

Sund, R.B. (1976): *Piaget for Educators*. $8 to $9 from Charles E. Merrill Publishing Company, 1300 Alum Creek Dr., Box 508, Columbus, Ohio 43216, USA. The best for all beginners. Explains how to identify a person's cognitive level of thinking. A slide presentation to accompany the book can be purchased at additional cost for teaching larger groups ($115), but is not really necessary. (The 1976 Sund edition has recently gone out of print and a 1983 revised edition is available. The new edition was completed after Sund's death and is more complicated and ambiguous.)

Gallagher, J. McCarthy and Reid, D.K. (1981): *The Learning Theory of Piaget and Inhelder*. About $17 from Brooks/Cole Publishing Company, Monterey, California 93940, USA. Excellent overall view with concrete examples. Good to read after Sund's book above.

Furth, H.G. (1970): *Piaget for Teachers*. $6 or $7 from Prentice-Hall Inc., Englewood Cliffs, New Jersey, USA. Written in the form of letters to teachers explaining how to use developmental learning theory. Good after the reader has basic understanding of Piaget's theories.

Innhelder, B. and Chipman, H.H. (Eds) (1976): *Piaget and his School*. Available in English and perhaps in French and German for about $18 to $20 from Springer-Verlag Inc. in New York or Heidelberg or Berlin. One of the best collections of articles by 9 different members of the Faculté de Psychologie et des Sciences de l'Education, Université de Genève. Each article discusses one of the main ideas in Piaget's developmental psychology. (In New York ask for book number: ISBN 0-387-07248-9 and in Heidelberg and Berlin, number: ISBN 3-540-07248-9).

# 8. Our responsibilities in patient education

J.CANIVET, J.-Ph. ASSAL AND M. BERGER

Since the DESG was set up in 1978 it has collected a mass of information on the most varied aspects of patient education from doctors, nurses, dieticians, psychiatrists, psychologists, educationalists and from diabetics, too; this information revealed all the difficulties encountered. Faced with this wide-ranging information, the following problem must be considered: as specialists in diabetes, we have an individual responsibility towards the patients and, as members of the EASD, we have a collective responsibility towards them. Is it possible, on these grounds, to outline a general policy for education and to suggest the best place in which to carry it out within the framework of our countries' medical services and health systems?

The overall aim of care for the diabetic is presumably to avoid complications and to give him a sense of well-being. No complications means the absence of acute accidents (diabetic coma, for instance) and long-term complications. For the patient to feel well, he must be in good clinical condition and capable of leading a normal life, despite the presence of diabetes and the constraints imposed by the treatment which have to be accepted as a necessary hardship.

We must be aware that this aim is not achieved: too many diabetics feel unwell and suffer too often from avoidable complications. This leads us to ask 2 questions: 1) what are the causes of this failure? and 2) how can matters be improved?

## CAUSES OF FAILURE

The lack of success may be due to 3 causes: (1) treatment of the diabetes is ineffective; (2) the treatment arranged by the doctor is inadequate; (3) the care procedures are incorrectly carried out by the diabetic. The term 'care procedures' is used comprehensively, i.e. to cover the administration of drugs, diet, exercise, monitoring, follow-up and also a certain style of life and appropriate conduct on the patient's part in relation to the events and vicissitudes of life.

1. It may be admitted that no ideal treatment exists, in that we cannot successfully mimic the endogenous secretion of insulin and eliminate the insensitivity of the peripheral tissues to this hormone. Nevertheless, thanks

to improved methods of treatment and monitoring and to the advance in our knowledge, it is possible to achieve satisfactory glycemic control and to curb any associated vascular risk factors. Despite its imperfections, diabetic therapy therefore still enables the goal mentioned above to be attained; proof of this is provided by the diabetics – far too few in number – who have led a normal life without complications.

2.   With some patients the treatment is inadequate and/or the follow-up is badly organized. This results in failures for which the responsibility rests with the doctors, and usually with those in general practice. These failures do not concern the DESG; they are a matter for the EASD, which each year organizes a postgraduate training course for general practitioners in one of the European countries.

3.   How the treatment is applied is up to the diabetic, who should carry out all the care procedures correctly and find a compromise between the therapeutic imperatives and a normal life. The cause of the great majority of failures lies in the application of care procedures and the patient is the person responsible.

The poor application of this care is apparent from various investigations conducted in different countries [1-4]; even when diabetics had been given the necessary instructions, these were too often poorly understood and not put into practice properly: thus, for instance, urine was not examined regularly, the diet was poorly followed or insulin injections carried out wrong [1-3]. The study conducted in Paris showed that even if the patients carried out these procedures correctly, they had not understood the implications for themselves and were not sufficiently motivated to implement all the aspects of care correctly [4]. The studies conducted in Geneva showed that too often the care procedures were poorly applied because they were explained at a time when the patient had not 'accepted' his diabetes [5].

The care procedures are poorly applied because of negligence on the patient's part. This may stem from 2 factors: (1) it may be due to the patient's character – this applies to the individual who will not or cannot carry out the treatment correctly even though he understands his illness and what he ought to do; and (2) it may be due to the patient's ignorance or lack of understanding, which means that he is not motivated to do things properly or that he does not know how to. So, too many diabetics feel 'overwhelmed' by a disease and a treatment which they do not understand and towards which they then adopt an attitude of resignation and irresponsibility which accounts for their lack of care.

The patient is not the only one at fault, however. In order to ensure that care is satisfactorily applied, he needs help from those around him, sometimes from other diabetics and always from the doctor and staff caring for him (nurses, dieticians); the doctor's help is essential, as he is, in the patient's eyes, the expert on diabetes and the risks involved and how to avoid them. Therefore alongside his role as therapist, the doctor has a fundamental responsibility to educate the patient.

The doctor, in fact, takes on this role. For a long time doctors, in their surgeries and in hospitals or clinics, have endeavoured to educate diabetics by supplying them with the information needed to carry out the treatment, so that they can learn to look after themselves properly and avoid acute metabolic accidents. Hence patient education is not something new; it has always existed and is carried out by those concerned to the best of their ability. We are therefore bound to observe that it has usually failed to achieve its purpose.

We may then wonder whether such education is really worthwhile. It is undoubtedly impossible to give a plain answer to this question at present. We know of 2 well-conducted experiments, however, which demonstrated that education could reduce the incidence of complications and hospital admissions [6, 7]. It can therefore be assumed to be worthwhile. The reasons why it too frequently fails must then be sought.

The causes may be due to the diabetic and/or the doctor. The diabetic: as mentioned above, some patients refuse to come to terms with their illness and others lack the will to submit to the constraints of their treatment. Failures resulting from the patient's character are difficult to overcome; however, they are not the most numerous. The doctor: the patient's carelessness is usually due to his ignorance or failure to understand, showing that the doctor's attempt at education has failed. This proves how difficult the teaching is, as shown by all the information collected by the DESG, and this undoubtedly calls for special training for the doctor.

The doctors consulted by diabetics are usually general practitioners whether in their private practice, at a health centre or in a hospital medical department. They have no preparation for the task of teaching and, in this connection, have one or more gaps, such as: (1) lack of expertise since they must know all the fields in medicine, and diabetes represents only a modest portion of all medical knowledge; (2) lack of experience, as diabetics constitute only a very small number of the total patients under their care; (3) lack of time, having no regard to the considerable attention required by diabetics; (4) lack of educational skills, which the universities do not teach their students. Even when patients attend a diabetes centre, the education is often not carried out by experienced diabetes specialists, who are too taken up by other tasks, but by temporary medical staff (housemen, residents) who are themselves at the centre for a training period and therefore also suffer from the gaps mentioned above. In some hospital systems the education is entrusted to the nurses and dieticians, who are well-qualified as regards everything within their competence (practical know-how, diet, how to cope with certain situations, such as hypoglycemic distress), provided that they have had a fair amount of experience with diabetics. These collaborators are valuable and essential but they also suffer from some of the deficiencies referred to above and cannot provide on their own all the information necessary for a complete education.

A special case and one not open to criticism is that of the diabetes specialist in private practice who instructs his patient himself over several consultations. This situation is not taken into account here as it concerns only a very small number of doctors.

## HOW CAN MATTERS BE IMPROVED?

We are all aware that this is very difficult. The individual effort made by each of us in his own sphere is important; everything that we have learnt and still have to learn in the DESG will enable us to understand and educate our patients better. But that is definitely not enough; we must also, by virtue of our responsibility, discover whether a policy for educating diabetics can be put forward.

The communications and discussions at DESG meetings have more clearly defined the needs of the patients, what they expect from us and what we must make them understand. The outcome is that patient education should have a threefold goal that may be outlined as follows: (1) To supply the practical skills necessary for daily care (diet, insulin injections, urine examinations, self-determination of the blood sugar, if necessary, and recognition and prevention of hypoglycemic accidents). This is generally done, more or less successfully. (2) To provide the theoretical knowledge required to motivate the diabetic to carry out the care procedures correctly, which can only be achieved if he has understood the significance of the medical strategy of care, i.e. of the treatment, monitoring and follow-up (for this purpose he must understand the implications for him of being a diabetic, the current and long-term risks, the reasons for the problems encountered in achieving and maintaining good control, the reasons for the follow-up and the various recurrent examinations). This is not often or inadequately done and not made clear to the patient. (3) To listen to the patient, as often and as long as necessary, and throughout his lifetime, as diabetes is a disease that is difficult to come to terms with. The constraints imposed by the care required are onerous and create problems which cannot be solved unless they have been explained and understood. For want of time and experience, this task of listening to the patient is poorly carried out and affords the diabetic little help.

How could patient education be adapted to fulfil this threefold goal?

Since the great majority of diabetics consult a general practitioner at his surgery or the doctor of internal medicine at a hospital or clinic, it might be suggested that they should acquire the knowledge, experience and educational skills that are essential. This is tantamount to saying that they ought to become experts on diabetes and education, which is manifestly impossible. It would nevertheless be desirable for some to attempt this and encouragement and help should be forthcoming.

Another way would be to set up independent units for educating diabetics on the lines of what has been done in Geneva. The advantages of this system are well-known. The difficulty would doubtless lie in convincing the responsible authorities of the various countries of their value.

Yet another method would be to use the diabetes centres already existing in most countries, which have the advantage of possessing the necessary expertise and experience. Not all of them would undertake such an onerous mission, as many are oriented towards problems of treatment, research, university teaching or other tasks. It would probably suffice, however, if only some of them in each country would accept this responsibility. It should be coupled with certain conditions: (1) the education should be carried out continuously over an extended period (a few years at least); (2) among the departmental medical staff one or more diabetes specialists should agree to contribute to and direct the patients' education; (3) the centre should be provided with or be able to provide itself with the necessary facilities (premises, diet kitchen, documentation, equipment, audio-visual system) and staff (nurses, dieticians, chiropodists, even a psychiatrist and psychologist) in a sufficient number so that, in addition to their other duties, they can devote the required time to education; it should also have a secretarial staff available that can, once the education has been completed, supply all necessary information to the doctors who have sent the patient and who treat him subsequently.

The way in which these centres would be appointed would depend on the customs in the country; it could be done by the health authorities, the university, the national diabetics' and doctors' associations or by any other means.

This latter pattern of education could be of advantage in establishing close relations between these centres and the doctors caring for the diabetics. This would benefit the patients, who would be better educated and yet still be looked after by their own doctors, and also the practitioners, who would thus be relieved of a task which they cannot undertake satisfactorily and who would, moreover, be helped by the centre's advice concerning the subsequent treatment and follow-up of their diabetic patients.

CONCLUSION

Too often the results of treating diabetics are disappointing. These failures are generally due to faulty application of the care procedures. This stems from too much carelessness on the part of the patient, because he has not understood the real implications for him as a diabetic and is consequently not sufficiently motivated to look after himself properly. The education given hitherto, in the majority of cases by medical practitioners, has therefore been largely unsuccessful. It has become apparent that this education is a difficult task calling for special skills. So, rather than trying to transform general practitioners into diabetes specialists and educators, which is an impossibility, it is proposed that we seek other solutions. This task could,

*J. Canivet, J.-Ph. Assal and M. Berger*

for example, be entrusted to certain diabetes centres, which already exist in all countries and which would, if necessary, have to equip themselves for this mission. Such a solution would enable the general practitioners to continue to care for diabetics, doubtless with better results.

## REFERENCES

1. Collier Jr, B.N., Etwiler, D.D. (1971): Comparative study of diabetes knowledge among juvenile diabetics and their parents. *Diabetes, 20*, 51.
2. Miller, L.V., Goldstein, J., Nicolaisen, G. (1978): Evaluation of patients' knowledge of diabetes self-care. *Diabetes Care, 1*, 275.
3. Wysocki, M., Czyzyk, A., Slonska, Z., Krolewski, A. and Janeczko, D. (1978): Health behaviour and its determinants among insulin-dependent diabetics. Results of the diabetes Warsaw study. *Diab. Metab., 4*, 117.
4. Larpent, N., Eschwege, E. and Canivet, J. (1981): Enquête sur les connaissances des diabétiques. *Diab. Metab., 7*, 35.
5. Gfeller, R. and Assal, J.P. (1979): Une expérience pilote en diabétologie clinique et en psychologie médicale: l'unité de traitement et d'enseignement pour malades diabétiques de l'hôpital cantonal de Genève. *Med. Hyg., 37*, 2966.
6. Miller, L.V. and Goldstein, J. (1972): More efficient care of diabetic patients in a county hospital setting. *N. Engl. J. Med., 286*, 1388.
7. Davidson, J.K., Alogna, M., Goldsmith, M. and Riley, T. (1976): Assessment of program effectiveness at Grady Memorial Hospital. In: *Report of the National Commission on Diabetes to the Congress of U.S.*, DHEW Publ. n° NIH 76-1018, p. 227. U.S. Govern. Print. Office, Washington D.C.

# 9. Therapeutical effects of diabetes education: evaluation of diabetes teaching programmes

MICHAEL BERGER AND VIKTOR JÖRGENS

## EDITORIAL

*The importance of patient education in diabetes therapy was recognized as far back as the 1920s, when insulin had to be injected several times a day, protection against hypoglycemic reactions had to be planned, and insulin doses had to be changed according to urine test results.*

*In nearly every country there have been enthusiastic, motivated diabetologists who have used their intuition to develop patient education as part of their therapy. This approach to diabetes treatment has only recently been seriously appreciated by physicians. It has taken almost 50 years for sound data to be presented showing the effects of educating and training the patient in diabetes care.*

*It is only by evaluating and correcting teaching programs for patients that this aspect of diabetes treatment might become a true therapeutical tool. The evaluation of a teaching program should help us to improve our methodology in teaching and training the patient. Research into this new therapeutical field is only just beginning. It is essential that whoever teaches patients tries to evaluate the effects of this approach on metabolic control, on long-term complications, as well as on the psycho-social implications of the disease. The following article presents some of the rare centers where such an evaluation has taken place. (The editors.)*

## INTRODUCTION

When reviewing the efficiency of patient education in the framework of diabetes therapy, one has to be aware of the fact that, of all the rapidly advancing areas of diabetes research, the treatment of diabetic patients has been somewhat neglected in recent decades; there has been very little progress in the actual care of diabetic patients ever since the insulin therapy was introduced 60 years ago – as we are increasingly told nowadays by patient-organizations, health-care politicians and sensible physicians, such as the late Franz Ingelfinger [1]. In this somewhat embarrassing situation, clinical diabetologists have rediscovered one important principle in the delivery of diabetes care, namely to involve the patient actively in the day-to-day management of his disease. It appears logical that, in order to keep track of his glucose metabolism on a continuous basis, the patient himself has to perform daily measurements of his glucose metabolism. Furthermore, it seems to be quite unescapable that the patient should be able to adapt his therapy immediately if his measurements indicate an unsatisfactory degree of metabolic control.

These simple considerations underline the paramount importance of the patient's active involvement in the treatment of his/her diabetes mellitus. The basis of any successful participation of the patient in the management of his disease is a thorough information achieved by an educational process, most often called a Diabetes Teaching Programme (DTP). To this end, various educational programmes and curricula have been designed, varying from center to center and from country to country. These educational programmes have, in fact, become in more recent years an integral part of the delivery of diabetes care in many hospitals. As for any other therapeutic measures, however, the long-term consequences of DTPs have to be evaluated – a necessity which has been consistently maintained by the Diabetes Education Study Group, right from the beginning of its existence.

This chapter deals with the problems and necessities concerning the evaluation of the educational process called DTP. Such an evaluation of diabetes education is obligatory because the DTP represents a therapeutic intervention. As for any other form of medical intervention, especially in relation to chronic diseases, the (long-term) effect of alterations of or additions to the conventional therapeutic strategy has to be scrutinized by appropriate evaluatory procedures. In essence, these procedures represent nothing but a 'quality control' of the therapy or certain aspects of it. One of the obvious principles of such a quality control has to be a precise definition of the respective goals of the therapeutic efforts. It appears rather trivial to demand an individualized treatment goal for any particular disease and any particular patient, but the explicit formulation of such an objective especially in the chronically ill seems to be the exception rather than the rule in nowadays medicine. Only on the basis of a comparison of the predetermined goal of the therapeutic attempt and the actual achievements of the therapeutic intervention can a valid appraisal be made of the effort-benefit ratio of a particular procedure. Those appraisals have to weigh the burdens involved in the treatment on the patient, on his relatives and on the health care system against the respective benefits as they appear from (long-term) follow-up studies in a representative group of patients. It is on the basis of evaluations like these that a therapeutic manoeuvre should be recommended as a routine procedure in the health care delivery systems or that its use should be discouraged. In surprisingly few instances, conventional or more recent therapeutic alternatives have been studied using such an evaluatory process.

As for the type-I diabetic patients without late complications, the goals of the treatment process may be summarized as follows: (1) attempting to normalize glucose homeostasis in order to prevent late complications and (2) minimizing restrictions in the patients' daily lives related to their disease. Thus, the ultimate objectives are to normalize metabolism as perfectly as possible with a quality of life as high as possible. The subjective components of these objectives are immediately apparent when patients with varying degrees of diabetic late complications and/or unrelated additional handicaps (intellectually, socially, emotionally, physically etc.) are included in these considerations.

## THE BACKGROUND OF ATTEMPTS TO EVALUATE DIABETES TEACHING PROGRAMMES

In essence, diabetes education is an integral part of any diabetes therapy; its ultimate purpose is not the distribution of diabetes- or diet-related knowledge, but its aims are directed towards the goals of diabetes treatment in general. In this context, evaluation of diabetes education is done by assessing the quality of diabetes therapy. Evaluation attempts should therefore include the long-term follow-up of a number of control parameters (Table 1). In contrast to evaluation procedures of purely pedagogic programmes or interventions, the evaluation of diabetes therapy has to take into account therapeutic measures unrelated to the educational objectives.

Table 1   *Parameters in assessing the quality of diabetes therapy*

| | |
|---|---|
| Metabolic parameters: | HbAIc, glycemia, glucosuria, ketonuria, incidence of acute metabolic complications such as hypoglycemia or diabetic ketoacidosis |
| Late complications: | Retinopathy, nephropathy, neuropathy, incidence of amputations, etc. |
| Psycho-social parameters: | Incidence of sick-leave, hospitalization, independence/restrictions in professional life, sexual behavior, family planning, sports activities, travel, general quality of life, etc. |

Furthermore, factors related to the patient – e.g. his social status, psychological or physical abilities, degree of diabetes complications, age and duration of diabetes etc. – will obviously influence the outcome of any therapeutic intervention quite profoundly, independent of the quality of the educational programme used. Thus, in any attempt to evaluate the effects of diabetes education, the characteristics of the patient population and the strategy of the 'medical treatment' have to be documented in order to make the conclusions (generally) applicable. For example, it would be misleading to evaluate a DTP delivered to a group of type-I diabetic pa-

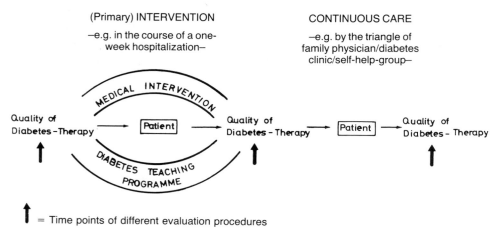

(Primary) INTERVENTION

—e.g. in the course of a one-
week hospitalization—

CONTINUOUS CARE

—e.g. by the triangle of
family physician/diabetes
clinic/self-help-group—

↑ = Time points of different evaluation procedures

Fig. 1   Scheme for potential time points of evaluation procedures with respect to the quality of diabetes therapy.

tients immediately following the manifestation of their disease on the basis of their metabolic control data when they are in remission, as compared to the results of a DTP in patients with brittle-type diabetes negative for C-peptide levels. On the other hand, it appears of little value to judge the efficiency of a DTP even in comparable groups of type-I diabetic patients if the strategy of the insulin therapy varies, e.g. between one injection of long-acting insulin per day and multiple daily injections of short-acting insulin preparations. In theory, the therapeutic intervention may be planned and its effect can be assessed as described in Figure 1. Any assessment of possible differences in the quality of diabetes therapy (Table 1) before and after the intervention has to take into account and to describe in detail the patients' characteristics, the medical treatment and the DTP. Once factors related to the patients and to the medical treatment have been taken into account, considering their potential consequences for the eventual quality of the diabetes treatment, the effects of diabetes education can be evaluated. During such an evaluatory process various positions have to be marked (Fig. 2).

In order to obtain an objective account of the effects of the DTP, there has to be a detailed description of the status quo ante (Fig. 2, A), i.e. the knowledge of the patients, the habitual diabetes-related behavior of the patients and the quality of the diabetes therapy (Table 1). Thus, the patient's knowledge has to be assessed, through interviews or questionnaires, via observations of the patients' behavior or based on the documentation of the patients' home blood glucose or glucosuria self-monitoring. Except for an assessment of the patients' initial knowledge by a questionnaire [2-4], attempts to describe the pre-curriculum attitudes and compliance

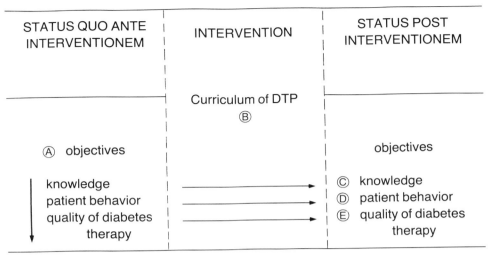

Fig. 2   Scheme of various items and details to be evaluated with respect to a Diabetes Teaching Programme.

rates to general or more specific principles of diabetes therapy have hardly ever been documented.

As to the judgement of the quality of diabetes therapy, any documentation of the degree of metabolic control before reproducible methods to measure $HbA_{1C}$-levels became available was next to meaningless. Therefore, earlier studies had to restrict their description of the pre-quality of diabetes treatment to incidence rates of sick-leave, hospitalizations, diabetic ketoacidosis, etc.

*The curriculum of the DTP (Fig. 2, B).* In other sections of this monograph, various forms of diabetes education curricula are described as pedagogic entities. In order to render any DTP assessable and thus improvable, it has to be planned and structured as to the relative importance of respective teaching objectives (teaching hierarchy). Thus, for any item a goal has to be defined, and appropriate teaching methods have to be developed in order to achieve this goal.

On the basis of such a standardized diabetes teaching curriculum, the knowledge transfer of the various items can be evaluated after the patients have been subjected to the educational process (Fig. 2, C). Again, the transfer can be assessed by questionnaires or by observation (e.g. by a video camera; see Chapter 11). Without a positive transfer of teaching objectives any alteration of the patients' behavior or any improvement of the quality of diabetes therapy may not be causally related to the DTP at all.

Furthermore, the diabetes-related behavior of the patients has to be evaluated and compared to the pre-teaching behavior (Fig. 2, D). Again, such an assessment may be based upon interviews or upon demonstration/

observation of certain behaviors. For example, it could demonstrate whether the patients do have some sugar (as hypoglycemia-treatment) with them on the day of the follow-up examination, or one could assess the frequency of meals/snacks, home blood glucose monitoring or the frequency of insulin dosis adaptations by the patients.

The ultimate context, however, in which all these criteria of knowledge (e.g. diet, diabetes pathophysiology etc.) and behavior (diet compliance, etc.) become relevant, is their importance to achieve a high quality of diabetes treatment (Fig. 2, E). In fact, the reason for assessing all these items is primarily to be able to improve the DTP, should the degree of diabetes treatment make such an improvement desirable. Thus, the most important part of any evaluation of DTPs is to assess the quality of diabetes therapy, based on the various goals of the care of the diabetic patient (Table 1).

In the following, we will review a number of more recent studies which have evaluated the effect of a DTP on various parameters of the quality of diabetes treatment.

## REVIEW OF STUDIES TO EVALUATE THE EFFICACY OF DTPs

In summarizing some of these studies, we have grouped them according to the evaluation system suggested in Figure 2, i.e. studies concerning the objectives at status quo ante interventionem (A), the quality of the DTP as such (B) and the evaluation of the efficacy of the DTP in achieving the 3 groups of objectives (C, D, E).

As mentioned above, there are very few studies reporting a valid assessment of the status quo ante interventionem (Fig. 2, A), i.e. the documentation of knowledge, behavior and quality of diabetes therapy before any (medical and educational) intervention is carried out. There are, however, numerous reports in the literature concerning the diabetes-related knowledge of various cohorts and population samples of diabetic patients. An interesting study was carried out recently by Dichmann et al. in East Germany: in particular, these authors have demonstrated that there was no apparent relationship between the diabetes-related knowledge of some 400 diabetic patients and the quality of their diabetes therapy, as judged on the basis of random blood glucose measurements [5]. This noteworthy investigation of the status quo ante underscores that the mere assessment of the patients' knowledge does not necessarily represent a valid reflection of the quality of the diabetes therapy. However, the examination of the diabetes-related knowledge in population samples might be rather helpful in planning a diabetes education curriculum. Thus, we have evaluated the basic knowledge related to diabetes as a disease state, its dangers and its therapy and various diet/nutrition-related items in a number of non-diabetic population groups, such as senior citizens, high school students, medical students, etc. This study revealed a surprising unawareness of diabetes-related problems, independent of the social class or the educational background of the various population groups [6, 7]. The study was helpful in the sense that it underlined the necessity to transfer very basic knowledge, at least in newly manifested diabetic patients – no matter what their educational background is. The study revealed in addition an almost unbelievable lack of diabetes-related knowledge in the senior medical students tested. The assessment of the knowledge at status quo ante provides the basis of any measurement of the transfer of knowledge offered in the course of a DTP.

Williams et al. [8, 9] and Watkins et al. [10] have published a series of studies on investigations of the behavior of diabetic patients on the basis of observations made in the homes of the patients. Again, it was found that knowledge did not correlate well with the patients' quality of day-to-day metabolic control, but there was a remarkable association between the patients' performance (i.e. behavior) and the quality of diabetes therapy. Finally, innumerable authors have demonstrated that the quality of diabetes therapy was profoundly unsatisfactory in their patients. In particular, the overall poor degree of metabolic control, as judged on the basis of $HbA_{IC}$ levels in unselected diabetic patients [11, 12], the incidence of hospitalizations [2, 13–15], severe hypoglycemias and diabetes-related amputations as well as the incidence of diabetic ketoacidosis [16, 17] has been amply documented. It is assumed that this inadequacy of diabetes therapy in general is the cause of the high rate of diabetic late complications and the overall increased morbidity and mortality in diabetic patients. In addition, the more recent literature contains investigations relating more refined parameters of the quality of life, such as the frequency of eating in restaurants despite being diabetic (of particular importance for French patients) as indicators for the quality of diabetes therapy [18].

It goes without saying that some immediate checks with relation to the efficacy of the DTP (Fig. 2, B) have to be performed in order to document the transfer of information to the patients. In fact, some of these checks have to be built into the educational process as an integral part of the teaching curriculum. Such feed-back enables the diabetes educator to justify a continuation or else a repetition of the learning procedures.

In addition, it becomes more and more essential to carry out appropriate evaluation procedures of the efficacy of certain teaching aids. Nowadays, diabetes teaching units are flooded with educational materials, such as booklets, video films, audiovisual aids, etc. Although some of these teaching aids are produced in a most professional manner, they have hardly ever been properly evaluated. Any adequate evaluation process has to involve testing the teaching aid in a large sample of diabetic patients – in this process the effects of the material on the patients' knowledge, behavior and (most importantly) the quality of the diabetes therapy have to be evaluated. Even though we appreciate that any such evaluation represents a major effort on the part of the producer, we are convinced that teaching materials which have not been scrutinized as to their effectivity with various groups of patients are of rather limited value. An example concerning the possibility to evaluate a certain teaching aid, i.e. a video film about the use of glucagon injections by patients' relatives, is given in Chapter 11.

Assessing the increase of knowledge is a rather easy and sometimes superficial method of evaluating the efficacy of a DTP (Fig. 2, C). Mostly this is done by asking patients to fill in a questionnaire before and immediately after the DTP. We suppose that such an evaluation procedure is in fact a direct test for the appropriateness of the teaching technique. Any valid assessment of the increase in knowledge provided by a DTP should be done a certain time period after the DTP. Again, many studies of this sort have been performed. Unfortunately, most authors have not extended their evaluation process further than a simple assessment of the change in diabetes-related knowledge. In our opinion, any demonstration of a change in knowledge is only helpful if it is directly related to respective (in)adequacies of patient behavior or the quality of diabetes therapy. Only in these cases can the documentation of deficient transfer of knowledge be used in order to improve the DTP and, hence, the quality of diabetes treatment. In other words, the demonstration of a specific deficit in diet/nutrition related knowledge is useless if it is not related to certain problems of metabolic control or specific impairments of the patient's quality of life.

Alterations in the patients' behavior (Fig. 2. D) are more difficult to assess. More detailed analyses of the patients' behavior and performance should be based upon observations of the patients at home or at work [9, 10, 19]. Only in certain instances may the assessment of behavior be done in a clinic setting, e.g. by checking the patient's home-blood-glucose-monitoring logs or by having him perform a blood glucose measurement under supervision. A simple but rather effective check is to ask the patients to prove that they are carrying sugar cubes with them. Thus, in the process of a follow-up investigation of insulin-treated diabetic patients 6 months after hospitalization (including a DTP or without a DTP), we have been able to document a substantial difference with respect to this particular aspect of behavior in direct relation to the DTP (Fig. 3). The most important investigations about the efficacy of DTPs represent a quality control of diabetes therapy (Fig. 2, E). By nature of the investigative protocols, these studies are focussed upon different aspects and parameters of the quality of diabetes therapy. L. Miller has clearly demonstrated the reduction of hospitalizations and sick-leaves in patients that have undergone an intensive DTP. These studies are, by now, considered as classics in the evaluation attempts of DTPs [13, 15]. In fact, the original findings of Miller and her associates have been repeatedly confirmed [14, 16, 20-22] (see also Chapter 34). Thus, Moffitt et al. found a substantial reduction of the bed occupancy by diabetic patients in their hospital in New South Wales as a result of the installation of a diabetes teaching programme [23].

The most impressive evidence of the efficiency of a DTP has been re-

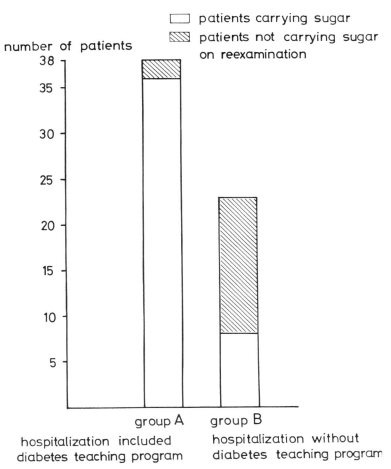

Fig. 3 Evaluation of insulin-requiring diabetic patients 6 months following discharge from hospital in order to improve diabetes control. Investigation of diabetes-related behavior. Did the patients carry sugar cubes with them on day of the evaluation procedure? Group A: 38 patients whose hospitalization included a standardized diabetes teaching programme. Group B: 23 patients whose hospitalization did not include any formal diabetes teaching programme. Taken from Jörgens et al. [27].

ported by Davidson [14, 16, 24] (see also Chapter 34). He has been able to reduce significantly the incidence of diabetic ketoacidoses and diabetes-related amputations as a result of his teaching activities. In addition, Davidson has produced most favourable cost-benefit analyses of his DTP [24]. He has introduced a rigid auditing system, with the consequence that changes in the health care delivery to his diabetic patients become readily apparent. On the basis of the outcome of continuous auditing efforts [25],

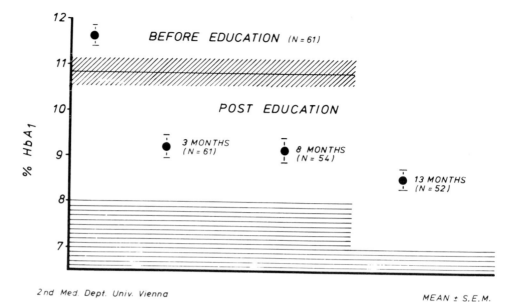

Fig. 4 Effect of a one-week diabetes teaching course on metabolic control in unselected type-I diabetic patients. Re-evaluation 3, 8 and 13 months after the in-patient diabetes teaching programme. The upper shaded area represents mean ± SEM HbA₁-levels of 90 unselected type 1 diabetic patients under out-patient care before the institution of a formal diabetes teaching programme. The lower shaded area depicts the normal range ($\bar{x} \pm$ SD) of the method to determine HbA₁-levels used. Taken from Mühlhauser et al. [26].

pitfalls and shortcomings in the intervention/education system can be identified without much delay, so that immediate corrections can be made if necessary.

Another type of investigation concentrates directly on the degree of the patients' metabolic control. Mühlhauser et al. [26] have been able to lower the HbAI levels in an unselected group of type-I diabetic patients as a result of an intense one-week in-patient DTP. In this study, 2 aspects are particularly noteworthy: the improvement of HbA₁ levels was not due to any systematic alteration of insulin- or diet-therapy but rather directly related to the DTP; and the improvement of the diabetes therapy was not a short-term effect, since it lasted for at least up to 13 months (Fig. 4).

Jörgens et al. have been able to relate the degree of the metabolic control to the institution of a DTP and to the compliance of the patients to the objectives of the programme (Fig. 5) [27, 28]. Only those patients who regularly practiced the self-adaptation of their insulin dosages were able to achieve a satisfactory degree of metabolic control 6 months after hospitalization. In addition, these data show that the self-monitoring of glucosuria by the patients – even if it was done quite regularly – did not help effectively

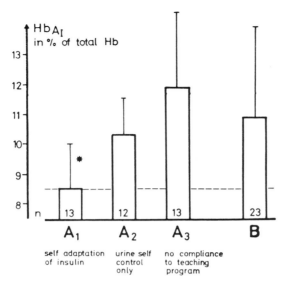

Fig. 5  HbA$_I$-levels (means ± SD) in insulin-dependent diabetic patients. Evaluation 6 months after discharge from hospital in order to improve diabetes control. Groups A and B as in Figure 3. Group A3 showed no compliance to the DTP, group A2 patients had performed glucosuria monitoring on a regular basis, and patients of group A1 had, in addition, adapted their insulin therapy regularly on the basis of glucosuria-monitoring. * = p < 0.05 for the difference between groups A1 and A2. The dotted line represents the upper range of normal HbA$_I$-levels. Taken from Jörgens et al. [27].

in improving control if it was not accompanied by immediate alterations of the insulin therapy by the patient in instances of unsatisfactory metabolic control.

On the basis of preliminary data from ongoing studies, we suggest that the quality of the continuing ambulatory care available to the diabetic patient after he has been subjected to a DTP is of profound importance for the long-term success in improving the quality of diabetes therapy. The continuous repetition of teaching processes through an outpatient clinic [19] or in the physician's office appears to be essential. According to the data of Basdevant et al. [18] from Paris, the provision of the necessary care in order to maintain the quality of diabetes treatment after the DTP seems to be superior in a specialized outpatient clinic when compared with the private physicians' efforts. These findings underline the importance of providing the possibility of a continuous high quality care for diabetic patients, including an ongoing educational process. These requirements could probably be most successfully met by a triangle of the family physician, a specialized outpatient clinic and a self-help group of diabetic patients. A definite demonstration of the usefulness of such a system (and its particular elements) has, however, to be based on an evaluation of the quality of the health care delivery to a large number of diabetic patients over an extended period of time.

## CONCLUSIONS

The success of any attempt to improve the quality of diabetes therapy depends on a number of interrelated intervention processes. The paramount effectivity of DTPs is, however, undebatable. In fact, there is no valid treatment of diabetic patients without a detailed, planned DTP. Its effectivity has to be proven by a specific evaluation process which should be carried out individually for every DTP. It is only on the basis of such an ongoing evaluation process that the DTP can be continuously monitored and improved and deviations can be discovered and corrected without much delay.

## SUMMARY

Diabetes Teaching Programmes have to be evaluated as to their effectivity in improving the quality of health care to diabetic patients; they are an integral part of the treatment of diabetes mellitus. A variety of different approaches to evaluate diabetes teaching programmes is discussed. In essence, any attempt to evaluate diabetes teaching programmes has to be regarded as a quality control of diabetes therapy as such. The effectivity of diabetes education in general has been proven by a large number of sophisticated studies. Nevertheless, every diabetes treatment unit should run its individual evaluation procedures in order to justify its particular programme and to be able to improve its efficacy on the basis of a continuous monitoring and auditing process.

## REFERENCES

1. Ingelfinger, F. (1977): Debates on diabetes. *N. Engl. J. Med., 296,* 1228.
2. Schurr, W.H.J., Minne, H.W. and Ziegler, R. (1981): Diabetiker-Ausbildung aus der Sicht des Patienten. *Akt. Endokrin. Stoffw., 2,* 114 (Abstract).
3. Geller, J. and Butler, K. (1981): Study of educational deficits as the cause of hospital admission for diabetes mellitus in a community hospital. *Diabetes Care, 4,* 487.
4. Graber, A.L., Christman, B.G., Alogna, M.T. and Davidson, J.K. (1977): Evaluation of diabetes patient education programmes. *Diabetes, 26,* 61.
5. Dichmann, R., Handreg, R., Libner, G. et al. (1981): Untersuchungen über die Bedeutung einer gezielten Patienten-Aufklärung auf die Güte der Stoffwechselführung in einer Kreisstelle für Diabetes mellitus. *Z. Gesamte Inn. Med., 36,* 491.
6. Arns, G. (1982): *Wissensstand ausgewählter Bevölkerungsgruppen über den*

*Diabetes mellitus*. Thesis, Medical Faculty, Düsseldorf University, FRG.

7. Wasser, K., Jörgens, V., Arns, G. et al. (1981): Knowledge about diabetes mellitus in the general population: a baseline of diabetes teaching. *Diabetes 30, Suppl. 1*, 12A.

8. Williams, T.F., Martin, D.A., Hogan, M.D. et al. (1976): The clinical picture of diabetic control studied in four settings. *Am. J. Public Health, 57*, 441.

9. Williams, T.F., Anderson, E., Watkins, J.D. and Coyle, V. (1967): Dietary errors made at home by patients with diabetes. *J. Am. Diet. Assoc., 51*, 19.

10. Watkins, J.D., Williams, T.F., Martin, D.A. et al. (1967): A study of diabetic patients at home. *Am. J. Public Health, 57*, 452.

11. Yudkin, J.S., Boucher, B.J., Schopflin, K.E. et al. (1980): The quality of diabetic care in a London health district. *J. Epidem. Commun. Health, 34*, 277.

12. Mühlhauser, I. and Schernthaner, G. (1982): Diabetiker-Schulung mit dem Ziel der Selbsttherapie – Grundlage jeder erfolgreichen Behandlung. *Österr. Ärzte Z., 37*, 263.

13. Miller, L.V., Goldstein, J. (1972): More efficient care of diabetic patients in a county hospital setting. *N. Engl. J. Med., 286*, 1388.

14. Davidson, J.K., Alogna, M. and Goldsmith, M. (1975): *Assessment of Programme Effectiveness of Grady Memorial Hospital*. A report of the National Commission on Diabetes Education for Health Professionals, Patients and the Public. Appendix DHEW Pub. (NIH) # 76-1031, vol. III PV., p. 225.

15. Miller, L.V., Goldstein, J. and Runyan Jr, J.W. (1976): Improving the organization of the care of the chronically ill. In: *Preventive Medicine*, p. 41. Fogarty International Center Series, DHEW (NIH) Publication, 76-854.

16. Davidson, J.K., Alogna, M., Goldsmith, M. and Borden, J. (1981): Assessment of program effectiveness at Grady Memorial Hospital-Atlanta. In: Steiner G., Lawrence P.A. (Eds), *E lucating Diabetic Patients*, p. 329. Springer-Verlag, New York.

17. Assal, J.P. and Gfeller, R. (1980): Diabetiker-Schulung. Wichtigkeit und Komplexität dieser therapeutischen Maßnahme. *Pharmako-Therapie, 3*, 233.

18. Basdevant, A., Costagliola, D., Lnöe, J.L. et al. (1982): The risk of diabetic control: A comparison of hospital versus general practice supervision. *Diabetologia, 22*, 309.

19. Nerup, V. and Folke-Larsen, D. (1982): Effects of home-visits on patient education, psycho-social adjustment and metabolic control. (Abstract.) *Diabète Metabol., 8*, 166.

20. Miller, L.V., Goldstein, J., Kumar, D. and Dye, L. (1981): Assessment of program effectiveness at the Los Angeles County-University of Southern California Medical Center. In: Steiner G., Lawrence P.A. (Eds), *Educating Diabetic Patients*, p. 349. Springer-Verlag, New York.

21. Legge Jr, J.S., Massey, V.M., Vena, C.I. and Reilly, B.J. (1980): Evaluating patient education: a case study of a diabetes programme. *Health Educ. Q., 7*, 148.

22. Schnatz, J.D. and Van Son, A. (1981): Diabetes Teaching Service – Buffalo. In: Steiner G., Lawrence P.A. (Eds), *Educating Diabetic Patients*, p. 289, Springer-Verlag. New York.

23. Moffitt, P., Fowler, J. and Eather, G. (1979): Bed occupancy by diabetic patients. *Med. J. Austr., 1*, 244.

24. Davidson, J.K., Delcher, H.K. and Englund, A. (1979): Spin-off cost/benefits

of expanded nutritional care. *J. Am. Diet. Assoc., 75,* 251.

25. Bryant, D., Can Son, A., Davis, P.J. and Segal, C. (1978): Computerized surveillance of diabetic patient/health care delivery system interfaces. *Diabetes Care, 1,* 141.
26. Mühlhauser, I., Kunz, A. and Binder, M. et al. (1982): A one-week in-patient teaching course improves metabolic control in unselected type-I diabetic patients for at least 8 months. *Diabète Metabol., 8,* 169 (Abstract).
27. Jörgens, V., Berchtold, P., Eickenbusch, W. and Scholz-Thielen, E. (1980): Beneficial effects of diabetes teaching. Importance of self-management by the patients. *Diabetes, 29, Suppl. 1,* 27A.
28. Kemnitz, J., Berger, M., Gösseringer, G. et al. (1982): Compliance zu den Lehrinhalten der Patienten-Schulung und ihre Auswirkungen auf die Einstellungs-Qualität bei 70 insulin-behandelten Diabetikern. *Akt. Endokrin. Stoffw., 3,* 70 (Abstract).

# 10. What patients should know

J. CANIVET AND J.-Ph. ASSAL

The responsibility for ensuring that a diabetic patient carries out the treatment correctly rests not just with the patient but with the doctor, too. The treatment covers all aspects of care, i.e. diet, exercise, drugs, routine checks, follow-up and also a certain lifestyle and appropriate conduct in various circumstances. The diabetic has to be educated in these matters. The problem is to determine what he needs to know.

Usually the education of diabetics has consisted, and still consists, in teaching patients: (1) the diet; (2) practical know-how (urine tests, estimation of blood sugar and, if necessary, insulin injection technique); (3) for insulin-dependent diabetics, the recognition and treatment of the symptoms of hypoglycemia. This information is imparted with more or less teaching ability and in more or less detail according to the time available. In most cases education has proved to be inadequate, because it does not motivate the patient to look after himself to the best of his ability. It is suggested that, in order to achieve this goal, the diabetic must have a clear understanding of the nature of diabetes, the risks involved, and how to set about avoiding them.

It therefore seems necessary to supplement the instruction usually given with much other information: (1) on the regulation of blood sugar so that the patient may understand and collaborate better in its proper control; (2) on the part played by certain associated anomalies (hypertension, hyperlipoproteinemia, obesity, smoking) that increase the likelihood of arteriosclerosis; and (3) on 'acute' and long-term complications. Thus the patient may co-operate better in the prevention of such complications and may understand the reasons for clinical follow-up.

This leads to the advocation of more intensive education. Besides the practical instruction, for which dieticians and nurses are especially well qualified, there should be some theoretical instruction. This should include talks with or without audiovisual illustration, given by doctors and designed to explain diabetes, the risks it involves, and ways to avoid the risks.

An example of the information that should be supplied is given in the appendix. It is set out in the form of a schedule intended to remind those responsible for these talks of what they should explain. For their greater assistance some concepts are dealt with in more detail than others because they relate to information which should be added to that usually supplied. This more detailed information concerns the general aspects of diabetes, the risks it involves, exercise, routine checks and follow-up. On the other hand, other concepts are dealt with in less detail as they are already imparted adequately (for instance, insulin therapy technique, care of the feet). It is the job of the 'educators' to explain the contents of the schedule simply and in such a way as to gain the diabetics' interest, which requires time, training and teaching ability.

To some it will appear that this schedule requires the patient to be taught too much. In reality, the aim is to provide strictly practical information in such a way that it enables diabetics to understand why the information is of importance to them.

It did not seem worthwhile to draw up different programmes according to age, treatment or the presence of long-term complications. Indeed, whatever the type of diabetes, the regulation of blood sugar is subject to the same physiological data; the risks are identical, and the routine checks and follow-up remain essential. It is, however, the task of the 'educators' to adapt this single programme to the type of patient: do not talk about insulin and possible accidents as diabetic coma to those not on insulin; do not talk about oral hypoglycemic agents to insulin-dependent diabetics; do not dwell on long-term complications with patients whose diabetes first appeared at the age of 75. All this is a matter of common sense. Nor was it considered necessary to set out here how to explain the practical know-how (urine tests, injections etc.) or to apply the dietary principles; it is the task of the nurses and dieticians to arrange these practical sessions according to the facilities of each centre. Finally, problems connected with pregnancy and contraception were omitted from the general schedule as it was considered that they are best dealt with by private interviews.

This programme may appear complex and difficult to execute; in fact it is workable and is carried out every week in the Diabetes Centre of Saint Louis Hospital in Paris, and in the Diabetes Unit of Hôpital Cantonal in Geneva. Of course, a team has to be formed and trained for this work and should have resources at its disposal; such problems do not come within the scope of this report. It is still too early to assess the results. Only prospective studies will indicate whether such an educational project is superior to what has been the norm hitherto.

## APPENDIX

### I. General concepts

*Part 1.   What is diabetes?*

A   –   *Definition*: diabetes is a state of chronic hyperglycemia.
B   –   *Blood sugar.*
B1  –   Blood sugar of the healthy person over 24 hours; point out its stability within certain normal limits.

B2   –  This stability is due to a balance between the intake and output of glucose in the circulation. Intake: exogenous sugar originating from food; endogenous sugar of hepatic origin (through glycogenolysis, through glyconeogenesis).
Output: for building up body tissue (glycoproteins etc.); for providing the energy necessary for the cell-life (glycolysis); for the deposition of reserves in the liver (glycogen) or in the fatty tissues (conversion into fat). Point out that in healthy persons there is no elimination in the urine.

B3   –  The maintenance of a stable blood sugar level is a necessity for the body. It is ensured by the action of certain hormones, particularly by insulin.

C    –  *Insulin.*

C1   –  Origin: it is produced by the pancreas; islets of Langerhans; B cells.

C2   –  Distribution: it goes straight to the liver which uses a large part of it; via the general circulation it then reaches all the tissues.

C3   –  Action: it inhibits the release of glucose from the liver into circulation; it promotes the penetration of glucose into all the peripheral tissues; it thus has a hypoglycemic effect. It also promotes the formation of proteins and fats.

C4   –  Secretion: this depends on the concentration of glucose in the blood (hence it rises after a meal and falls some time after the meal), which ensures the automatic regulation of the blood sugar.

D    –  *Diabetes.*

D1   –  In such a carefully regulated system the break-down that causes chronic hyperglycemia, i.e. diabetes, can be defined as (1) a deficiency (total or partial) of insulin (hence insulin-dependent diabetes) in the pancreas, or (2) insensitivity of the tissues to the action of insulin (hence non-insulin dependent diabetes), or (3) a combination of these 2 factors. Diabetes is due to a deficiency of insulin in the pancreas or the loss of action of insulin on the tissues; or the association of these two causes.

D2   –  Consequently the symptoms observed in diabetes are: glycosuria, polyuria, polydipsia and, in the event of insulin deficiency, loss of weight and ketonuria.

D3   –  Diabetes is not a single entity. Two main types are insulin-dependent diabetes and non-insulin dependent diabetes (the differential characteristics).

*Part 2.   What risks does diabetes involve?*

These risks must be known in order to be avoided.

E    –  *Acute risks.*

E1   –  Diabetic coma: it occurs in insulin-dependent diabetes and is due to a complete or relative insulin deficiency.

E2 – Usually induced by: discontinuation of insulin injections or an intercurrent disease (especially infection) which causes or aggravates this deficiency.

E3 – Glucose is therefore no longer able to penetrate into the cells: fat is then extensively broken down and this results in the formation of ketone bodies.

E4 – Thus a biological sign appears and heralds diabetic coma, *ketonuria*.

E5 – A doctor must be consulted immediately and the diabetic admitted to hospital, if necessary.

E6 – Hyperosmolar coma; observed especially in non-insulin dependent diabetes and in the elderly.

E7 – Predisposing circumstances: an intercurrent illness (infection, burns), the ill-considered use of certain medicines (diuretics).

E8 – Loss of water and dehydration ensue.

E9 – It is heralded by tiredness and polyuria; there is pronounced glycosuria and a very high blood glucose level.

E10 – A doctor must be consulted immediately or, failing that, admission to hospital secured.

E11 – Diabetic coma and also hyperosmolar coma can be avoided by proper control of the diabetes.

F – *Delayed risks*: long-term complications. These may occur in all types of diabetes. Some are peculiar to diabetes and due to the harmful effects of hyperglycemia on the small blood vessels and on certain tissues.

F1 – Retinopathy: this impairs vision and may progress to blindness.

F2 – Nephropathy: this may extend to fatal renal failure.

F3 – Neuropathy: this may cause pain in the lower limbs, foot ulcerations, difficulty in walking.

F4 – These complications generally appear after several years of hyperglycemia, tend to become worse, and can be treated only by palliative measures.

F5 – Diabetics must therefore be subject to a regular follow-up with a clinical examination, eye examination and tests of renal function, and they must ensure that the blood sugar level is normal.

F6 – Indeed, statistics show that proper control of diabetes can avoid these complications.

G – *Other complications* are accidents which may occur to anyone but are more frequent in diabetics than in non-diabetics.

G1 – Angina pectoris and myocardial infarction.

G2 – Cerebrovascular accident.

G3 – Arteriosclerosis of the legs with the danger of gangrene of the foot.

G4 – Moreover, certain anomalies are often observed: obesity, hypertension, hyperlipidemia; smoking predisposes towards these accidents.

G5 – The diabetic must therefore be followed up if necessary with regular examinations to correct these latter anomalies and thus avoid such accidents.

H — *Other complications* need only be mentioned: cataract, urinary infection, mycosis of the feet.

I — *Permanent good control* of the metabolism, with certain complementary treatments if necessary, can prevent these complications.

## II. The treatment of diabetes

The object of this is: 1) to ensure proper control in order to avoid any acute or delayed risk; 2) to find the best possible compromise between the necessities of treatment and a life acceptable to the diabetic.

The treatment comprises: 1) a suitable diet; 2) a certain amount of physical exercise; 3) hypoglycemic drugs when necessary; 4) the treatment of associated complications or anomalies (hypertension, hyperlipidemia, obesity) if necessary.

### 1. Diet

This is a fundamental element of the treatment, always necessary and in many cases adequate in itself. The aim is (1) to achieve or maintain an ideal weight; (2) to attain good metabolic control by restricting certain foods whilst ensuring that the diet remains balanced and compatible with a normal life; (3) in the case of diabetics on insulin, apportionment of the food to assist in good regulation of the blood sugar.

The diet therefore differs according to the diabetic.

J — *In non-insulin dependent diabetics with obesity* it is essential to eliminate the excess weight; indeed this will cause the insensitivity of the tissues to the action of insulin (endogenous) to vanish and will in many cases lead to good control of the diabetes.

J1 — The diet must be low in calories, hence restrictive.

J2 — The restrictions must refer to carbohydrates and fats, the foods from which the body manufactures its own fat, the excess of which is precisely what we are seeking to eliminate.

J3 — The aspects of the low-calorie diet, related in such a way that the diabetics can themselves organize and adhere to it.

J4 — It is hard to keep to a restrictive diet and adhere to it without fail; willpower and perseverance are required.

K — *In non-insulin dependent diabetes without obesity* the normal weight must be maintained, therefore no weight put-on.

K1 — The diet must be 'normal', that is to say without excesses in regard to carbohydrates and fats.

K2 — The aspect of the 'normal diet', explained as in J3 (with the aid, as in J3, of tables showing the composition of the principal foods, equivalences and rapidly absorbed sugars).

L   – *In insulin-dependent diabetes* the normal weight must be maintained by a 'normal' diet (as under K) and the diet must also be apportioned in relation to the insulin injections (so as to avoid postprandial hyperglycemia and hypoglycemia some time after meals).
L1  – The aspects of a 'normal' diet.
L2  – The apportionment of the food: meals and intermediate snacks.
M   – *The information* supplied in this way should be supplemented by meals organized for self-service, in the course of which the diabetics would work out their own menus, taking their personal tastes and usual activities into account, with the help of a dietician.

## 2.   Exercise

This is one of the elements of treatment. In fact, muscular hyperactivity enhances glucose to penetrate into the muscle, hence a reduction in the blood sugar level. Sports (with exceptions) are permitted. Failing these, walking or cycling are exercises to be encouraged. However, there must be no striving after performance and the exercise must never be exhausting.

Exercise must be subject to certain rules, however, especially in the case of the diabetic on insulin:

a.   It is forbidden for the poorly-controlled diabetic. Indeed, since poor control is due to an insulin deficiency (complete or relative), it means that there is not enough insulin to cause the glucose to penetrate the muscle tissue; on the other hand this very deficiency fosters the release of glucose into the circulation by the liver (through glycogenolysis); the consequence of this is hyperglycemia. There is also the possibility of ketonuria as the hyperactive muscle uses (in order to obtain its energy) fatty acids provided by the breakdown of body fat, also encouraged by the insulin deficiency.

b.   It is recommended for the well-controlled diabetic (hence appreciably normoglycemic) since he has enough insulin to cause the glucose to penetrate into the muscle. But the reduction in blood sugar level may become excessive (hence hypoglycemia) when the exercise is prolonged or if it brings into action the muscles in the region where the injection was given; in such cases carbohydrates must be taken during and after the exercise.

## 3.   Oral hypoglycemic agents

In diabetics who do not need insulin, whose weight is normal or who have returned to normal with an appropriate diet and in whom control of the metabolism has not been achieved, oral hypoglycemics may be used.

These agents consist of 2 types: sulphonylureas and biguanides.
N   – *Sulphonylureas.*
N1  – They act principally by stimulating the secretion of insulin in the pancreas.

N2 – Mention the various types of sulphonylureas: the choice and dose are fixed by the doctor.

N3 – They are well tolerated, they cause side-effects only in exceptional circumstances (leukopenia) but, after the ingestion of an alcoholic beverage, they sometimes cause a flush.

N4 – In elderly persons and those with renal or hepatic disorders, however, they may cause severe hypoglycemia with coma.

O – *Biguanides.*

O1 – They have no effect on the pancreas and act by curbing the absorption of sugars by the intestine and the production of glucose by the liver (glyconeogenesis).

O2 – Biguanides used: metformin.

O3 – They sometimes cause gastric or intestinal disorders. They do not involve the risk of hypoglycemic accidents.

O4 – However, in elderly persons or those with cardiac, renal, hepatic or respiratory insufficiency, they predispose to a very serious accident: lactic acidosis.

4. *Insulin*

Insulin is inactivated by the digestive tract, hence the need to resort to injections.

It has a hypoglycemic effect (recall its action: see General Concepts, Part 1, C3).

P – *The injection of insulin.*

P1 – The different types of insulin: rapid-acting, intermediary, long-acting; purified insulins; human insulin.

P2 – The site of injection: the various regions; the need to vary the site of injection.

P3 – The number of injections per day; the time of injection.

P4 – The injection technique: the syringe and how to fill it; the injection; possible minor mishaps (accidental puncture of a blood vessel etc.).

P5 – Explain that insulin injected in this way (exogenous) causes the blood glucose to fall in relation to dose and duration of action independently of the level of the blood sugar of the diabetic; this is where it differs from the insulin (endogenous) of the pancreas of the normal individual which is secreted in response to the level of blood sugar.

P6 – Hence the precautions to be taken as regards: 1) diet (to be apportioned) 2) exercise (ingestion of sugar).

Q – *Accidents of insulin therapy.*
  There is virtually only one: hypoglycemic attack.

Q1 – This is explained by what was recalled in P5.

Q2 – Signs of hypoglycemia – to be explained; if the attack is not attended to, it may end in a coma.

Q3 – Therefore symptoms must be recognised immediately and eliminated by the ingestion of sugar in a rapidly absorbed form (granulated sugar, chocolate, confectionery). If the diabetic is unable to replace the blood sugar himself because he has become confused or semi-comatose, someone present must give him an injection of glucagon. Failing this, glucose solution must be administered i.v. by a nurse or doctor.

Q4 – When the hypoglycemic attack has been treated, the cause must always be sought (in order to avoid a recurrence): 1) an injection mishap (into a blood vessel); 2) an inadequate or badly distributed diet; 3) unaccustomed physical exertion.

Q5 – The diabetic must always carry several lumps of sugar on him. Other accidents of insulin therapy (allergic accidents, lipodystrophy) are only to be explained if necessary.

## III.  Routine checks and follow-up

The objective of the treatment is for the diabetic (1) to feel well, and (2) not to have any complications now or later.

1.  To feel 'well' like a non-diabetic means that he has to adopt a certain life style which is acceptable and accepted despite the constraints of treatment. To this end it is advisable:

a.  to live a regular life
b.  to avoid alcohol and tobacco
c.  to take special care of the skin (dermatoses, cutaneous injections) and the feet (sores, ulcers)
    – looking after the feet
    – foot hygiene (washing and drying; the nails; perspiration, calluses, footwear) to be explained.

2.  To avoid complications, good control of the diabetes is needed.

R1 – The criteria of good control.
R2 – The laboratory analyses (glycosuria, glycemia, glycosylated hemoglobin).
R3 – The urine tests carried out by the diabetic (glycosuria, ketonuria): the methods, the commercial kits that can be used, frequency and timetable of these tests, their significance.
R4 – Self-determination of blood glucose: method.
R5 – The teaching of how to do these tests and to check that they are properly carried out.

3.  A regular follow-up of the diabetic is essential if he wants to keep well and avoid any accidents. Regular medical examinations are therefore necessary.

S1 – For the diabetic to be able to explain his problems and difficulties (hypoglycemic attacks, dietary problems and those relating to his working or family life, travel, car-driving etc.) and to be helped to overcome them.

S2   – For the doctor to check that all is well or to be able to suggest the corrective measures necessary:

    – by examining the results of the tests (urine, blood) carried out by the diabetic (note-book) or the laboratory for the control of the diabetes;

    – by observing the absence or appearance of a complication: by a clinical examination and examinations repeated at certain intervals: examination of the eyes, of renal function, of the nervous system, of the vascular system (blood pressure, electrocardiogram) or others;

    – by checking for the absence or onset of an associated anomaly (hypertension, hyperlipidemia, weight gain);

    – by instituting treatment of the complications or associated anomalies.

4. Thus through collaboration and regular supervision on the part of diabetic and doctor, the diabetic will be able to lead a normal life free from disabling accidents.

# 11. Educational objectives in diabetes teaching. The need of defining objectives and the evaluation of teaching objectives

V. JÖRGENS, L. HORNKE AND M. BERGER

## EDITORIAL

*In order to both standardize a diabetes teaching programme and to render it transferable and eligible for evaluation procedures, diabetes education has to be planned, structured and defined as to its specific objectives. Based on a number of practical examples, this article describes how to define operationalized objectives.*

*In the second part, the authors present a particular educational goal, i.e. the instruction of patients' relatives to inject glucagon in case of a severe hypoglycemia, as to the definition of its particular objectives, the planning of the educational process and its evaluation. As in other sections of this volume, the necessity to evaluate teaching materials and treatment equipment is underlined. In fact, it is a primary responsibility of the diabetes teaching team to define the objectives, to develop the teaching methods and aids and to evaluate their efficacy in a large number of diabetic patients.*

*The article presents one impressive example for such a series of educational processes in detail in order to encourage an operationalization and evaluation effort concerning the entire diabetes teaching programme. (The editors.)*

## INTRODUCTION

Most of the physicians, nurses and dieticians that are confronted with the task of patient education are not professional teachers. The question is, do they need to become professional teachers? Can good teaching be studied and learnt? All of us have had good and bad experiences with teachers during our school years – some of us remember excellent teachers, but also some we 'did not like', whom we did not accept as good teachers. But what is a good teacher? Which criteria decide whether a teaching process is effective or not? And how could those criteria be evaluated?

In each teaching process, the teacher defines objectives before he is going to teach, even if he does not know what this term means in education. The teacher defines the 'goals' of his teaching, and he knows (or believes) that a certain change in the knowledge or in the behavior will bring the student nearer to the main goal of the teaching process.

60

## WHY CAN IT BE USEFUL TO ATTEMPT A PRECISE DEFINITION OF OBJECTIVES?

1.   It is necessary to define educational objectives for an efficient communication of the teaching team. Each member of the team must have a defined task in the teaching process and defined responsibilities in the teaching programme.

2.   The precise definition of objectives makes it possible to plan a teaching programme, to think about an efficient syllabus and to choose adequate means for the instruction.

3.   Based upon defined objectives, it becomes possible to evaluate the educational process. Thus, critical points of the educational process can be identified and the time of instruction or the methods and means can be changed with respect to each particular objective in order to improve the efficacy of the educational programme.

4.   Furthermore, the general efficacy of the teaching programme has to be evaluated, i.e. the overall changes in the patients' behavior which are intended by the teaching objectives need to be measured in an acceptable percentage. Those changes in behavior should lead to the main goals of the teaching programme – i.e. good metabolic control and better quality of life.

## KNOWLEDGE AND BEHAVIOR

*'Gesagt ist nicht gehört,*
*gehört ist nicht verstanden,*
*verstanden ist nicht einverstanden,*
*einverstanden ist nicht angewendet,*
*angewendet ist noch lange nicht beibehalten'.*
*(K. Lorenz)*

The more objectives of the teaching programme are well defined, the easier it becomes to differentiate between the knowledge how to do something, the motivation to do it and the real behavior.
   There is a world between the decision to do something and to actually do it, as W. Shakespeare lets Brutus say:

*'Between the action of a dreadful thing*
*and the first motion, all in the interim is*
*like a phantasma, or a hideous dream'.*

What our patients have to do should not be all that 'dreadful' (in our

61

opinion), but for them injections, self-monitoring or diets might very well create 'phantasmas and hideous dreams' before they actually go about doing these things.

But we can learn from Shakespeare even more: Brutus and his friends represent a perfect example of a team that failed to define well the main objective of their programme of action: once the well-defined short-term objective was achieved, disagreement within the team (and unexpected reactions of the public) occurred and at the end, even the achievement of the short-term objective had lost its purpose. Our teaching approaches in patients should not only attempt the short-term objectives, e.g. increase in dietary knowledge, but should be directed to achieve the main goals of diabetes management as such.

## SINCE IT SEEMS USEFUL TO DEFINE TEACHING OBJECTIVES, HOW CAN WE DEFINE THEM?

Asked about the objectives of his patient education programme, a teacher might answer that he tries to enable the patient to manage his diabetes independently, based upon a certain knowledge about the disease in general, daily self-monitoring and the adaptation of diet and insulin dosage corresponding to the results of metabolic self-monitoring.

Such a 'goal' of education seems self-evident and will be generally accepted. But it can not be called detailed information about the 'content' of a teaching approach. This 'long range goal' is in the eyes of the patients 'something to move foreward, it gives him something to want to work for' (Kappel).

It must therefore be translated into a schooling programme and educational activities. The particular behavior-patterns which will help the patient to achieve this main goal must be defined well enough to guide instruction and to make an evaluation possible.

How to define a schooling programme for diabetics? One possible way to define it might be the following list.

The diabetes educator must explain:
self-monitoring of glucosuria
interpretation of the results
consequences of bad results
adaptation of the insulin dosage
and so on ...

This list describes actions of the teacher; it is a teacher-centered approach and not a student-centered one.

The aim of patient education, however, is to change the patients' behavior; therefore the desired changes in the patients' behavior should become the primary focus for the definition of the objectives. 'Teacher activities are means to an end and not ends to themselves; otherwise they could be performed in the absence of the students' (Bloom). The reason a teacher carries out any teaching activity is to help the students change in some way, to assist them in developing new abilities. This is the ultimate aim for which teachers plan, demonstrate, read lectures, etc.; it is the change in the student that is the real aim, the objective of any of the teacher's activities.

Another method to state objectives is to compile lists of detailed subjects such as:

urine testing
complications
insulin injection
muscle exercise
and so on ...

This way of describing objectives is nothing but a list of contents which are to be 'covered' by the teacher. The content by itself, however, might be meaningless, if there is no description of what the patient should be able to know and to do after having participated in the lessons. The teacher might have the feeling that he has fulfilled his task when he has covered all the items on his list of contents; his task, however, is to check knowledge and behavior during the course of the teaching process.

**The definition of 'operationalized objectives'**

A way to define objectives, focussed on the intended behavior, is the 'operationalized' objective. This 'operationalization' leads from a teacher-oriented 'theme' to a precise definition of the goal of the teaching process.

An operationalized objective includes:
1. the 'operation';
   for example: 'the insulin-dependent diabetic should carry sugar';
2. the condition;
   in this case: any time and everywhere;
3. and a 'measure', i.e. a test (situation) proving the efficacy of the teaching process; in this case: to check whether the patient carries sugar with him.

The formulation of the objectives of diabetes teaching in their particular patient education program leads the teaching staff to a better way of planning, practising and evaluating their teaching curriculum.


EVALUATING OBJECTIVES IN DIABETES EDUCATION

Some evaluation of operationalized educational objectives in diabetes education should be part of the daily routine in order to check and, if need be, improve the results of the teaching procedure. On the other hand, a detailed scientific evaluation of the educational problems of an objective in diabetes teaching requires – as a basis – the analysis of the educational objectives.

## 1. The evaluation of educational objectives in the daily routine. What should be checked at what time and by whom?

Cross-checks as to whether the behavioral objectives of a teaching curriculum have been achieved by a patient should be included in any teaching program. It should be planned within the teaching team who evaluates in what way and at which step of the teaching program.

An example for a bad timing of evaluation: in a one-week teaching curriculum, patients are learning Monday evening how to test their urine and Tuesday evening how to measure their glycemia with strips.

The chief physician – full of enthusiasm for patient education – asks the patients about their results of blood glucose monitoring on Tuesday morning – but they have not yet learnt how to do it. His questions confuse the patients – they are just proud to have measured their glucosuria for the first time this morning and now they are questioned about glucose monitoring.

How to solve the problem? List the patients' skill according to the course of the teaching program, for example in a one-week in-patient teaching program:

> Teaching items:
> self-monitoring and insulin injection.
> Monday morning.
> The patient measures preprandial glucosuria 3 times per day.
> He prepares and injects his insulin under supervision of a nurse.
> Tuesday morning.
> The patient begins to measure preprandial glycemia with a strip (supervision necessary).
> Wednesday morning.
> The patient has written his results of self-monitoring in his booklet correctly. He should be able to prepare and to inject mixtures of insulin alone, etc.

If the patients' skills are defined and listed like this, every member of the team should know what he can and should 'evaluate' at a certain time.

The head physician – on his usual ward-round on Tuesday morning – can ask the patients for the results of their glucosuria testing; on Wednesday morning, the physician can have a look at the results of the patients' glucose monitoring and ask for eventual problems and so on.

The more clearly the objectives and their short term evaluation process are defined within the curriculum, the lesser the patient becomes confused during an educational program. In addition, the evaluation should already take place during the lessons of the patients. An ineffective attempt to evaluate during a lesson would be the following question: 'Has everybody got it now!? Which alcoholic drinks you should not drink being diabetics!? Yeah!? Then we can go on! Well, let's discuss saccharin now!'

This is an attempt to evaluate; but trying to evaluate like this, a dietician could teach all her life without becoming aware of the inefficacy of her teaching approach.

How to improve this? The *objective* of the dietician is the following one: During a party, my patients should be able to identify alcoholic drinks containing a lot of sugar. They should be able to identify alcoholic drinks that they can drink in moderate amounts.

The *condition* would be: The patient is in front of 10 bottles with alcoholic drinks, and he wants to drink 2 glasses of one of those. The *test situation* would be that the patient actually chooses the right bottle during the party.

It would be a nice job for our dieticians to go to all the parties of our diabetics in order to evaluate the teaching objective. However – within the teaching curriculum – this objective can already be evaluated under less demanding conditions:

A party is simulated; every patient gets 10 cards displaying alcoholic drinks; he is then asked to eliminate those which are containing too much sugar and to turn those cards upside down. If the backside of these cards is red versus a green back of cards displaying drinks suitable for diabetic patients, the success of the patient in having achieved this objective is easily demonstrated. The teaching curriculum can continue to the next objective.

Looking at our daily teaching routine, we should introduce these relatively easy possibilities of evaluation. The more we are doing it, the more our patient education becomes a patient-oriented teaching and the less the teacher is feeling as a preacher in a desert.

Trying to use educational techniques in patient teaching does not mean developing a more and more sophisticated computerized teaching program in which each step is scrutinized and in which one can measure at any time what the patient knows and does. Patient educators differ in one crucial point from a professor of medicine in a university: the professor has to evaluate not only in order to improve his teaching but also to *eliminate* unsuccessful students who are unable to follow the curriculum and who would eventually do harm to their patients after becoming physicians.

A patient educator, however, cannot prevent a diabetic to leave the hospital as a diabetic! He can not eliminate any patient as a result of the evaluation process; he must find methods to enable most of his students to live independently with their disease.

That is why the methods of evaluation must strictly avoid situations scoring or frustrating the patients, showing them how little they know and can! In contrast the evaluation of patients' knowledge and behavior has to be done in such a way that the patient feels: 'evaluation is done to help myself to learn better'.

*V. Jörgens, L. Hornke and M. Berger*

## 2. Scientific approaches to evaluate objectives in diabetes teaching – a way to identify educational problems and how to solve them

The number of studies describing the results of educational objectives in diabetes teaching is quite limited – it seems that more efforts should be invested in this field.

As an example of a method how precisely to evaluate the teaching of a precise objective in diabetes education, we will discuss a study performed in our unit.

In a follow-up-study, we have measured various compliance rates in 70 insulin-dependent diabetics 1 year after they had followed a 1-week diabetes teaching programme. 34 of the patients' relatives had been taught to inject glucagon in case of a severe hypoglycemia. In 4 patients severe hypoglycemias had occurred during the follow-up period: in 3 of them glucagon was administered effectively by the patients' relatives, thus avoiding hospital admissions.

In order to teach more patients' relatives how to use glucagon and to analyze the educational problems of this objective, we planned the following study:

Evaluation of the objective: the diabetics' relatives should be able to inject glucagon in case of a severe hypoglycemia. Evaluating this objective, we were interested in the following questions:

1. Which results can be achieved?
2. Which educational problems can be observed?

The study was performed in the following way:

a. We wanted to develop a 10-minute video film demonstrating the handling of the NOVO Glucagon Set. This includes the parts of a syringe which have to be prepared to be ready for use, the solution fluid already being incorporated in the syringe and a vial with cristalline glucagon.

Thus, a task analysis was necessary: we had to define the sequence of behavioral steps, necessary to make the Set ready for use. Those steps are:

A: from opening the set ------ to ------ completely unpacked
B: from endpoint A ------ to ------ caps removed
C: from endpoint B ------ to ------ needle fixed and plunger pulled off
D: from endpoint C ------ to ------ plunger screwed in
E: from endpoint D ------ to ------ solution fluid injected
F: from endpoint E ------ to ------ glucagon vial shaken
G: from endpoint F ------ to ------ solution drawn into the syringe

b. Not only the handling, but also the injection procedure and the site of injection must be taught.

c. Furthermore the patients' relatives should learn that sudden unconsciousness in insulin-dependent diabetics should always be treated with glucagon because the probability of hypoglycemia being the underlying cause is very high.

## DEVELOPMENT OF A STANDARDIZED TEACHING MEANS: A VIDEO FILM

The video film about the glucagon injection begins with a physician explaining the necessity of a glucagon injection by the patients' relatives in case of severe hypoglycemia. The symptoms and eventual origins of hypoglycemias are demonstrated in the film with a patient. Then, the content of the Glucagon Set is displayed by a patient, who subsequently demonstrates the handling, the first time very slowly. Thereafter, an unconscious patient lies in his bed at home; his wife immediately prepares the Glucagon Set and injects intramuscular. The patient wakes up and his wife gives him some carbohydrates to eat. Finally, in a trick version the preparation of the Set is repeated once more.

*Formative evaluation.*
A first version of the film was demonstrated to 20 diabetologists, nurses and dieticians. Various episodes of the film were changed according to their comments and suggestions.

*Summative evaluation.*
To this end the film is shown to a representative sample of diabetic patients; thereafter the various objectives are evaluated.

*Knowledge.*
The objectives of the film related to the transfer of knowledge are assessed using a multiple choice questionnaire to be filled in before and after the film.

*Behavior.*
The behavioral objectives are assessed using the video media: the subjects are video-taped trying to prepare the Glucagon Set. Since the glucagon injections have to be performed by laypersons we asked 40 non-diabetics (mean age 15-36 years) to watch the video film. Immediately thereafter, they had to prepare the Glucagon Set as correctly and as fast as possible under video supervision.

Especially the results of the behavioral assessment might be interesting: 60% of the subjects arrived successfully at the endpoint of the procedure. For these the mean time to prepare the Glucagon Set was $42 \pm 124$ seconds. On further analysis of the video tapes, we found out that drawing the solution into the syringe seems to be the most critical step during the procedure to make the glucagon syringe ready for use. Secondly it became apparent that the steps D and G (see above) were particularly time-consuming.

In practice, the glucagon injection technique can be trained with the subjects until they have learned to prepare it themselves. But the above analysis of the teaching objective permitted us to make some particular suggestions in order to improve the results of the teaching process. These suggestions are related both to the teaching approach and to the material used.

Thus, the video film should be directed more specifically to the critical points of the handling procedure. Appropriate additions and repetitions should be made at the end of the film.

On the other hand, the video taping technique made apparent that the material of the Glucagon Set can and should be improved. Certain steps require simplification. These improvements – very easy to introduce – could diminish the number of behavioral steps. Thus, the number of objectives to instruct could be diminished; and more time could be spent to instruct the most difficult step, namely drawing up the solution into the syringe (step G).

Concluding the results of this little study, we proposed the described improvements in the Glucagon Injection Set in order to make it more useful for laypersons. Material for patients and their relatives should be evaluated using a standardized educational procedure in order to achieve better results in the teaching procedure. Who would evaluate the problems due to the materials utilised in diabetes education if it is not done by the teams teaching diabetics?

## EPILOG

In a recently-published booklet for diabetic patients, T.M. Flood of the Joslin Diabetes Center cites a poem of A.L. Gordon to describe how he would like patients to deal with their diabetes and accept their being diabetics:

*'Question not but live and labour*
*Til your goal be won,*
*Helping every feeble neighbor,*
*Seeking help from none;*
*Life is mostly froth and bubble*
*Two things stand like stone:*
*Kindness in another's trouble,*
*Courage in our own'.*

In contrast, patient educators MUST question, they MUST evaluate the effects of their teaching; if they don't, 'the goal' might never 'be won'. Helping the 'feeble' diabetic does not mean keeping him dependent on the medical staff. Exactly the opposite is the goal: based upon the objectives of diabetes teaching, he should be able to act independently, so that he feels a little less 'froth and bubble' living with his disease. Finally, we should be aware of the fact that – even with the most excellent teaching –

the patient needs a lot of 'courage' in his 'own'; not all of his problems will be solved by our treatment and education.

## SUMMARY

The treatment of diabetic patients must include patient education in order to achieve efficient care of the disease. It has been proven that patient education can limit the costs due to hospitalization and sick-leave of diabetics, and there is no doubt that self-management by the patients is necessary to achieve the main goals of diabetes treatment – good metabolic control and a high quality of life.

If patient education is accepted as one of the most important parts of diabetes treatment, the medical team needs to develop qualities of a professional teacher, a role which is unusual for physicians and nurses. In this article we summarize the advantages of a precise definition of the objectives within a diabetes teaching curriculum, and we describe some methods to evaluate teaching objectives both in research and in the daily routine. This might be helpful for physicians and nurses on their way to become professional patient educators.

## REFERENCES AND LITERATURE ABOUT PATIENT EDUCATION

1. Steiner, G. and Lawrence, P.A. (Eds.) (1981): *Educating Diabetic Patients*. Springer-Verlag, New York.
2. Etzwiler, D.D., Hess, K., Hirsch, A. and Morreau, L. (1978): *Education and Management of the Patient with Diabetes Mellitus*. Ames Company, Elkhart, Indiana.
3. Green, L.W. (Ed.) (1980): *The Professional and Scientific Literature on Patient Education*. GALE Research Company, Detroit, USA.
4. Bloom, B.S., Hastings, J.T. and Madaus, G.F. (1971): Handbook of Formative and Summative Evaluation of Student Learning. McGraw-Hill Book Company, New York.
5. Speers, M.A. and Turk, D.C. (1982): Diabetes Self Care: Knowledge, Beliefs, Motivation and Action. *Patient Councel. Health Educ., Vol 3*, 144.
6. Jörgens, V., Dopatka, H., Mulders, A. et al. (1982): Glucagon injection by the patients' relatives; evaluation of an objective of diabetes teaching using the video media. *Diabetes 31, Suppl. 1*, 18 A (Abstract).

# 12. Educational aspects of pump treatment in type-I diabetic patients

G.E. SONNENBERG, E.A. CHANTELAU AND M. BERGER

## EDITORIAL

*This article outlines a specific diabetes teaching programme for patients treated with continuous subcutaneous insulin infusion (CSII). This programme represents an advanced course for particular patients who have already become familiar with the teaching objectives of general diabetes education. For this particular group of patients, a highly sophisticated teaching programme has been developed by the authors. In fact, they state repeatedly that the advanced technology of portable insulin pumps can only be used to its best advantage and without introducing additional risks if an effective teaching programme can be delivered to the patients. It appears that the more advanced the therapeutic techniques become, the more important the proper training of the patient becomes to use them. On the other hand, the authors describe but one example of the necessity to deliver particular, advanced diabetes teaching programmes for particular needs such as for pregnant diabetic ladies, diabetic patients on chronic ambulatory peritoneal dialysis or diabetic top-level athletes and sports professionals. The performance of these patients in their particular environment will largely depend on whether or not they had the chance to participate in a particular teaching and training programme. (The editors.)*

## INTRODUCTION

The special teaching protocol for patients on insulin pump treatment presupposes their prior participation in the education programme for diabetics, described in greater detail elsewhere in this volume. Knowledge and comprehension of this general diabetes education programme is the basis for any training in pump treatment. For example, the patients have to be informed about the physiology of insulin secretion, the effects of short- and long-acting insulin, the exact carbohydrate content of their nutrition as well as blood glucose self-monitoring.

Further to this general information on diabetes treatment, the patients have to learn the differences between conventional insulin injection therapy and continuous subcutaneous insulin infusion treatment with portable pumps (CSII).

70

# THE PRINCIPLE OF CONTINUOUS SUBCUTANEOUS INSULIN INFUSION (CSII)

CSII represents a new approach to insulin therapy in type-I diabetic patients. In approximation to the physiological secretion, short acting insulin delivery is maintained at a constant basal rate; in addition, insulin is administered in premeal doses 15 min before meals to prevent postprandial hyperglycemia by carbohydrate absorption. The diabetics have to control the rates of insulin supply themselves, since CSII represents a so-called 'open loop' system without any feedback regulation of the insulin supply according to automatically measured blood glucose levels. That is why it is important for the patients on pump treatment to learn themselves to 'close the loop' by measuring their daily blood glucose levels and adjusting the insulin infusion rates accordingly.

The main objective of CSII treatment is to achieve a stable and normoglycemic or near-normoglycemic metabolic control in type-I diabetic patients. In consequence, CSII treatment is expected to be effective in preventing or delaying the development of diabetic late complications. In addition, patients appreciate the substantial improvement in their quality of life during CSII treatment, as it affords far greater flexibility in their dietary habits and general daily schedule.

# WHAT KIND OF PATIENT QUALIFIES FOR PUMP TREATMENT?

CSII treatment is only suitable for highly cooperative, interested and well-informed type-I diabetic patients. The patients must be so motivated towards achieving optimal diabetic control that they are willing to endure the discomfort of wearing the pump at all times. Furthermore, they have to check their blood glucose levels 3-5 times a day, record their progress in a daily log, and come to the out-patients department at regular intervals (during the first 2 months of CSII treatment at weekly or biweekly intervals). Only on these premises can CSII treatment be effective and free of risk.

Our experience of CSII treatment in 61 patients over the last 2 years indicates that the patients initially selected along those lines turned out to be very cooperative indeed. Especially in the early stage of pump treatment, the patients themselves gave us many practical hints which we were able to pass on to other diabetics treated by CSII. Thus, they pointed out optimal ways of wearing the pump (either on a belt or concealed under their clothing). Also, our patients on CSII turned out to be very active in organizing self-help groups for diabetics.

G.E. Sonnenberg, E.A. Chantelau and M. Berger

FIRST INTERVIEW

If a well motivated and educated type-I diabetic patient is interested in pump treatment, he comes for his first interview to the out-patients department. There, he is informed about this new kind of treatment by a specially trained physician and by other patients already being treated with CSII. First of all, the differences between pump treatment and the conventional insulin injection therapy are explained. The patient should be well informed about the advantages and disadvantages of pump treatment. He should understand that pump treatment is not a simple and easy matter; on the contrary, it requires the patient's meticulous co-operation.

During the first interview various types of insulin infusers are demonstrated and explained in detail.

At first, most patients are worried about the idea of catheters being continuously inserted in the subcutaneous tissue of the anterior abdominal wall. At this stage it is helpful to have another patient who has been on pump treatment for some time to set the newcomer's mind at rest by showing him the position of the catheter, ways of wearing the pump and pointing out that every day life is not unduly impeded.

This patient-to-patient talk seems to be extremely useful and effective for the diabetic patient with regard to his attitude towards the pump and his subsequent decision.

EDUCATIONAL PROGRAMME DURING THE INITIAL PHASE OF PUMP TREATMENT

## 1.  Pump handling

In our experience a short hospital stay of only 4-5 days is necessary to initiate pump treatment. On the first day the patient is introduced to all the technical details of the particular pump that has been selected as being the most suitable for him. The function of all the buttons, switches etc. on the pump are explained. Further operating instructions are: filling the syringe with short-acting insulin in a special dilution with saline, the loading procedure of the syringe, the insertion of the catheter into the subcutaneous tissue, changing the battery, and inserting the battery into the pump. Also discussed are various ways of wearing the pump. After some time, most patients find individual solutions which are often quite surprisingly effective. Frequently, several patients are put on pump treatment at the same time so they can help each other during their stay in hospital with such tasks as filling the syringe, inserting the catheter and handling the reflectometer for blood glucose monitoring.

## 2.  Adjustment of the insulin basal rate

In consultation with the patient, the physician works out the individual insulin requirement. The initial insulin basal rate is estimated at about 50% of prior daily insulin requirement. During the remaining 3-4 days in hospital, the basal insulin rate should be adjusted to actual requirements.

The patient is taught that the fasting blood glucose value, the bedtime value and the 3 a.m. value are important for adjustment of the basal rate. Since the 3 a.m. value is often very low, the fasting blood glucose level should not drop below 90 or 100 mg/dl to prevent hypoglycemia during the night. For the same reason, patients are advised to take a small amount of carbohydrates, if their bedtime value is below 100 mg/dl.

The patients are instructed that the insulin basal rate may decrease after 3 or 4 weeks of pump treatment, as the insulin sensitivity increases with (near-) normoglycemia.

## 3.  Adjustment of premeal insulin dosages

One of the most important tasks the patient has to master during his hospital stay is the adjustment of the preprandial insulin dose administered 15 min before each meal. The patient must be taught that the premeal insulin dose depends on the amount of carbohydrates, the actual blood glucose value and the time of the day. The early morning insulin requirement per unit of carbohydrate is significantly higher than any other time of day. In order to check their individually adjusted premeal dosage, patients are instructed to determine their blood glucose levels 15 min before and 60 min after each food intake. In this way they learn about the effect of the insulin in relation to the carbohydrate absorption.

During their hospital stay, the patients should keep a special record sheet noting the time of the day, the blood glucose level, the premeal dose (by turning the button, e.g. one 'click' on the Mill Hill Infuser), the ingested carbohydrates and any special remarks. The physician and the patient discuss the record sheet several times a day to check whether the patient has administered the additional rate correctly. The blood glucose values monitored by the patients are occasionally double checked by laboratory determination.

On the basis of this discussion, guidelines are worked out which, to begin with, apply to the normoglycemic range between 80 and 140 mg/dl. The patients should also learn to adjust the premeal insulin dose if the actual blood glucose values are not within the normal range. One example: A patient had achieved good diabetic control using the following regimen: breakfast 12 clicks per 3 BE (Bread Exchange, 1 BE = 12 g of carbohydrates), elevenses: 4 clicks per 2 BE, lunch 6 clicks per 3 BE, tea time: 2 clicks per 1 BE, supper: 9 clicks per 3 BE, late snack: 4 clicks per 2 BE. Table 1 indicates the changes the patient has to perform if the preprandial

G.E. Sonnenberg, E.A. Chantelau and M. Berger

Table 1  *Adjustment of premeal insulin doses (Mill Hill Infuser, basal insulin infusion rate 20 U/day)*

| Time of day | Blood glucose (mg/dl) | 'Clicks' | BE (= 12 g carbo-hydrates) | Special remarks |
|---|---|---|---|---|
| 7.00 a.m. | 93 | | | |
| 7.45 a.m. | 105 | 12 | | |
| 8.00 a.m. | | | 3 | |
| 9.00 a.m. | 135 | | | |
| 9.45 a.m. | 160 | 4 + 1 | | 1 more click! |
| 10.00 a.m. | | | 2 | Diet demonstration at supermarket |
| 11.00 a.m. | 115 | | | |
| 11.45 a.m. | 106 | 6 | | |
| 12.00 noon | | | 3 | |
| 1.00 p.m. | 122 | | | |
| 2.15 p.m. | 102 | 2 | | |
| 2.30 p.m. | | | 1 | Educational session |
| 3.30 p.m. | 99 | | | |
| 5.00 p.m. | 90 | | | Walk |
| 6.15 p.m. | 72 | 6 | | |
| 6.30 p.m. | | | 3 | 3 fewer clicks |
| 7.30 p.m. | 110 | | | |
| 8.45 p.m. | 122 | 4 | | |
| 9.00 p.m. | | | 2 | |
| 10.00 p.m. | 116 | | | |
| 3.00 a.m. | 98 | | | |
| 7.00 a.m. | 109 | | | |

blood glucose values are outside the normal range.

The patient had chosen the premeal dose correctly: he had turned one more click during the morning, because of a higher blood glucose level (160 mg/dl) and he had lowered the number of clicks by 3 before supper because of the low blood glucose level of 72 mg/dl.

The basal rate also appeared to have been adjusted correctly: the 3 blood glucose values at bedtime, at 3 a.m. and the fasting value of the following morning remained within a stable range.

Such frequent blood glucose determination as well as frequent meal intake should be practised only during hospital stay to get the patient used to pump handling. Later, during the out-patient stage, dietary restrictions can be lifted by varying the number and distribution of meals over the day as well as the amount and distribution of carbohydrates over their meals without having to worry about a deterioration of metabolic control. Yet, despite the general liberalization of the dietary regimen, it is extremely important that the patient should be able to accurately gauge the amount of carbohydrates in his food.

From all these factors it becomes clear that the complete pump education during hospital stay must be exceedingly thorough and demanding for both the patient and the physician. On leaving hospital, the patients should be so well-trained that they are able to adjust without help their insulin basal rate and varying premeal dosage.

## GUIDELINES FOR SPECIAL SITUATIONS

### 1. Concomitant illnesses

The patients are instructed that in the case of feverish illness their basal insulin requirement is raised. Consequently, they have to increase the basal insulin rate gradually while closely checking blood glucose values. In extreme situations with ketoacidotic deterioration, patients should administer additional insulin doses via subcutaneous injections in accordance with the guide lines of conventional insulin therapy.

### 2. Sports activities

Physical exercise is a further factor upsetting the glucose homeostasis. That is why we recommend that patients check their blood glucose levels more frequently. During strenuous sports activity the pump should be removed, and the additional dosage before the previous meal be reduced. In case of less strenuous exercise, the pump remains in place and the basal insulin rate can be reduced. The patient should be made aware that his insulin requirement can remain low for several hours after physical exercise so he may have to eat some additional carbohydrates to prevent hypoglycemic reactions.

### 3. What to do if blood glucose suddenly rises?

If the blood glucose suddenly rises without any apparent cause, the patient is advised to check the functioning of the pump and the catheter. For that purpose he should consult the checklist he has been provided with (see checklist).

Checklist (for patients using the Mill Hill Infuser)
1. Is the *pump* working correctly?
   Is the motor humming as usual, and is the lamp blinking every 4 seconds?
2. Is the *battery* empty?
   Place the reserve battery and check the functioning of the motor.

3. Is there still enough liquid in the *syringe*?
   Please remember that the last 3 graduations cannot be emptied (only while using Omnifix® syringes with Luer lock).
   Has the correct amount of insulin been drawn?
   If necessary, refill the syringe.
   Are there any large air bubbles in the syringe?
   If necessary, refill the syringe.
4. Is the *catheter* lying correctly in the subcutaneous tissue? If not, reinsert.
   Is the catheter tightly connected with the syringe?
   Is the catheter bent?
   Is there any pressure of clothing against the catheter (for example a belt)?
   Does the insulin flow back from the area where the catheter has been placed?
   If so, reinsert the catheter.
   The butterfly catheter should be replaced at least every 3-4 days.
5. Is the *reflectometer* functioning correctly?
   Repeat the blood glucose determination and compare with Haemoglucotest 20-800 test-strip.

If you have not discovered any reason for the high blood sugar value going through the check-list or if you cannot correct it, please contact us. In the meantime, you should inject insulin in the conventional manner subcutaneously, i.e. Actrapid® insulin in adequate doses, according to the blood sugar value.

If the patient can neither discover nor repair any fault in the apparatus, he must contact our department. There is a round-the-clock telephone service in operation, where specially trained physicians give advice.

## WHAT ARE THE PATIENT'S TASKS AFTER DISCHARGE FROM HOSPITAL?

In line with instructions during his hospital stay, the patient keeps a daily log in which he enters the following data: 3-5 blood glucose values monitored at home, the insulin basal rate, the amount of premeal insulin dosage, the number of meals and the amount of carbohydrates. The patient has been handed his special logbook which also provides space for entries, such as hypoglycemic reactions, sports activities, changes in the basal rate as well as any possible complications involving catheter and pump, etc. Keeping this log not only serves the physician's convenience, but helps the patient to gain security about his metabolic control and to learn how to better adjust his treatment on the basis of past experience. The daily log provides the basis for consultation with the physician on regular visits to the out-patients' department.

On these occasions, the actual blood glucose is measured by the laboratory and compared on the spot with the patient's reflectometer reading to check its proper functioning.

A blood sample is drawn for the determination of hemoglobin $A_{IC}$ Thereafter, physician and patient jointly inspect the daily log, and discuss the level of the basal rate and the ratio between the premeal insulin dosage and the carbohydrate intake. Also checked is whether the patient has reacted properly to special situations.

## SUMMARY

Continuous subcutaneous insulin infusion (CSII) with portable pumps is a new approach to insulin therapy in type-I diabetic patients. CSII treatment represents an effective tool in order to achieve normoglycemia or near-normoglycemia and is expected to prevent or delay the development of diabetic late complications. CSII treatment is only suitable for highly motivated and cooperative type-I diabetic patients.

The general diabetes education programme run by our department should be the basis for the special training protocol for patients on pump treatment. This special training protocol is conducted during the short (4-5 days) hospital stay for the initiation of pump treatment. Main points of instructions are: pump handling with all its technical aspects, adjustment of the insulin basal rate and the premeal insulin dosage, and the keeping of a daily log. Furthermore, the patients are given guidelines for special situations, such as concomitant illness and sports activities; they are also instructed how to confront sudden unexplained hyperglycemia by means of a check list.

In conclusion, in view of the intricacy and demands of the pump treatment, the education programme has to be exceedingly thorough. Only if the patient's knowledge and comprehension are fully activated can CSII treatment be effective and free of risk. In fact, the efficacy of the specific diabetes training programme is one of the cornerstones of the success of the CSII therapy.

# 13.  Difficulties encountered with patient education in European Diabetic Centers

A report of 6 workshops conducted by the DESG

J.-Ph. ASSAL AND S. LION

EDITORIAL

*This article provides a unique collection point and channeling of the thoughts and concerns of physicians directing medical teams in the treatment of patients with diabetes mellitus throughout Europe. The major difficulties in patient education for these physicians are identified through their own discussions and selections during workshops of the Diabetes Education Study Group with the results presented in order of importance.*

*With the primary difficulties well identified, the approach to finding the solutions is clearly opened to the entire medical community. For the improvement of some of the leading concerns of the physicians, the findings reported in this article indicate that considerations from fields outside medicine may be needed for issues like: (1) the systematic analysis and evaluation of all elements of patient education; (2) the study of techniques in management and education to aid directors and personnel functioning in medical teams; and (3) psychological understanding of methods for the improvement of doctors' attitudes towards working with patients whose disease is chronic. (The editors.)*

One of the first activities planned by the Diabetes Education Study Group (DESG) of the European Association for the Study of Diabetes (EASD) was an inventory of the difficulties encountered in patient education and diabetes control in several diabetic centers throughout Europe. Our objective was to organize several workshops in which members of different medical teams could express and discuss the difficulties experienced in their daily practice.

6 workshops were held from November 1980 to July 1982. 5 were organized in Geneva for the Western European countries and 1 in Bucharest for the Eastern European countries. 166 participants, mainly physicians with some nurses and dieticians, attended. Each workshop lasted for 3 days. The number of participants oscillated between 25 to 45. A total of 23

European countries were represented. 135 physicians, who were in charge of a diabetic center and collectively responsible for more than half a million diabetic consultations a year, attended.

The discussions during these workshops were probably representative of the clinical situations that occur, at least in part, in European diabetic centers. Although the participants could easily describe the structure of their centers (e.g. size, number of collaborators, number of patients and consultations per year, etc.), they had much more difficulty describing the many problems encountered with patient education and those experienced with the medical team.

An inventory of these problems is an important first step towards finding solutions for better patient education and management of the medical team. In order to clarify these problems, we used a discussion technique which favored interaction between participants. (See Chapter 24.)

The 4 main difficulties encountered in the practices of the physicians who were present were analyzed within the different groups of physician participants according to the following criteria:
1.  language affinity and/or geographical vicinity (Table 2);
2.  a general European level, regardless of country (Table 3);
3.  Northern and Southern Europe (Table 4);
4.  Eastern and Western Europe (Table 5).

The discussions helped the participants to define sectors to which efforts should be directed to improve diabetic treatment and patient education. Common basic difficulties were cited by all participants in their groups: poor motivation of patients, the need for guidelines and objectives for training the health care team in patient education, difficulties in evaluation of a teaching program, poorly adapted attitude of doctors, nurses and dieticians to the chronical condition of diabetes and lack of equipment and supplies.

## I.  GROUP DISCUSSIONS AND INVENTORY OF THE DIFFICULTIES ENCOUNTERED IN THE DIABETIC CENTERS

The same person, one of the authors (JPA), was the moderator throughout the 6 workshops. Each group discussion was structured in 3 phases:
1.  Each participant had to answer a standardized questionnaire about his or her Diabetes Center. Questions to be answered were: number of collaborators, type of teaching programme, description of teaching equipment, number of patients under the care of the center, number of medical visits performed in each center yearly (Table 1). Each participant had also to answer an open question: *Which are the 2 main problems you have in your Center concerning patient treatment and/or patient education?*
2.  The next phase in the workshop was for the moderator to group similar difficulties together on a tackboard and to give a title to each grouping (Fig. 1).

3. Finally, the participants discussed each group of difficulties.

At the end of the discussions, partipants were asked which difficulty listed on the board interfered the most with the treatment of patients. To clearly label his or her answer, each participant received 3 adhesive dots that could be put on the tackboard next to the difficulties for which he or she wanted to vote as the most important (Fig. 2). At the end of the voting, the moderator summed up the dots for each difficulty and listed them in a rank order (Tables 2 to 5). In each workshop about 8 to 12 difficulties were listed. In this paper, however, only the 4 most frequently mentioned problems will be discussed. These problems will be ranked from 1 to 4 in order of importance.

Table 1   *DESG workshops*

| Country | Participating physicians in charge of DM Center | Number of patient-visits per year in the partici- pating Centers |
|---|---|---|
| Austria | 2 | 6,000 |
| Belgium | 5 | 19,000 |
| Bulgaria | 1 | 1,000 |
| Czechoslovakia | 2 | 1,200 |
| Denmark | 6 | 29,000 |
| Finland | 5 | 10,000 |
| France | 14 | 64,900 |
| E. Germany | 5 | 60,000 |
| W. Germany | 10 | 16,800 |
| Great Britain | 8 | 37,800 |
| Greece | 4 | 12,100 |
| Hungary | 4 | 3,100 |
| Israel | 1 | 5,000 |
| Italy | 17 | 86,400 |
| Netherlands | 6 | 21,500 |
| Norway | 5 | 8,500 |
| Poland | 4 | 8,200 |
| Portugal | 4 | 17,500 |
| Rumania | 10 | 59,700 |
| Spain | 5 | 49,900 |
| Sweden | 7 | 25,800 |
| Switzerland | 5 | 10,000 |
| Yugoslavia | 3 | 12,700 |
| TOTAL: 23 countries | 133* | 566,100 |

* 31 nurses and dieticians also participated, which makes a total of 164 participants in these workshops.

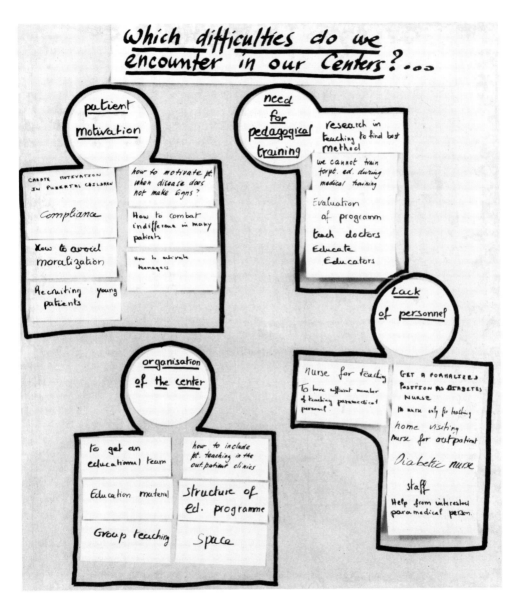

Fig. 1   Grouping of similar difficulties headed by a common topic heading.

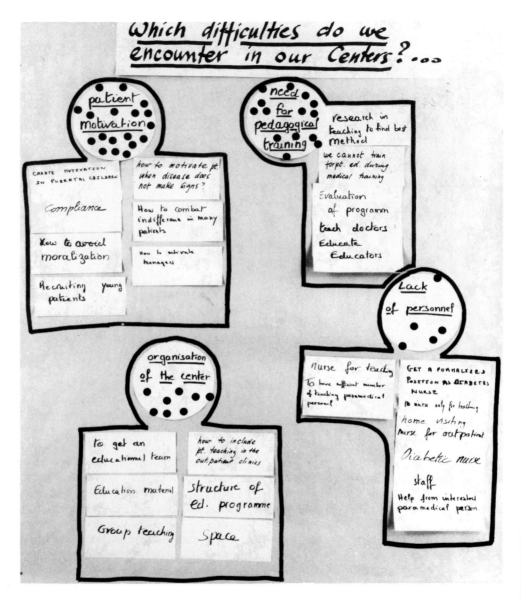

Fig. 2   Voting results on participants' greatest difficulties. Each black dot represents 1 vote. Each participant had 3 votes.

Table 2   *Difficulties[1] encountered in diabetic centers grouped by regions*

| Groups of countries | Score* |
|---|---|
| **Group 1:   ITALY – YUGOSLAVIA – GREECE** | |
| 1.   Attitude of doctors | 25 |
| 2.   Lack of training in patient education | 13 |
| 3.   Poor patient motivation | 9 |
| 4.   Insensitivity of public health administration | 4 |
| **Group 2:   BELGIUM[Δ] – FRANCE – PORTUGAL – SPAIN** | |
| 1.   Organization of center for integrating patient education with treatment | 19 |
| 2.   Lack of training in patient education | 11 |
| 3.   Evaluation of patient education (methods and results) | 10 |
| 4.   Psychological support for the patient | 9 |
| **Group 3:   AUSTRIA – WEST GERMANY – SWITZERLAND[□]** | |
| 1.   Evaluation of patient education (methods and results) | 18 |
| 2.   Poor patient motivation | 11 |
| 3.   Poor motivation of the health care team | 8 |
| 4.   Lack of training in patient education | 6 |
| **Group 4:   DENMARK – FINLAND – NORWAY – SWEDEN** | |
| 1.   Poor patient motivation | 21 |
| 2.   Lack of personnel and time | 19 |
| 3.   Lack of training in patient education | 17 |
| 4.   Evaluation of patient education (methods and results) | 7 |
| **Group 5:   NETHERLANDS – UNITED KINGDOM** | |
| 1.   Poor patient motivation | 13 |
| 2.   Evaluation of patient education (methods and results) | 12 |
| 3.   Organization of center for integrating patient education with treatment | 11 |
| 4.   Lack of training in patient education | 7 |
| **Group 6:   BULGARIA – CZECHOSLOVAKIA – EAST GERMANY – HUNGARY – POLAND – RUMANIA** | |
| 1.   Poor patient motivation | 24 |
| 2.   Attitude of doctors | 22 |
| 3.   Lack of equipment and supplies | 14 |
| 4.   Heterogeneity of patients | 5 |

[1]   Ranked in order of importance out of 8 to 12 problems.
*   Results of 3 votes from each participant on his most pressing difficulties.
[Δ]   Only French-speaking participants attended.
[□]   Only German-speaking participants attended.

## II. PROBLEMS ENCOUNTERED IN DIFFERENT EUROPEAN REGIONS

In order to improve the quality of the interaction between participants, workshops were organized according to language affinity and/or geographical area of participants. Workshops were held in English, French, German and Italian. The 6 workshops grouped the physicians of the following countries:

Group 1: Italy, Yugoslavia (26 participants)
Group 2: Belgium, France, Greece, Portugal, Spain (22 participants)
Group 3: Austria, West-Germany, Switzerland (25 participants)
Group 4: Denmark, Finland, Norway, Sweden (32 participants)
Group 5: Netherlands, United Kingdom (22 participants)
Group 6: Bulgaria, East-Germany, Hungary, Poland, Rumania, Czechoslovakia (39 participants)

Table 2 shows the 4 main difficulties (out of 8 to 12) experienced by participating physicians in their diabetic centers. The problems identified by participants from the different diabetic centers ranged from lack of medical equipment and supply (group 6) to the unadapted attitude of the physicians when they have to treat chronic diseases (group 1 and 6). Concern about poor motivation of patients was found in 5 groups (groups 1, 3, 4, 5, 6). Need for training the medical team was expressed in groups 1, 2, 3, 4 and 5. Particular concern for the evaluation of the teaching methods and the medical effect of patient education were expressed by groups 2 and 3.

Table 3   *Difficulties[1] encountered in diabetic centers as identified by all European participants*

| Problem | Score* |
|---|---|
| 1.   Poor patient motivation | 78 |
| 2.   Lack of training in patient education | 54 |
| 3.   Organization of center for integrating patient education with treatment | 53 |
| 4. – Attitude of doctors, nurses or dieticians | 47 |
|       – Evaluation of patient education (methods and results) | 47 |
| 6.   Lack of equipment and supplies | 14 |
| 7.   Lack of personnel | 11 |
| 8.   Psychological support of the patients | 9 |

[1]   Ranked in order of importance.
*   Results of 3 votes from each participant on his most pressing difficulties.

## III. PROBLEMS ENCOUNTERED AT A EUROPEAN-WIDE LEVEL

The problems encountered during all the 6 workshops are listed in a decreasing order of importance (Table 3). By far the most important problem observed was poor patient motivation (score of 78). Then came a group of 4 problems with scores between 47 and 54:
- lack of training for patient education,
- evaluation of the teaching approach,
- attitude of doctors toward patients with a chronic disease,
- organization of a center where integration of patient education could best be made with the classical medical approach.

Finally, lack of equipment and supplies, lack of personnel and need for psychological support for the patient were also considered.

The 5 problems most frequently encountered by the physicians in their diabetic centers (Table 3) are discussed in more detail below.

### 1. Poor patient motivation

This important problem involving long term success in treatment of diabetes has been a major concern during almost all workshops. Some expressions of physicians about the poor motivation of the patients are illustrated by the following remarks: '1 out of 2 of my diabetics is not motivated'; 'How do we fight indifference in so many patients?'; 'How can I modify attitudes in adolescents and in adults?'; 'How can the attention of the patient be kept open?'; 'They may not be motivated because we are too negative and moralizing'; 'It is easy to motivate them while in a teaching unit, but after they go home, how can we maintain this motivation?'; 'Anyhow the adult is not motivated to go again to school for his diabetes'. These statements reflect a climate of sadness and resignation among the physicians. During the discussions, only a few solutions for improving the motivation of patients were suggested. Future workshops will be necessary to study more systematically the various aspects involved in motivation.

### 2. Lack in training for patient education

This was the second important problem which was brought to light. The participating physicians determined that if patient education plays a key role in the treatment of diabetes, then the physicians need more training in order to improve their skill for teaching diabetics. Several advantages which could be gained from such a training were identified to include the following: knowledge of some teaching methods to help the physician, the nurse and the dietician to select more appropriate techniques for specific patients and situations; simplified teaching; saved energy for those who teach; and easier exchanges between teachers from one diabetic center to another.

## 3. Organization of the medical center integrating patient education with treatment

Another problem raised was how to really integrate patient education in the classical medical care of diabetics. Several examples were given of the difficulties encountered in the organization of a diabetic center. Patient education constantly has to fight for a correct place in the treatment scheme. There is a lack of trained teaching nurses and stable personnel. Lack of adequate space for patient education was cited: in many centers the classroom was nothing more than a busy floor. Lack of time and no official recognition of the need for patient education by the public health administration completed the list.

## 4A. Attitude of doctors, nurses and dieticians

The discussions between physicians also revealed concern about the attitude of health care professionals. Helping the patient with a chronic disease requires the members of the medical team to display an attitude other than that which is often observed. Specifically, there is no time to listen to the patients, often resulting in inadequate information which does not sufficiently take into account the patient's personal experience with the disease. The participants wanted to find ways to adapt more to the patient's psychological and social profile.

The next problem identified by the participants received the same number of points and is listed below as item 4B.

## 4B. Evaluation of patient education: methods used and results

Another difficulty expressed was how to evaluate the correct choice and efficiency of the methods used for patient education and their effects on diabetes control, long term complications and psycho-social well-being. One factor which may interfere with the interest of the medical team for patient education is the difficulty to obtain immediate, clearcut results of the education of the patients. Other difficulties are the lack of appropriate knowledge of doctors for testing methods and results of teaching patients.

## IV. ARE THERE DIFFERENCES IN DIFFICULTIES ENCOUNTERED BY DIABETIC CENTERS BETWEEN NORTHERN AND SOUTHERN EUROPE?

Although there is an arbitrary separation between North and South in our workshops, many physicians thought that there would be major differences between the 'Latin' countries and Northern Europe. The list of major difficulties encountered in the diabetic centers shows that there are in fact

Table 4   *Difficulties[1] encountered in diabetic centers: differences between Northern and Southern Europe*

| Northern Europe (Groups 3, 4, 5) | Score* | Southern Europe (Groups 1, 2)▫ | Score* |
|---|---|---|---|
| 1. Poor patient motivation | 45 | 1. Attitude of doctors | 25 |
| 2. Evaluation of patient education (methods and results) | 37 | 2. Lack of training in patient education | 24 |
| 3. Lack of training in patient education | 30 | 3. Organization of center for integrating patient education with treatment | 23 |
| 4. Organization of center for integrating patient education with treatment | 30 | 4. Poor patient motivation | 18 |

[1]   Ranked in order of importance out of 8 to 12 problems.
*   Results of 3 votes from each participant on his most pressing difficulties.
▫   French-speaking participants were put in this group.

many common problems (Table 4). The participants of the Northern countries seemed more preoccupied with evaluation of the teaching process than the Latin European participants. The latter seemed more preoccupied with the attitude of the doctor dealing with a patient with a chronic disease.

## V.   ARE THERE DIFFERENCES IN DIFFICULTIES ENCOUNTERED BY DIABETIC CENTERS BETWEEN EAST AND WEST EUROPE?

Both groups of countries had in common their most important problem: the poor motivation of patients (Table 5). Like Southern Europe, the participants of East European countries thought that the attitude of physicians should be modified to help patients who have chronic diseases. Lack of medical supply, mainly reagents for glucose measurement, was a concern. The need of training for patient education was not so outspoken as in Western European countries.

## CONCLUSIONS

Among the topics and activities which occurred during the workshops of the DESG, the inventory of problems encountered by physicians in diabetic centers was the most appreciated by the participants. The clarification of the problems will help the participants and other involved health care professionals to find better ways to study and organize improved training for

Table 5   *Difficulties[1] encountered in diabetic centers: differences between Eastern and Western Europe*

| Eastern Europe (Group 6) | Score* | Western Europe (Groups 1-5)□ | Score* |
|---|---|---|---|
| 1. Poor patient motivation | 24 | 1. Poor patient motivation | 54 |
| 2. Attitude of doctors | 22 | 2. Lack of training in patient education | 54 |
| 3. Lack of equipment and supplies | 14 | 3. Evaluation of patient education (methods and results) | 47 |
| 4. Heterogeneity of patients | 5 | 4. Organization of center for integrating patient education with treatment | 30 |

[1]   Ranked in order of importance out of 8 to 12 problems.
*   Results of 3 votes from each participant on his most pressing difficulties.
□   Includes Yugoslavia for reasons of internal group logic.

physicians, nurses and dieticians who work with diabetics.

This report was based on the difficulties experienced by physicians, nurses and dieticians in diabetic centers of 23 European countries. Many of the 135 physicians participating in these workshops of the DESG were responsible for important diabetic clinics. They represented a medical power of about 567,000 diabetic consultations a year. The major problems these physicians faced with diabetics in their centers were identified in this article. These problems are directly related to the medical practice and are often the causes of inefficiency in treating diabetes.

From this inventory based on daily experience with medical practice, guidelines might be drawn for research and training programs for the health care team. Guidelines might be developed on how to motivate patients; what is needed to train the doctors, nurses, and dieticians to teach patients, and how to reorganize diabetic centers for a more integrated medical and teaching approach of the patients. The difficulties of medical practice in diabetes are all different from one another; however, they are also linked together because they all involve the doctor-patient relationship.

## SUMMARY

The difficulties encountered by physicians in their Diabetic Centers were discussed during 6 workshops of the DESG. 166 participants attended, mainly physicians who came from 23 European countries and represented centers which provided more than half a million diabetic consultations a year.

In decreasing order of importance, the problems which the physicians indicated and concerned them most were as follows: (1) poor patient motivation, (2) no training for patient education, (3) unadapted organization of diabetic centers to patient needs, (4) unadapted attitude of doctors toward patients with chronic disease, (5) poor evaluation of the effect of patient education, (6) lack of equipment and supplies, (7) lack of personnel, and (8) lack of psychological support for patients.

# 14. Diabetes patient education: problems we encounter

J.L. DAY

EDITORIAL

*The different workshops organized by the Diabetes Education Study Group all devoted at least one day to the discussion of problems which physicians, nurses and dieticians encounter when teaching patients. The difficulties in opening a teaching center for patients or continuing to run such a center efficiently, are manifold: the health-care system is not accustomed to alternative therapeutic methods including the education and training of patients. As far as therapy is concerned, the thinking and behavior of the medical profession is currently more attuned to the use of drugs, surgery and physical therapy.*

*Another group of difficulties is related to new pedagogic needs: educating patients is different from educating students. The method used by health-care providers is unfortunately too often that of a traditional, vertical school system, where the teacher is active and the student is passive. Further problems arise concerning the correct use of teaching material, particularly audiovisual equipment. For a more global, bio-psycho-social handling of the diabetic patients, an interdisciplinary approach is needed: new management techniques are therefore required.*

*The analysis of these difficulties is a prerequisite for a more structured and rational approach to diabetes therapy. (The editors.)*

We all appreciate that diabetic patients are unlikely to achieve satisfactory self-control of their diabetes without a deep understanding of their disorder and its management. Attempts therefore have been made to examine the application of educational theory to the teaching of the diabetic patient. All of us involved in the diabetic patient workshops have, in an analysis of our own experience, recognized a number of common important definable problems in the area of patient education. Diabetics, especially those who are insulin dependent, need to acquire new knowledge, new skills, and, of course, different motivation if maximal control is to be reached. Application of the standard educational paradigm:

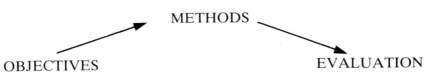

is, however, fraught with many difficulties not encountered in standard educational practice.

Firstly, the 'students' are patients. Their attitudes to the learning process are quite different therefore from those usually encountered. Unlike traditional adult learning situations there is a compulsion to learn certain basic skills and facts. In addition, however, the learning process may be hampered by the emotional difficulties associated with the change from previous 'fit and normal' to the acceptance of having developed a chronic lifelong disorder. Under these circumstances much educational effort may be wasted, since the patients' fears and worries for their future may make effective learning impossible.

Secondly, whereas most courses of tuition are designed with some knowledge and expectaction of the degree of student homogeneity, i.e. previous academic achievement, knowledge and experience, as for example for different courses at school and university, in the case of diabetic tuition there can be no such prediction. The students are completely heterogeneous, encompassing all ages, both sexes and a complete diversity of intellectual ability, previous knowledge and attainment. Furthermore, the diabetic student requires to achieve different levels of training according to the individual nature of his disease; most obviously the insulin and non-insulin dependent diabetic differ in this respect. Any course of teaching for the diabetic must in necessity therefore provide for the individual to a far greater extent than traditional teaching methods. In these DESG workshops that have been conducted to date, these particular problems have been highlighted. We have had the opportunity to analyze a variety of teaching methods, their objectives and achievements in relation to our experience of the management of diabetes and their application to the problems outlined above. The methods analyzed have included:

1. individual tuition/counselling/consultation;
2. group tuition, (a) structured, (b) open;
3. tape slide programmes/books/pamphlets.

As a result of this analysis a number of additional problems have been identified. Clearly tape slide programmes, being difficult and time-consuming to produce, are often expected to reach as wide an audience as possible. In many instances they take little account of the heterogeneity of the audience referred to above, and are often applicable only to small sections of the diabetic population, or so broad in the aims with multiple concepts, as to be incapable of achieving any specific objectives. Books and pamphlets may suffer the same criticism. Recognizing this, the British Diabetic Association has very recently decided to update all their pamphlets, not only to provide more comprehensive information for all groups of diabetics, but also to write quite different sections for insulin-dependent and non-insulin dependent subjects. Because of the problems inherent in all productions of this kind, it must be realised that written or audio-visual material can only be used as an aid to more individual tuition.

It would seem that individual tuition with the doctor caring for the patient – teaching during the consultation procedure – would be ideal. However, problems do arise in potential conflicts between consultation and tuition. In the workshops the most common initial reason given for teaching failures was lack of time. However, closer examination of the process of the consultation reveals that the attitudes of the patient to the doctor as a medical advisor differ somewhat from the tutor/pupil relationship. Secondly, it is difficult to structure the consultation to be comprehensive from an educational point of view. Time constraints may limit discussions to medical problems. Postponement of important items may lead to their omission. The structure may be imposed not by the tutor/doctor, but more by the physical needs of the patient.

Group tuition has been examined in some detail by a number of workers and in many instances offers very useful alternatives. This can be highly structured and organized as in the formal lecture or more didactic teacher-led group or less structured or open ended in free group discussion. In the more didactic situation the attitudes of the patients may debar effective learning. Unless these can be exposed and examined the content of the discussion may not be acceptable to the participants. This is only possible in open groups. In such groups it might be thought that if patients (or parents in the case of children) determine points to be discussed, important areas might be omitted. In practice we have found this not to be the case. The group leader, who preferably should be medically qualified, can allow free discussion, but may need to summarize, highlight and return the discussion to points with high priority within his agenda, but maximize the use of patients' own experience. Within 6 separate hours of discussion, say with a group of 8 to 10 patients, all important areas of diabetic management can be fully discussed. Although apparently time-consuming, the effectiveness of such discussions are very often greater than an equal duration spread over a number of consultations with 1 individual. In terms of 'behavioral change', the ideal of the educationalist, the group process seems more effective than individual one to one consultation in achieving change, due to the support given to individuals by their peers. For example, the effectiveness of certain manoeuvres can be greatly reinforced when shown to have worked by others with the same problem (for example insulin dosage change).

Having discussed the heterogeneity of patients, we must remember that as doctors we also embrace a wide diversity of attitudes to teaching and in particular are not necessarily comfortable with particular methods. It is impossible therefore to force an individual to adopt a particular method,

but rather each individual should chose that with which he is most comfortable. However, awareness of different procedures and their relative effectiveness should become more widespread.

Further problems arise from the number of individuals involved in the
teaching process, doctors, dieticians and, increasingly in the U.K., teaching
nurses, all of whom may need some instruction in how patients learn.

I refer finally, perhaps paradoxically, to objectives and the evaluation of
their achievement. It is because of the difficulty we have encountered of
acceptance by most clinicians of the discipline of behavioral objectives,
which often appears trivial and obvious, that discussion is frequently omitted or introduced belatedly only when its need is accepted. Overtly all our
objectives are the same, best expressed as 'better control of the diabetes',
but practically, unless these goals are broken down into formally stated
simple objectives capable of some form of evaluation and similar interpretation by all, especially in multi-disciplinary teams, the education of the
diabetic will remain far from complete. Perhaps future workshops might
devote some time to the definition of statements which can be accepted by
all. If this can be achieved, then the methods of evaluation will automatically follow. Examination of the success and definition of particular
methods highlight these needs.

# 15. Problems encountered with patient education as seen from the point of view of institutionalized and centralized diabetes education

C. BÖNINGER

## EDITORIAL

*This article represents a comprehensive attempt to discuss systematically the problems encountered in diabetes education. Thus the problem areas are specified as those arising from the patient at various stages of the educational process, as those of the medical team and its interactions amongst themselves and with the patients, but also as those that are more directly related to the course of the disease and to organizational difficulties. The views presented are based on experiences in a centralized diabetes hospital, a form of diabetes education/treatment which appears to have a particular tradition in Germany. Thus, some of the problems listed – such as the discontinuation of the diabetes care on leaving the institution and the difficulties to incorporate the patients' families in the educational process – are specific to this type of Diabetes Hospital. However, the great majority of the difficulties described are inherent to any diabetes education program. Therefore, the solutions offered by Dr. Böninger to some of the problems – headlined as 'Observation-Information-Activation-control' – are to be considered of great importance to any treatment center focussing on diabetes education. (The editors.)*

By means of diabetes education we want to enable the patient to carry out such therapeutical measures as his doctor may advise and to control their effectiveness. At the same time, he should be able to live according to his own wants and needs as far as possible.

As blood-glucose-controlled insulin-application will not be available to the majority of diabetics for a long time, the regulation of spontaneous activities will remain part of all types of diabetes therapy. Most patients experience some part of such a regimen as uncomfortably restricting. Education should help them accept therapy. Problems arise from often quite simple hopes and desires which the patient may have, but which are inappropriate to his environment. Recognizing and evaluating such problems are the first steps to their solution. This education can only be successful, however, if the therapy is adjusted concurrently. Education in isolation

94

teaches only abstract knowledge, giving the patient little opportunity to develop an idea of how the more practical skills are employed day to day.

As diabetes education is a lifelong process, everybody in the patient's social environment is involved. The person closest to the patient in this process is the doctor or the institution, which, according to the national system, takes care of the diabetic.

In West Germany, this is usually a general practitioner or internal specialist. Since diabetes became a specialty, it has been recommended that therapy should be centralized [1]. As early as 1906 there were diet-cooking courses and stays in clinical institutions. In 1930 a specialized institution (*Diabetikerheim Garz auf Ruegen*) was founded by Gerhardt Katsch, whose new concept [2] of diabetes treatment included education (*Schulung und Erziehung*). This successful institution has been existing up to now and is still working in Karlsburg (DDR) under the successors of Katsch.

Following this tradition and parallel to the development taking place in different sections of medicine from 1950 onwards, several specialized hospitals for diabetics (*Diabeteskliniken*) started working. After they proved to be useful, there have been established in recent years growing numbers of smaller diabetes units (up to 40 beds) in general hospitals and departments of internal medicine of university hospitals. This type of unit was known previously because some were already in existence before the Second World War (H. Reinwein sen., Kiel; F. Bertram, Hamburg). Education of the patient has been part of the treatment in all these different kinds of institutionalized diabetes care.

The Diabetesklinik Bad Oeynhausen was opened by an independent holder in 1965 as a hospital with 200 beds. Improvement of general care and enlargement to 240 beds followed in 1976, when a second building was added. Personnel and technical equipment and cooperation with a neighboring general hospital allow treatment of diabetes of all types and complications of the disease. The costs of treatment are paid for by national schemes and private insurance companies. Other people who are close to the patients can stay for a few days for instruction.

Education of all patients is included in the clinic's concept, and this is made clear to the patient by stressing that it is part of the treatment according to the rules of the house, which every patient has to sign on admission. Instruction of all types is offered to all patients, and they are asked to participate, but this is not checked.

The problems we encounter in diabetes education are different from those of other institutions only in quantity but presumably not in quality.

This article should outline and analyze daily problems of teaching diabetics. They will be described as
- the patient's problems,
- the teacher's (medical team's) problems,
- problems of the doctor at home,
- problems arising from the disease and

C. Böninger

– problems to be solved by administrative authorities.
In conclusion there will be short remarks on how we try to solve some problems.

## I. The patient's problems

These may be grouped by the time they occur: problems on admission, during teaching and on discharge. Many variations arise with differences in diabetes duration, foreknowledge and personality of the patients. Only a few typical issues are listed here from a very great number of problems which occur.

A. *At the time of admission* the patient has wishes, expectations and hopes. The confrontation with the reality of the clinic (Table 1) may change

Table 1   *The diabetic patient on hospital admission*

| Wishes and hopes | Reality |
|---|---|
| to live (eat, drink etc.) as before | calculated diet |
| to loose fear of blindness and black toes (and of irritation and impotence) and ... | to meet blind and amputated people, to suffer with the neighbor from noctural paresthesia, to hear about lost partners ('diabetes is to blame for this?') |
| to loose fear of hypoglycemia | become aware of oligosymptomatic hypoglycemia |
| less regimentation | more regimentation, perhaps even more subtle |
| to understand diabetes | to become aware of what diabetes really means to a person (getting afraid of it) |
| daily help (for example with cooking) | help to be independent (for self-help) |
| is what my neighbor told me right? | are diabetics' stories all true? |
| to train recommended behavior | to understand rules and keep them in mind |
| my husband (wife) likes me looking well nourished | 'You have to loose weight?' |
| I know how to cook a nice meal! | 'How many bread exchanges are on your meal plan?' |
| I never miss the visit at the doctor's surgery every 4 weeks! | 'Don't you know any more figures (blood sugar/urine sugar)?' |
| I know my injection technique (have been practicing it for 15 years after all!) | 'The longer diabetes lasts, the more often we find errors in insulin dosage!' |

his mental attitude. Depending on his or her personality and the situation, the reaction of the patient may range from a smile, a feeling of uncertainty and fear, to resistance. These sudden changes in mental attitude may have an important influence on motivation and cooperation – for example in attending lectures or taking tests at the beginning.

B.  *Problems during teaching* are of a more technical kind:
1.  The understanding of *technical terms* will increase with diabetes duration (they should always be explained!).
2.  The *quantity of information* is more often too great than too small.

> For example: the handing of long exchange lists to older people with simple and regular meal habits, or extensive information on self-control, concerning type II-diabetes, given to a young person with type I-diabetes.

Oversaturation and/or boredom are caused by the excessive supply of information.
3.  Incorrect *choice of information* will occur in case of insufficient evaluation of the patients needs:

> A 19-year-old girl had frequent episodes of bad control during a diabetes duration of 16 years. Many hospital admissions for ketoacidosis had been necessary. A few days after admission she seemed to have diet-problems. Objective evaluation showed an almost complete lack of knowledge on diet, but she was quite good in the fields of pathophysiology and epidemiology, as well as complications.

In this situation discussion on regulating diet according to muscle work should take place only after repeated fundamental diet instructions, which she really needed. This deficiency is often overlooked as diabetic children are becoming adult diabetics.
4.  By the incorrect *choice of time* for certain information the patient may become demotivated and even fatal situations may follow:

> Teaching and training of semiquantitative methods on measuring urine sugar according to a usual scheme, up to 4 times a day during partial remission, may cause discontinuation of urine testing, as the patient is feeling ineffective because he produces only negative (although good) results. He may thereby fail to recognize the end of his remission phase.

5.  Delivery of *written material* as external information storage (exchange lists, rules on footcare, brochures) has to be done at the correct moment and reconfirming the part that they play in the therapy. By careless selection and handling, those patients who are not used to working with written material independently will not profit by it.
6.  *Information on medical recommendations* (for example to use dressings

mixed without oil; self-control) is ineffective without giving the opportunity to try the result (taste dressings without oil; adapt the next insulin
dose according to the protocol of urine tests).
7. *Rules of action according to certain requirements* ('wenn-dann-Regeln')
will only be followed by the patient if he can relate them to his own
situation ('if I had known I had to take sugar with the first signs of
hypo, I would not have gone unconscious'). Using them immediately
will be the most effective way to remember them later ('if your evening
test shows sugar 3 times, raise your morning dose of long-acting insulin').
8. Opportunities for *personal contact with the 'teacher'* will increase the
patient's readiness to participate (amount of involvement) and promote
understanding. (For example the use of audiovisual media.)

> The participation in discussion about problems seen in a film the day before
> will be more active if a doctor gives a short introduction to the film, attends
> its performance and asks the patients to think about problems in preparation
> for a discussion.
>     The amount of knowledge gained by working on programmed texts is
> higher when working in open groups with a member of the teaching-team
> present, who is ready to talk in a friendly way, than by working in isolation
> after getting the brochures from a nurse or a clerk.

Showing sympathy and giving the opportunity to discuss acute problems
seem to raise motivation in such circumstances.

C. *At the time of discharge* technical and organizational problems on
further management come into the foreground. Besides these, uncertainty
about one's own staying power and fears concerning the confrontation with
the private environment may affect the pleasure of getting home and also
diminish the hopes for a further favorable course of the disease. The actual
weight of uncertainty and fear is influenced, among other factors, by diabetes duration, because with time the patient usually gets experience in
some way or another. Articulation of resistance sometimes takes place for
the first time in this situation.
    As there are many points for consideration, some of them are listed in
Table 2.

## II.   Problems of the medical team

Staff problems are usually seen as quantitative. These are most important,
but from our point of view it is a matter the administrative authorities have
to deal with. Problems occurring in the teaching team should be watched
very carefully. There may be problems arising from the individual situation
of staff members or problems arising from organizational aspects.

Looking at this means finding out first of all whether or not the problem occurring as one of the second group has in reality its origin in the first group and therefore might require a completely different approach, instead of only some sort of organizational recommendation.

A few weeks after a young doctor had started his work, a growing number of complaints on frequent hypoglycemia occurred on hectic rounds ('I could not even tell that I was hypoglycemic at 10 last night!'). Maybe the advice given here would be to discuss insulin-dosage with a more experienced person (nurse!). But at the same time he should be given the chance to get more experience in working with patients who have their own first experience with insulin; in this way both doctor and patient may learn some rules of dosage together.

A.  *Problems of the staff-members, which arise from their own professional situation*

1.  Problems concerning *knowledge of diabetes* are predominant with high staff-fluctuation, especially amongst younger staff members. Lack of experience in handling the disease and improper familiarization can produce inappropriate behavior (Table 1, right column (reality)). Frustrations may be produced in this situation by negative patient reaction, and these may block further motivation on the side of the personnel both to teach and – more important – to learn.
    a.  Ignorance of physiologic tolerances and thereby of the necessary accent in treatment are followed by excessive information supply:

    Diet-instruction in type I-diabetics stresses carbohydrates; in type II-diabetics it gives information mostly on nutritive values, which are far more important.

    b.  With increasing knowledge, staff-members sometimes change from an attitude of uncertainty to one of authority. The desired attitude of partnership develops only with much experience.

2.  Staff who lack *training in educational methods* are well known and often discussed nowadays. This is true especially with the medical professions (doctors and nurses), somewhat less with dieticians.
    This may lead to:
    a.  Language problems. Unhelpful behavior in this situation may result in a prejudice like this: 'He does not understand me – his IQ is too low'.
    b.  A preoccupation with theoretical ideas instead of practical training. This may happen if the teacher does not clearly point out the target of the lesson (for example: 'the patient shall be able to inject insulin correctly' instead of 'insulin and its modes of application').
    c.  Very often confusion occurs with facts being *important* and *interesting* at a certain level of teaching:

Table 2   *The diabetic patient on discharge from hospital*

Problems and uncertainties

I cannot read the handwriting on the meal plan...

The syringe I got from the pharmacy looks different from that I used in the hospital.

There is nothing that I am allowed to eat for supper at home...

Tomorrow I shall take a long walk with my grandchildren – may I (am I able to) do that?

I wonder whether my doctor really knows
  a. about the facts I learnt in hospital?
  b. what he should prescribe (I am sure he will do everything for me he can...)?
  c. how he can really help me (help for self-help)?

Do I really know enough to explain hypoglycemia to my colleagues (friends, family), and will they help me quickly and in the right manner, in case I cannot do it myself?

Shall I really manage with all that and hold out?

How can I find other diabetics in my town?

How can I avoid too many people's knowing of this disease I have?

At Christmas I shall certainly eat plumpudding with my family!

My people don't actually know all about the difficulties you have to cope with, being diabetic.

After a hospital stay you really become aware of being sick as a diabetic! (Diabetes duration 0-3 months).

I really am glad being fully instructed and trained now – so it will be easier for me to manage daily life than during the first months of being diabetic (diabetes duration of 3 months to 2 years).

Patients usually are fascinated by the idea of a renal threshold for glucose. During practical training lessons, the teacher should presume this term to be known and not discuss it further. In this situation this term is not important, though it might be interesting to discuss.

d.   The personal attitude of the staff towards patients with long duration of the disease is very demanding on the didactic experience. The patient is used to living with his or her diabetes and in general needs no more instruction (although interest and sympathy are needed). Finding out the facts to produce information which might help him requires a great amount of experience with diabetes, knowledge of the patient's own history and aptitude in one's own profession. At least during the first phase of personnel training, this should not be left to inexperienced people without help.

B.  *Staff organization problems*

1.  A main assumption for effective teaching in the field of diabetes is *knowledge of the patient's individual situation.*
    a.  Knowledge of social background (which also means knowledge of lifestyle):

    > Are people in his region used to eating potatoes or farinaceous products? At what time (late?) does Mr. M. who is 75 years old and lives alone, get up in the morning?

    b.  Knowledge of the influence that the patients labour environment has:

    > In a laboratory it may be forbidden for security reasons to take any food during working time. Knowing this, the patient's resistance to a snack at 11.00 a.m. seems likely, although he gets hypoglycemic quite often before noon.

    c.  Knowledge of therapy:

    > A blood-glucose-stix-value of 60 mg/dl causes the nurse in charge to react differently, depending if patients are on insulin or on biguanides.

2.  *Availability of knowledge* about all influencing factors from a patient's personal situation is one precondition for effective education. It is extremely difficult to meet these requirements in a system with most personnel working in shifts. If it is really impossible to have the same people responsible for the same patient's care, there is, in our experience, no chance of all the necessary information being passed from one shift to the next.
3.  From the necessity to form small units, problems arise concerning '*common philosophy*' in handling educational needs.
    a.  The contents of all lectures, etc., must be exactly defined.

    > During a practical Clinitest-training a patient insists on not being ready to try it himself. He argues that Dr. M. has told the patients during a lecture that there was a strip now available with the same accuracy, but which was much easier to handle. The teaching nurse did not know this information.

    b.  The topics should be strictly planned in relation to each other. Otherwise unintentional repetition causes boredom which might even surprise the teacher.
4.  An atmosphere of *intolerance* between the different *professional groups* may easily take place if changes in this direction are not carefully watched and treated at the roots. Personal contact when passing messages is a good means to prevent this problem.

5. With *numerous staff-members* all those persons who are in contact with patients should acquire the knowledge we expect the diabetic to have.

> The boy dialing one figure on the telephone again and again for 3 minutes will get sugar (and thereby help) instead of being scolded by the worker, who was watching him and knew that hypoglycemia might cause strange behavior.

## III.   Problems of the practitioner

Sometimes on admission the patient has with him a protocol with blood glucose values found on different occasions. This is better than nothing. It would, however, be very impressive for the patient if there was a free flow of information in both directions: between the doctor and the hospital. The idea of the necessity for continuous treatment would be established more easily, and continuous diabetes education could take place as well. To further this, the information given to the practitioner from the hospital must be very specific and include all aspects of diabetes treatment and education, unless there are standards that both partners have agreed on.

The keeping-up-to-date of a protocol on self-control, that became an object of discussion with the doctor at each consultation is a great help for patient and doctor. A call on the practitioner at the moment of discharge of the patient from hospital will improve cooperation on both sides and prevent the patient from being the only bearer of news on his treatment and educational state.

## IV.   Problems arising from the course of diabetes mellitus

1. We do not know the individual prognosis of most patients, and it is necessary to apply some kind of fundamental instruction and training at the beginning  and correct contents and style of education according to the aims of treatment, which may vary during the further course of the disease. Therefore, it should be ensured that the education process does not stop at different occasions during the patient's life.

> If good control is said to be the only means to prevent complications from diabetic microangiopathy, it may be rather difficult to make the patient keep good control at the first finding of proliferative retinopathy.

2. Each diabetic has his very own experience in handling his or her diabetes from the first day of manifestation. It is sometimes a difficult task making out the events which happened in the course of the disease and distinguishing them from accidents depending on the patient's behavior (for example: likeliness of hypoglycemic reactions).

## V. Problems to be solved by the administrative authorities

The administrative authorities have to accept education as a part of diabetes treatment, including information, training and evaluation. It must be understood that the education of the patient:
1. competes with nursing him,
2. is not dependent on the technical equipment of a hospital but needs special technical aids on which agreement should be reached before buying them (perhaps a round table instead of a square one is more useful for group sessions),
3. does not include mainly lectures and brochures,
4. must be considered by the whole medical staff,
5. requires quite a lot of time, especially preparation time, which must be taken into account,
6. is in urgent need of a pleasant atmosphere among the whole staff.

### Some ways out of the dilemma

During 16 years of diabetes education some modifications of structure and organization took place to improve efficiency.
1. The importance of a lecture course was diminished by stressing lessons with small groups of patients,
2. Instructions on diet are given in as many personal interviews as can be arranged by 2 to 3 dieticians.
3. By producing a series of programmed textbooks for patients (on 'Blood-sugar and urine sugar' – 'Insulin' – 'Hypoglycemia' – 'Diabetes decom-

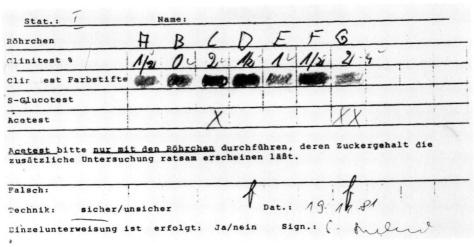

Fig. 1 Documentation of urine-test check-up, signed by the nurse (the patient has to test solutions with unknown glucose concentrations under supervision and control of a nurse).

pensation' and 'Diet in diabetes mellitus (5 brochures)') [3] we arrived at the following objectives:

a.  the medical staff keeps to the contents of the brochures when teaching patients,

b.  the booklets can be used like building-bricks in an instruction system which allows close adaptation to the patients' needs,

c.  by having patients work through 1 or 2 booklets together with others, we can build up open groups under supervision and evaluate these group members if necessary.

4.  Participation of nurses, dieticians and technicians in patient teaching enables us to stress training situations for self-control, injection-technique, diet cooking etc.

We learned to act as teachers according to the sequence ORIENTATION – INFORMATION – ACTIVATION – CONTROL [4], and we mostly succeeded in building up the learner's motivation by this.

The need for *information* can be evaluated by personal talks or by questionnaires. Information is offered and applied by group sessions, informal lectures, demonstrations, working with programmed textbooks and sometimes audiovisual media. A good idea is to use the daily rounds for individual patient teaching, which is the most effective teaching after all. The possibility that the doctor will adopt this suggestion depends on his own experience and certainty, because in one-to-one situations the problems of teaching become apparent to teacher and learner (and the long-term diabetic may well estimate the staff's experience).

The *activation* of the patients, which seems to optimize learning, starts with the first talk by asking him for his views on therapy, by visualizing therapeutical effectiveness by means of protocols of self-control or/and announcement of missed questions in the questionnaire [5]. As soon as *control* of the techniques is documented (Fig. 1, Fig. 2) and diet is adapted to mealtimes at home (Fig. 3) as well as to known individual difficulties of the blood glucose profile, the patient's attention is directed to self-management as far as is possible and convenient. During this phase group discussion is

**Spritztechnik:** <u>schräg</u> / senkrecht

**Umgang mit Spritze:** sicher / <u>unsicher</u>

**Spritzstellen:** *Oberschenkel, Oberarm*

**Fehler:** *Alkohol, zieht ungenau auf*

**Überprüft:** <u>18. 12. 81    Reiners</u>

Fig. 2  Documentation of correct injection-technique (injection with own syringe takes place under supervision of a nurse).

Ernährungsanamnese, Injektionszeiten

| | 20.12. | 21.12. |
|---|---|---|

5⁰⁰ 🦅 Depot Hoe (

| 5⁰⁰ 118 | 5⁰⁰ 122 |
| 8⁰⁰ 134 | |

1.F. 5⁴⁵ 4 BE

| 12⁰⁰ 102 | |
| 16²⁰ 132 | |

2.F 9⁰⁰ 5 BE (Brot

| 20⁰⁰ 130 | 18⁰⁰ 116 |

Mittag 12⁰⁰ 3 BE

Vesper 15⁰⁰ 1 BE (A

| ⊘ | |
| 800 | 1200 |

Abend 18⁰⁰ 5 BE

Spät 21⁰⁰ ~ 3 B

| 04 2 | 0,2 2 |
| 330 | |
| 140 | |

~ 220( 160

3450

**Diabetesklinik Bad Oeynhausen**

Ärztliche Verordnu

**Diät** — Stationärer Aufent

Kostplan

**1. Frühstück** — Brot
um 5³⁰ Uhr — Aufschnitt (mager)
5+1 BE — Käse (mager)
Magerquark
Streichfett
Diabetikermarmela

**2. Frühstück** — Brot
um 8⁰⁰ Uhr — Aufschnitt/Käse (n
4 BE — Streichfett
Obst
Milch/Joghurt

**3. Frühstück** — Brot
um 11⁰⁰ Uhr — Aufschnitt/Käse (n
2 BE — Streichfett
Obst
Milch/Joghurt

**Mittagessen** — Kartoffeln
um 12³⁰ Uhr — Gemüse/Salat
5 BE — Fleisch/Fisch (ma
Kochfett
Obst

**nachmittags** — Brot
um 15⁰⁰ Uhr — Aufschnitt/Käse (n
3 BE — Streichfett
Diabetikermarmela
Obst

**Abendessen** — Brot
um 18³⁰ Uhr — Aufschnitt (mager)
5 BE — Käse (mager)
Magerquark
Streichfett
Obst
Gemüse/Salat

**Spätmahlzeit** — Brot
um 22⁰⁰ Uhr — Aufschnitt/Käse (r
3 BE — Magerquark
Streichfett
Obst
Joghurt/Milch

**Injektionstechnik** (Injektionsareale, Spritzentyp)

| | 5+1 |
| | 4 |
| | 5 |
| | 3 |
| | 6 |
| | 3 |
| | 21+1 |

Oberschenkel /

Hautkomplikat

**Berufs-, Sozial-Anamnese:** (wird versorgt durch:)

Gelernter Maurer

Seitdem als LK

Schl.-Halstein,

Jetztiges Arbeits

Arbeitsgeber w

Bescheid u. ist

Hat auch Ne

**häusliche Essenszeiten:**
1. Frühst.: 5²⁰ Uhr
2. Frühst.: 8⁰⁰ Uhr
3. Frühst.: 11⁰⁰ Uhr
Mittag: 12³⁰ Uhr
Vesper: 15⁰⁰ Uhr
Abend: 18³⁰ Uhr
Spät: 22³⁰ Uhr

**Gesamtmenge:** Kohlenhydrate
Eiweiß
Fett insgesamt

**Gesamtnährwert:** (Joule/Kalorien)

arbeitsunfähig seit:

Schwerbeh.-A (ein) ___%)

**Insulin** ~ 5⁰⁰ Uhr
Uhr
18⁰⁰ Uhr

**Ta** morgens
mittags /
abends

*Doctor* *Nurse* *Dietician*

Fig. 3 Documentation of diet-adaption steps: history taken by the doctor (left), adaption of mealtimes during the stay in hospital by the nurse (middle), diet-prescription on discharge by a dietician (right).

a valuable instrument, as patients can discuss their own practical difficulties.

The aim of diabetes education and treatment is keeping up good control. Evaluation has to show our success in attaining this. Apart from this, it may help to improve definite parts of the instruction program or to watch the efficiency of groups within the whole staff. Good results may even counteract frustrations coming from longstanding routine which has not produced visible success. Results and their origin must be discussed, therefore, with the whole staff in regularly planned meetings.

A great problem in all institutions with planned education is the fact that all our endeavours only focus on younger insulin-dependent diabetics. It is known from publications [6] that therapeutical success in type-II diabetics depends partly on the early recognition of the patient's tendency to be dependent. We might therefore be able to transfer experiences in educating younger people to the instructional requirements of one of the older groups (those seeking independence), modifying the methods according to more life experience and changed learning abilities of the learner. Beside this we are considering developing objective learning materials in a similarly adaptable system (Bausteinsystem).

## SUMMARY

The daily problems we encounter in running institutionalized diabetes education are listed and analyzed. They derive from the patient, from the teaching staff, from the disease itself and in addition those that have to be dealt with by administrative authorities. Some of the problems are discussed and illustrated by examples, and means to avoid or overcome such problems are outlined.

## REFERENCES

1. Van Noorden, C. (1912): *Die Zuckerkrankheit und ihre Behandlung*, p. 347. August Hirschwald Verlag, Berlin.
2. Katsch, G. (1930): Produktive Fürsorge für Zuckerkranke. *Dtsch. Med. Wochenschr.*, 56, 1941.
3. Steinberg, H., Böninger, Ch. (1981): *Lernprogrammserie über den Diabetes mellitus (Zuckerkrankheit)*. Diabetesklinik Bad Oeynhausen (Ed.).
4. Steinberg, H. (1977): Die Motivation des Diabetikers zu einer konsequent therapiekonformen Ernährung: notwendige Maßnahmen mit motivierender Wirkung. *Aktuel. Ernährungsmed.*, 4, 160.
5. Miller, L.V., Goldstein, J., Nicolaisen, G. (1978): Evaluation of patients' knowledge of diabetes self-care. *Diabetes Care, 1*, 275.
6. Alonga, M. (1980): Perception of severity of disease and health locus of control in compliant and noncompliant patients. *Diabetes Care, 3*, 533.

# 16.   The role of a diabetes teaching nurse in a hospital

K. WASSER-HEININGER AND V. JÖRGENS

## EDITORIAL

*The authors give a detailed job description of the diabetes teaching nurse working in the department of medicine of a general hospital. The various obligations and duties of the diabetes teaching nurse are listed. Based upon personal experience (K.H.-W. was the first diabetes teaching nurse in West Germany), a number of potential difficulties are discussed as well. By nature of her job, the diabetes teaching nurse will soon have more knowledge and experience of the treatment of diabetes mellitus than most physicians in the hospital. On the other hand, she is working in a rather privileged position compared to the nurses on the wards. This particular situation might create personal problems within the complex interactions of the medical and paramedical personnel of a hospital setting. Only on the basis of a mutual understanding of the necessity of the team approach in the care of diabetic patients can such difficulties be avoidable. The authors conclude that the installation of well-trained and qualified diabetes teaching nurses appears to be one of the most important prerequisites for the urgently needed improvement in the general quality of the care of diabetic patients in our countries. (The editors.)*

## INTRODUCTION

During the last years, clinical diabetologists have become more and more convinced that patient education has to be an integral part of any treatment of any form of diabetes mellitus. Especially insulin-dependent diabetics need to learn and adopt a considerable number of measures, if the treatment of their chronic disease is to be successful. In fact, the primary goals of modern diabetes therapy, i.e. normoglycemia and a high degree of personal independence from the physician, can only be achieved by an intensive diabetes teaching programme.

The main problem concerning patient education is the discrepancy between the large number of diabetic patients in need of specific educational programmes and the apparent lack of adequately trained personnel prepared to deliver such education. Structured patient education programmes for inpatients in general hospitals are almost non-existent, at least in this country. In order to provide adequate care for diabetic patients, the delivery of diabetes teaching programmes is, however, obligatory. Therefore, manpower, facilities and adequate administrative conditions have to be provided wherever diabetic patients are treated. Based on our experience, it appears to be optimal to have a diabetes teaching nurse and a dietician deliver the educational programme for diabetic patients in general hospitals.

In the following we will describe the diabetes teaching programme as it is used in our department for inpatients with insulin-requiring diabetes – as a possible alternative with proven effectivity.

## Why don't physicians teach the patients?

The actual role of the physicians in the process of teaching diabetic patients is quite limited: in most European countries, physicians in a general hospital have neither the opportunity nor the motivation to spend the time necessary for patient education, due to the fact that the younger physicians need to fulfil their curriculum for their specialization, for example, in internal medicine, and the already specialized senior physicians and heads of departments are unable to devote sufficient time for patient education because of their various other commitments. In addition, physicians have hardly ever learnt how to teach groups and, in general, they will have only very limited experience with the transfer of diabetes-related knowledge and behavior to patients. Unfortunately, very often they will not even be able to handle the relevant materials and methods, such as insulin syringes, glucosuria tests, etc. The time a physician can spend on diabetes during his medical education might be sufficient to learn enough about the disease, but very rarely will he have the chance to learn and practice methods of adult education. Thus, one basic obstacle for the institution of a diabetes teaching programme is the question of who is going to do it.

Theoretically, there are at least 2 possible ways to fill this lack of specialized personnel for diabetes education:
1. to motivate more physicians for patient education or
2. to make a specialized profession of the education of diabetes – the diabetes teaching nurse.

Based on our experience, it is the second alternative which appears to be the most promising approach.

## Conditions for efficacy of a diabetes teaching nurse programme

Nowadays, nobody could imagine a school-teacher without a class-room or a professor teaching individually rather than in groups. During the last century, when education was restricted to a small part of the population, individual teaching was the rule; however, when teaching became a general need and offer, it had to be done in groups, because teaching in schools was and still is the only practicable system. In analogy, it seems unrealistic to offer individual teaching for all our diabetic patients: if every patient were to receive 13 hours of teaching, one nurse could teach no more than 3 patients per week. Thus, it is clear that there have to be adequate classroom facilities available for group teaching.

It is not only the cost-benefit relationship which leads us to recommend the group approach in teaching diabetics, but also the possible benefits of interaction between the learning patients, which can be used as an important part of the teaching process.

In order to establish a teaching curriculum for inpatients, these conditions seem to be basic prerequisites for any effective work of a diabetes teaching nurse in a hospital.

## Job description of the diabetes teaching nurse in a hospital

As an example of the organization of a teaching programme for insulin-dependent diabetics, we will describe the 1-week teaching curriculum as practiced in our department. This teaching programme is carried out by a diabetes teaching nurse and a dietician. Control of transfer of knowledge as well as long-term results in the compliance of the patients seem to indicate that this way of teaching diabetics can be efficient.

### Teaching the patients

The main obligations of the diabetes teaching nurse are to organize and deliver this 1-week teaching curriculum (Table 1). All patients who are able to attend the programme are admitted to this curriculum: patients who cannot participate in the programme, e.g. due to additional diseases or handicaps, receive bedside teaching, or one of their relatives is asked to join the programme. In our hospital the diet-related objectives of diabetes teaching are instructed by a dietician, even though the diabetes teaching nurse should be able to answer questions concerning the diet as well.

On Monday morning, before the beginning of the programme, the diabetes teaching nurse is informed by the physician about the characteristics of the patients who are participating in the week's curriculum. This information is necessary in order to define the educational goals of every single patient. For example, patients suffering from advanced stages of diabetic complications would need an individualized discussion about the goal of their particular treatment; patients with abnormalities of the renal glucose threshold must be taught self-monitoring of metabolism in a special way, etc.

On Monday afternoon, the resident of the metabolic ward opens the teaching programme and introduces himself, the dietician and the diabetes teaching nurse. He asks each patient to introduce him/herself by name, age, how long the diabetes has been known, how the disease has been

Table 1  *Diabetes teaching course – time table*

| Time | Monday | Tuesday | Wednesday | Thursday | Friday |
|------|--------|---------|-----------|----------|--------|
| 8.00<br>9.00 | | | | excursion to<br>a super-market | |
| 10.00 | introduction<br>why educa-<br>tion? | | | | |
| 11.00 | | diet I | diet II | | diet III |
| 12.00 | lunch – calculation and assessment of the diet with the dietician | | | | |
| 13.00<br>14.00 | | hypoglycemia | exercise<br>driving, travel | reduction of<br>insulin dose | augmentation<br>of insulin<br>dose |
| 15.00 | self-<br>monitoring | | | | |
| 16.00<br>17.00 | | insulins<br>insulin-injec-<br>tion | disease<br>late complica-<br>tions<br>foot care | contraception<br>pregnancy | |
| 18.00 | | | | | |

treated and the reason why he/she came to this hospital. Afterwards, the physician gives a short review of the pathogenesis, prognosis and treatment of type I and type II diabetes.

The dietician explains the diet-related objectives in a pragmatic way. Together with the patients she weighs the food they eat on the ward. During their visit to a supermarket, the dietician demonstrates how to identify carbohydrate in the foodstuffs, she shows the special diet nutrients and discusses when and how these should be used in the diabetes diet.

The first lesson of the diabetes teaching nurse concerns urine and blood glucose monitoring. After this lesson, metabolic self-control of glucosuria is performed by each patient already during their stay on the ward. The diabetes teaching nurse and the patients compare the results of these urine tests with the values of glycemia, which are measured in the laboratory as a control of the correct performance and to find out abnormal renal thresholds. This active participation of the patients demonstrates to them the importance of the metabolic self-control.

The correct injection of insulin is practised in the next lesson and should also be performed by the patients themselves supervised by a nurse. For patients with newly discovered diabetes, the 'know-how' of insulin injection can be practised with the diabetes teaching nurse, using a special doll.

Once these basic subjects are understood by all patients, the more complicated objectives can be discussed. The adaptation of the insulin dosage can be introduced by some easy rules. The reduction and increase of the insulin dosage is demonstrated by every-day-life examples on the blackboard.

The last lesson of the week includes a general repetition, either in form of a written questionnaire or by questions asked by the diabetes teaching nurse. Due to this repetition, the diabetes teaching nurse gets an overview of the topics which are not quite clear with the patients, and there should be enough time left to repeat and discuss these.

In addition to the group teaching sessions, the diabetes teaching nurse should offer the opportunity to discuss problems individually. At these occasions, patients might discuss questions that could be embarassing if brought up in public, such as questions concerning family planning. Birth control methods and problems concerning pregnancy should be explained to all young diabetic women. Also competent genetic counselling must be offered to patients and their relatives. Furthermore, the diabetes teaching nurse should explain particular problems of late complications of diabetes, such as impotence or frigidity. In addition, patients should be made familiar with certain social aspects of their disease, such as choice of a job, tax reductions, social benefits, restrictions in driving a car, etc. With a newly discovered diabetic, individual conversations concerning the changes in every-day-life are necessary to reduce their fears and anxieties.

In some patients additional instructions and explanations are needed after the group lessons.

These individual conversations require a lot of time and effort on the part of the diabetes teaching nurse, but in many cases the teaching programme is completely useless if the patients do not get a chance to discuss their individual problems.

## Teaching relatives and friends of diabetic patients

Relatives of all insulin-treated diabetic patients should learn the treatment of severe hypoglycemic reactions with glucagon injections.

There should be a special teaching programme for relatives of patients who are not capable of participating in the teaching programme because of an additional disease or handicap.

When diabetic patients are too young or too old to take over the responsibility of their own treatment, their relatives have to be actively involved and, therefore, have to be instructed accordingly. In fact, special educational programmes have to be compiled for friends, teachers or colleagues of diabetic patients. This is especially important with respect to team-mates and trainers of diabetic patients involved in sport activities, outings, mountaineering, etc. Thus, the diabetes teaching nurse has to be able to adapt her educational approach to the specific situation of teaching non-diabetic individuals who are in some way related to a diabetic patient.

## Participation in the out-patient clinic

Twice a week our diabetes out-patient clinic takes place in the evenings so that the patients do not have to miss school or work. At these clinics the diabetes teaching nurse is always present, and since she is known by every patient, she has a personal approach to their individual problems. At these occasions, the diabetes teaching nurse will check compliance with the teaching programme and has the opportunity to evaluate metabolic self-control and the insulin adaptation by the patients. She can attempt to improve upon the patient's compliance and deal with some topics that might have remained unclear. On the other hand, patients will discuss their problems with the disease often more readily with her than with the physician.

## Participation in the ward rounds

The diabetes teaching nurse should be actively involved in the ward rounds in order to get familiar with the clinical aspects of the diabetic patients. In addition, quite often the diabetes teaching nurse will act as a patient's advocate in the process of medical demonstrating.

### Co-operation in defining insulin therapy

Every evening, the residents of the ward discuss the insulin dosages for the next day with the patients. Since these physicians rotate from ward to ward every 3 to 6 months, the diabetes teaching nurse must be present during the discussions of the insulin dosages in order to give advice when necessary and avoid errors. On this occasion, the diabetes teaching nurse transfers the results of the patient's metabolic self-control into the diabetes charts. After the adaptations of insulin dosage have been discussed in class, the patients have to be actively involved when their insulin dosage is discussed for the next day.

Besides these obligations, the diabetes teaching nurse is responsible for the diabetes education of the personnel on the ward. Every nurse, nurses' aid, student nurse, physician, professor and student who works with the diabetic patients has to be familiar with the aims and objectives of the diabetes teaching programme. Therefore, the staff also has to participate in a complete teaching course, or the diabetes teaching nurse must arrange some lessons especially for them.

### Work of the diabetes teaching nurse that is not concerned with the patients in hospital

The work of the diabetes teaching nurse does not only require the care of patients in the hospital or outpatient clinic but should also be concerned with diabetics outside the hospital:

a. The diabetes teaching nurse answers written questions of diabetic patients from outside the hospital and provides counselling over the telephone.
b. The diabetes teaching nurse participates in postgraduate courses for physicians and allied health personnel in the field of diabetes. In addition, she is actively involved in distributing diabetes-related information to lay organisations of diabetic patients. Together with the other members of the medical team, she is prepared to provide assistance for self-help-groups of diabetic patients on special demand.
c. The diabetes teaching nurse also participates in all postgraduate and scientific projects that are carried out in the field of diabetes education and its evaluation.

**Integration of the diabetes teaching nurse into the medical team**

The position of the diabetes teaching nurse represents a substantial enlargement of the traditional role of the hospital nurse in a way that she plays a primary role in the treatment of diabetic patients (Lancet Editorial, Lancet I: 145-146, 1982). Since this represents a rather new concept, problems in the interactions of the diabetes teaching nurse with other members of the health care team might arise. In order to minimize such difficulties, each member of the diabetes teaching team has to be informed about and accept the particular role of the diabetes teaching nurse, i.e. her rights and duties in the delivery of health care to diabetic patients. In a general hospital department, it will become readily apparent that the diabetes teaching nurse's knowledge and competence with regard to diabetes mellitus will exceed that of many physicians quite substantially. This discrepancy has to be acknowledged and used in order to improve the training of the doctors, both in the field of diabetes and with regard to the necessary cooperation within the team approach in health care delivery.

CONCLUSION

In our experience, the diabetes teaching nurse plays an essential part in the psychological and pedagogic basis of the therapy of diabetes patients. Therefore, we suggest that the creation of the position of diabetic teaching nurses should be regarded as essential in the overall improvement of the health care delivery to diabetes patients, which remains a burning necessity to date.

K. *Wasser-Heininger and V. Jörgens*

## SUMMARY

Practical problems with regard to the institution of a diabetes teaching programme in general hospitals are described with particular emphasis on the difficulties in recruiting appropriate personnel for the delivery of continuing high-quality diabetes education. The necessity to install a diabetes teaching nurse as the principal diabetes educator within a teaching and treatment team together with the physician, the dietician and the technician is delineated. Subsequently, a job description of the diabetes teaching nurse working in a department of medicine of a general hospital is given. The various duties of the diabetes teaching nurse are listed, her interactions with other members of the diabetes teaching team are described. It is concluded that the incorporation of a diabetes teaching nurse in the system for diabetes education appears to be one of the most important prerequisites for the urgently needed improvement in the quality of the care for diabetic patients.

# 17. Which objectives? Listening to patients! Why rationally analyze our methods in patient education?

'Results begin on the drawing board'

J.-Ph. ASSAL

## EDITORIAL

*The following article is an adapted version for publication of a talk given at the Opening Session of the Second European Symposium on Diabetes Education, June 1982, which was designed to strongly interject the need for educational dimensions in medical thinking concerned with patient education. The speech addresses 3 topics which the author asserts would greatly improve the effectiveness of patient education. One topic, 'Listening to patients', is discussed in more detail in the article 'Active listening' (Chapter 29). The other 2 topics concerning 'Educational objectives' and 'The rational analysis of the teaching methods within patient education' are only discussed in this paper and represent the vitally necessary framework needed to increase the rate of success in patient education programs. (The editors.)*

## WHICH OBJECTIVES?

During the several workshops that the Diabetes Education Study Group (DESG) has organized over the last 2 years, 3 concepts were repeatedly brought up by the 240 participants: (1) which type of teaching objectives are appropriate for our patients; (2) what are the effects of listening to patients; and (3) why should we rationally analyze all our methods in patient education? Most of these participants were physicians, along with some nurses and dieticians, who represented a broad and important clinical experience. We have calculated that the physicians attending the workshops had supervised, as a group, around half-a-million diabetic consultations a year!

The importance of each of these concepts will be illustrated by examples from a non-medical field (industry) to show that the situations we have to face with patient education are not specific for medicine only. Solutions have to be sought for similar problems in other fields.

J.-Ph. Assal

## WHICH TYPES OF TEACHING OBJECTIVES ARE APPROPRIATE FOR OUR PATIENTS?

Historically, the use of short, intermediate and long-term objectives was widely propagandized by those who organized the industrial development at the beginning of our century, when it was required to switch from an empirical, intuitive, individual organization to a more analytical, scientific approach.

This scientific drive mainly started at the beginning of the century in the United States. One of the pioneers of the American Industry, Mr. Henry Ford, scientifically organized the assembly line of his car. This type of production was based on a whole range of very practical, short-term objectives called 'operational objectives'. We know the result of this systematic approach: the tremendous development of the car industry symbolized by the famous Model T-Ford. This car became popular about the same time that Banting and Best discovered insulin.

Henry Ford wrote the famous sentence which symbolized the scientific, as opposed to empirical, organization of labor: 'Sales begin on the drawing board'. He meant that to attain the maximum efficiency, production had to be organized and planned in advance. The product had to be very precisely engineered, the industrial production had to be planned. The next requirement was to have clear ideas about how to sell the product, under which conditions and within what period of time. Finally, it was mandatory to evaluate how these various objectives could be reached. Furthermore, in the case problems occurred, it was necessary to rapidly modify either the product, its production or its marketing. It is quite certain that part of the success of economic development and efficiency observed in industrial countries results from the systematic use of operational objectives in management: what has to be done, how it has to be done, under which conditions it has to be done and how to evaluate what has been achieved [1].

For years, and even now, education has been mainly concerned with the acquisition of knowledge. There has been, in fact, little teacher concern for training students in the practical application of knowledge. It was only in the 1950's that a man named Tyler, who was a specialist in education, introduced the concept of technical 'know-how' which then became part of the teaching process.

Tyler was a professor of education at the University of Chicago School of Managers. His responsibility was to train industrial managers in the technique of using efficient methods (system analysis) for their professional activities. Emphasis was not only placed on what the students had to know, but especially on what the students had to do *in practice* at the end of the learning period. In Tyler's program, the 'know-how' quickly became the cornerstone of teaching: the teacher not only wanted the student *to know* specific things at the end of the teaching period, but the student also had to *know how to do them*. In the general field of education, the concept of

116

achieving this 'know-how' has been presented *in the change of behavior produced.*

## OPERATIONAL OR EDUCATIONAL OBJECTIVES

These objectives are defined as what the students should be able to do (visible activity) at the end of a learning period and what test or criteria the teacher will use to examine if the student can demonstrate the new learned behavior [2].

But what have patient education and therapy to do with these operational or educational objectives? Even more, we must first translate educational objectives into medical terms. In training members of a medical team, the educational objective would be what the doctor and/or the nurse should be able *to do* at the end of a learning period. For the patient, the objective would be what he or she should be able *to do* for his or her treatment at the end of a learning period. The action and ability resulting from the successful completion of the objective will be something the learner did not know or did not realize he or she knew before undertaking the work of the objective.

Please remember that knowledge is not the culminating point of patient education. The culminating point is therapeutical action and changes in behavior. To know all the symptoms of hypoglycemia is not a direct therapeutical action. However, to know the symptoms and to be prepared to take a snack 3 times daily containing 15 to 20 grams of CHO and to carry 3 cubes of sugar in one's pocket are examples of short-term educational objectives in therapy which could be used and easily evaluated by the medical team.

Let us now switch to another aspect that is always defined as crucial by clinicians: *listening to patients.* Listening to patients helps both the physicians and the patients. The physician who takes into account what he has learned from his patient will be in a better position to adapt the treatment to his patient. He will also be in a better position to plan educational objectives.

As we have seen, educational objectives for patients not only define what a given patient has to know, but also what the patient has *to do* in order to improve his or her treatment. Each patient faces different problems with his or her health and it is only through active listening that the physician, nurse or dietician will be able to adapt the teaching program to each individual. A patient who can freely express feelings to his or her doctor and whose doctor *listens*, can usually cope better with the disease and, consequently, compliance with the treatment will improve. The effect of this more active doctor/patient relationship will be marked by improved control of the disease and the psychosocial well-being of the patient. Listening is not just remaining silent. Real listening means trying actively to understand what

117

the person who is speaking really means by trying to take into account what has been expressed.

Active listening has not only beneficial effects in medicine. There are also examples from the field of industry. In 1922, in Chicago, the Western Electric Company went through a production crisis. This company was one of the best organized and most scientifically planned industries in the USA. Assembly lines were very efficient, but gradually the level of absenteeism increased. The search for the reasons proceeded in a scientific manner. Specialists analyzed the equipment and found that the tools and machinery were adequately adapted to the kind of work required. Questions were asked concerning the speed of the assembly line etc., but experts could not find the reasons to explain exactly what was wrong.

Finally, a psychologist, Elton Mayo, was called in to observe the working process. He started his analysis by having discussions with the workers. In a few weeks absenteeism dropped. It was observed that when the workers were able to express themselves to someone who really was interested in their problems, the degree of absenteeism dropped by 80%. This occurred even without any modifications in the assembly line process.

This notable observation at Western Electric in 1922, which took into account the human dimension in the production line by listening to workers, stimulated the motivation to work. It showed quite clearly that the technical organization of work was not sufficient, in itself, to ensure optimal production. Although this observation was a matter of common sense, it was the first time that the effects had been evaluated. The workers' motivation was enhanced by active listening, exactly as in medicine where motivation of the patient to follow the treatment is not directly related to the pharmacological power of the drug, but is more dependent on the doctor-patient relationship.

Another question which was frequently asked by physicians during our workshops was: 'Is it really so important to analyze rationally what we do when teaching patients?' So our third concept was the question, *why rationalize or rationally investigate our actions?*

To rationalize can be understood as a dynamic process involving several steps: (1) an observation of what has been done; (2) a systematic analysis of what has been observed and (3) a plan of the new course of action. To rationalize may be seen as a circular model based on observation, analysis and planning a new improved activity. Any given medical treatment is the result of such a dynamic procedure.

On the premise that patient education is part of the therapeutical arsenal, a systematic analysis of the teaching process is implied. For instance, we should analyze if our patient education program really helps the patient to improve his treatment! Teaching patients to measure urine glucose and not training them to modify their treatment according to glucosuria is pointless. Millions of urine tests are carried out daily and are useless because the patients have not been trained to modify their treatment accordingly! This is a therapeutical failure. As medical teachers, we are not sufficiently trained in educational techniques to teach patients how to modify their treatment with methods that produce real understanding.

What about those physicians who are 'self-made educators' with a long experience in patient education? Maybe nothing is more conductive to efficiency than daily practice and experience. However, I would like to counter this statement by giving an example from industrial history. Henry Ford insisted on systematic, scientific analysis of routine, everyday activities. His analyst, Taylor, studied most routine activities in Ford's factories and wrote in 1905 that simple activities or apparently simple activities, such as transporting bricks from hand to hand along an assembly line, were never accomplished spontaneously in the most efficient manner. Systematic analysis of these routine activities would improve efficiency of the workers; one could produce more in less time and the worker would spend less energy and be less tired.

Taylor described the following story to illustrate the importance of rational analysis. One man who was never trained and ignored the technique of cutting metal sheets was able, through the simple fact of systematically analyzing the problems involved in cutting metal, to work 3 to 9 times more rapidly than an 'experienced' worker who had performed the same activities for more than 10 years. Taylor further explained that the practitioner, even the good one, who works routinely at the same job is not able to analyze what he does for the simple reason that he has 'his nose stuck in his daily routine'. This example shows us that an outsider, acting as an observer and analyst, could develop a more efficient strategy than the practitioner who is too close to his activities and cannot be sufficiently objective.

The previous industrial example taken from the beginning of the century may well reflect the present situation faced by physicians, nurses and dieticians when teaching patients. Being too close to the daily routine of patient education may be the problem of self-taught educators who may have a certain amount of intuition, but waste a lot of energy and often lack efficiency. There is an urgent need to analyze what we do and to ask for the assistance of professionals in pedagogy and psychology who can help us to improve our efficiency.

## CONCLUSION

Hopefully, these examples will help us to be aware of the importance of analyzing what we do when instructing patients. Pedagogical objectives should serve to activate patients, rather than simply provide knowledge: 'What the patient has to do' rather than 'what he has to know'. *Active listening* to the patient could be one of the strongest stimulants to motivate the patient and thus help him to cope optimally with his diabetes. With the application of diabetic educational programs of these 3 principles in advanced planning and active involvement, perhaps Henry Ford's perceptive statement, slightly modified, would serve as well: 'Results begin on the drawing board'.

## SUMMARY

3 concepts from fields other than medicine – the beneficial use of educational objectives; the influence of active listening on patients and the importance of careful, rational analysis of all teaching steps included in any educational approach – are presented with an explanation of how their application can improve the effectiveness of patient education programs. The development and use of 'objectives' are traced in the history of the Model T-Ford and then converted into use on the 'production line' of a diabetic teaching center. Active listening is shown to have reduced the absenteeism in industry and is suggested to have a positive effect on patient motivation towards compliance in following a prescribed medical treatment. The need for a rational analysis of all teachers' actions in any diabetic patient education program as well as a third-party, objective analysis by a person outside the daily teaching routine is explained in the third concept. All 3 concepts can be used to improve the effectiveness of a medical team's diabetic education program.

## REFERENCES

1.  Drucker, P.F. (1974): *Management: Tasks, Responsibilities, Practices.* Harper & Row, New York.
2.  Mager, R.F. (1962): *Preparing Instructional Objectives, 2nd ed.* Fearon Publ., Lear Siegler Education Division.

## SUGGESTED READING

1.  Assal, J.Ph., Gfeller, R. and Ekoe, J.M. (1982): Patient education in diabetes in recent trends in diabetes research. In: Bostrom, H, Ljungstedt N. (Eds.), *Skandia International Symposia*, pp. 276-290. Almquist and Wiskell Intern, Stockholm.
2.  Assal, J.Ph., Gfeller, R. and Kreinhofer, M. (1981): Stades de l'acceptation du diabète. Leur interférence avec le traitement, leur influence sur l'attitude de l'équipe soignante. *J. Ann. Hôtel Dieu, Flammarion Med. Sci.*, 223.
3.  De Montmollin, M. (1981): *Le Taylorisme à Visage Humain.* P.U.F., Paris.
4.  Freud, S. (1917): Trauer und Melancholie. In: *Gesammelte Werke, Vol. 10*, 428.
5.  Guilbert, J.J. (1982): *Educational Handbook for Health Personnel.* World Health Organization (Ed.), 2nd ed., Geneva.
6.  Hamelin, D. (1979): *Les Objectifs Pédagogiques en Formation Initiale et en Formation Continue.* Edition ESF, Paris.
7.  Kübler-Ross, E. (1969): *On Death and Dying.* MacMillan, New York.

# 18. The circle of effective communications in patient education

M.O.C. JANUARY AND N. GAY

## EDITORIAL

*Acceptance of the thesis of this article by the reader hinges on 2 premises; firstly, that education of patients with diabetes is an accepted element of normal therapeutic treatment and secondly, that interpersonal communications between health provider and client is a basic element of education. If we accept the first premise, then it follows that some basic knowledge of education and educational techniques might turn out to be a useful tool in attempts by health providers to meet a number of objectives such as increased effectiveness of time spent in patient contact, better adjustment of patients in coping with a disease, increased patient compliance, and reduced numbers of medical crises and traumatic incidents, to name a few. If the second premise, that interpersonal communication is an essential element of education, is accurate, then nurturing existing skills and adding new and additional communication skills should greatly enhance the impact of the health providers in their role of patient educators.*

*This article briefly examines a model of the basic person-to-person communication and serves as a foundation for further examination by the reader of techniques of effective interpersonal communication. In a similar manner to that in which the physician modifies treatment based on feedback (lab results, visual observations, patient responses), the educational 'treatment' is adjusted based on feedback in the communication process. The article is provided with a glossary of terms. (The editors.)*

## INTRODUCTION

To speak is not to be heard. To write is not to be read with understanding. Only through the receipt of feedback information can we be assured that the spoken or written message has been received and acted upon. Our body provides us transmitters such as mouths, as well as receivers such as ears, eyes, and fingers. All of our impromptu messages are transmitted through these few means. Given advance preparation, messages may be prepared ahead of time with printed materials, audio cassette tapes, video tapes, slides, filmstrips, photographs, or other media. However, the vast majority

121

of physician/patient interaction during treatment and most often in patient education takes place through oral interaction. Thus, complete communications are absolutely essential for successful treatment and patient education.


## ASSUMPTIONS

For the purposes of this paper, the following assumptions are made:
1.   The patient needs to be a part of the health care team. In the treatment of a chronic disease such as diabetes, the patient must perform health maintenance activities with the physician, nurses, and dietician intervening in crises.
2.   Therefore, patient education must be an integral part of the treatment of diabetes.
3.   The patient must provide feedback to the other members of the health care team to ensure that treatment information in patient education is understood and properly acted upon.
4.   The physician and other members of the health care team need to elicit information (feedback) from the patient in order to make the correct decisions concerning the treatment and education of the patient.


## THE NATURE OF COMMUNICATIONS

Is not just telling a patient something enough? No! Speaking is only one part of the communication process. The purposes of speaking can be information giving, two-way interpersonal communication, training, or education. Information giving is the one-way broadcast mode in which the information is dispensed, much like medicines from a pharmacy or theater posters or television advertisements. No immediate feedback.

Two-way interpersonal communication, as discussed in Chapter 29, implies immediate feedback with a constant modification of the message based on the feedback. In communication terms, constantly using the response of your listener(s) to modify the next transmission of your message results in a 'feedback loop'. It works much the same in improving the effectiveness of the assimilation and accommodation of the message by other people as the 'closed loop' insulin-delivery system in which the amount of insulin delivered is based on the feedback from the body about the blood glucose levels, as opposed to the 'open loop' system in which the pump delivers rates of insulin without an internal monitoring device for feedback.

'Training' is by definition a process to teach a particular skill such as self-injection of insulin or home blood-glucose testing. 'Patient education' implies a larger, more general scope of increased learning by the patient to act upon available information in a responsible, dependable and productive way. Both patient education and training become more effective by using the 'feedback loop' model of interactive communication.

Advertising agencies receive feedback to television and radio advertisements through public opinion and market research polls as well as through consumer purchasing of the advertised products. Politicians receive feedback through votes cast in elections. However, physicians and other patient educators are in a position to receive immediate feedback from their patients.

## THE MODELS

In the open loop or broadcast model mentioned above, the emitter, like a radio transmitter, merely broadcasts the message in all directions. No indication is present that the message is received. Everyone might have their radio receiver turned off. A concrete example might be the physician who quickly announces that the diabetic must get better control of his blood glucose level, gets a short nod of the head from the patient and moves on to the next patient.

The closed loop or feedback loop model (Fig. 1) demands a recognizable response from the patient that confirms to the physician or educator that the patient has in fact received and understood the message. The closed loop system model discussed below is a model of the communications/training/education process. The feedback loop process is repeated until the health care professional concludes that the message is received and a new message can be formulated and transmitted, or until the patient terminates the process. In this process there is an enlargement of the patient's (and often of the physician's) previously gained knowledge. Thus, the use of the closed loop or feedback model of communication is helpful both to the patient and the patient educator.

### Formality

A formal step by step process need not be thought out and analyzed for each and every act of communication between educator and patient. The educator, however, must grasp the essential concept of the closed loop communications model, so that just a short time of conscious practice can lead to continual use of the model. Recognition of the communication patterns and recognition as to when the closed loop is being broken by the patient or educator are the critical desired skills.

### The closed loop model explained

1. *Input stimulus* is the event that causes the emitter to prepare and transmit a message. The stimulus could be a question from a patient, lab tests results, patient records analysis, or a part of a formalized education scheme.

123

The need of the emitter (sender) to want to send a message can affect the message – the urgency of the situation, the preconceived notions of the emitter, or the emotional state of the emitter. For instance, if a physician is extremely angry or upset because the patient has been in a ketoacidosis state, the emotional factor can shape the very words and, certainly, the style and mode of delivery.

2.   *Prepare/select the message* based on the input stimuli and the information available, the emitter may generate an entirely new and original message or select whole or partial messages from a repertoire of preplanned and often used messages. These 'stock' messages can be extremely useful in delivering information that is common, often needed, or for eliciting a response from a patient. Audio-visual media can be used to deliver stock messages – how to clean the feet or how to give an injection – for many of the 'how to's'. The disadvantage of stock oral messages is that a message quickly selected may not apply to the stimulus situation. The ease in the use of stock messages can lead to quick, off-the-cuff responses to stimulus situations that in reality demand a more thorough analysis.

3.   *To encode the message* is to translate the prepared/selected message from the thought of the emitter into a 'set' of transmittable outputs which

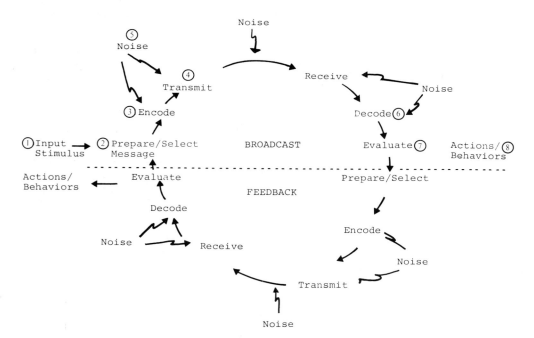

Fig. 1   The closed loop or feedback loop model of interactive communication.

it is hoped can be received and decoded accurately by the receiver. The term 'set' is used because the message may be transmitted orally, visually, tactile, or even by taste, singularly or in any combination. The emitter encodes the message in the choice of words and/or visual or other cues used in the transmission of the message. The encoding of the message as well as the transmission is greatly influenced by the perceptions and preconceived notions of the emitter. What perceptions could possibly influence the encoding and transmission of the message? The emitter's perception of himself, the receiver, the situation, the message itself, the stimulus – in short, the entire environment creates a complex set of variables which influence the creation and transmission of the message. For example, many patients might well agree that physicians have an extremely strong self-concept. This perception may be encouraged by physicians through word and deed. On the other hand, the physician might view the patient in any of a number of ways: serious, frivolous, intelligent, dumb, ill-informed, incapable, or eager. Certainly the physician's view of the patient will influence the way in which the physician encodes and transmits the message. These perceptions may be based on fact, assumption, or preconceived notions. Perceiving that the patient is stupid will influence not only the choice of words to be used, but also the message itself.

Perceptions can also lead to the 'self-fulfilling prophecy'. If the patient is viewed as stupid, the message can be encoded by word and gesture so that the patient tends to respond in a stupid way, fulfilling the prophecy that he is stupid.

4.   *Transmitting the message* is sending the encoded message by one or a number of transmission media. How often have we said, 'I was quoted out of context' or 'I did not mean it the way it sounded'. There may be more to a message than mere words. Messages can be transmitted in a number of ways: primarily orally (speech, music, audio tapes), but also visually (printing, graphics, television and films, photographs, and body language). Of course the senses of taste and smell can enter into message transmission, but they are less common. The message in spoken form can be transmitted not only by words, but also by voice inflection, tone, speed and volume. The most pleasant words can be spoken in a most unpleasant manner, conveying a different message than the words alone. Body language (body positions, movements, and gestures) often can reinforce or deny the spoken message. Visual expressions, stance, and hand motions can all convey the same or different messages as the spoken word. A smiling face and supportive gestures do not correlate with harsh words. The other cues derived from the multiple transmission media can reinforce or detract from the intended message. Consistency of message and transmission media in a manner to reinforce the intended message is highly desirable.

5.   *Noise* is any factor which can cause confusion in the message or distort the intended message to the emitter, the receiver, or anywhere in the trans-

mission of the message. The Shannon-Weaver mathematical model of communication stressed the importance of considering noise in any form of communication. Patient/physician communications are as subject to the noise phenomena as any other communication.

In a popular party game, a simple message is whispered from person to person throughout the room. The object is to compare the original message transmitted by the first person with the final message received by the last person in the chain. The results can be amusing and illustrative of the noise factor in our interpersonal communication.

Noise that takes place in the patient/physician relationship can be both external and internal. External noise includes physical background noise, distance, twists in messages passed by third parties (receptionists, aides, family members), or time constraints, to name just a few. Internal noise can include preconceptions which block the ability of the emitter or receiver to even conceive of the central idea carried in the message (such as home blood-glucose monitoring is impractical). Other noise can include learning disabilities, verbal and interpretative skills of the receiver and emitter, reading abilities and developmental level of the patient, previous bad information (knowledge founded on incomplete or erroneous data).

6. *Decoding the message* is the reverse process of encoding the message. Noise can also be introduced into the communication process at this stage. The same factors that influence the encoding and transmission of the message can influence the decoding process. Such faults might include verbal abilities, developmental levels, intelligence, physical hearing difficulties and the vocabulary level. Perceptions which may cause faulty decoding might include the patient's view of the physician or health educator, the disease, himself or herself, the setting, the quality of treatment, and the physician's perception of the patient. The emotional state of the patient can affect the decoding as well.

7. *Evaluation of the message* occurs when the receiver perceives the meaning(s) of the message based on his or her background experiences, knowledge, and current emotional state. The evaluation stage is the decision-making stage in which the receiver decides what the next action will be.

8. *Actions or behaviors* are those actions and behaviors which result from receiving, decoding and evaluating the message. From the behaviorist viewpoint, this is the end result of the message and is possibly observable and measurable. If observable and measurable, the emitter can best judge the accuracy of the receiver's receipt, decoding, and evaluation of the message as well as the quality and accuracy of the intended message. These actions can be as extensive as tighter blood glucose control, evidence of blood glucose control such as log books and journals, fewer insulin reactions, reduced number of hospitalizations, weight control, verbal reports

and blood tests results. The most immediate feedback is the verbal and visual cues (body language) of the patient. This brings us to the feedback or closed loop. The other half of the loop is the mirror image of the physician to the patient side of the model.

## The closed loop

On the basis of the evaluation, the receiver can formulate messages (oral, written or visual) to transmit back to the emitter. The receiver becomes the emitter and the communication process is repeated with the roles reversed. Now the physician as receiver receives feedback from the original message transmission. Based on the feedback (verbal, visual or written), the physician can take one of the following actions:
a.  take specific actions or exhibit certain behaviors;
b.  modify the message or transmission techniques and start the cycle again;
c.  start a new message cycle;
d.  terminate the process.
The closed loop based on feedback will be repeated again and again until the physician is sure that the proper message has been received or until the patient cuts the loop and withdraws from the conversation. In this model the physician and patient continually flip-flop roles of emitter and receiver. Is this process more difficult and time consuming? Yes! Is this process more productive and accurate? Yes!

Without the feedback, the physician is merely in the open loop or broadcast model. Very efficient in time, but not necessarily very effective. There is no feedback – no assurance that the proper message has been received.

## How to test your communication

Can we be sure that we are sending out the right message and that the message has been accurately received? Immediate feedback can be obtained using the 'Active listening' techniques discussed in Chapter 29. The key lies in ensuring that positive feedback is obtained by asking questions that require more than a mere 'yes' or 'no' answer. If the patient can repeat the meaning of the message, then there is a reasonable probability that the emitter did a good job of transmitting and the receiver did a good job of receiving. The true test is for the receiver to restate the message in his own words. Try it. You may be amazed at the results.

CONCLUSION

Communication, specifically in diabetic patient education and treatment, is more effective when using the closed loop (feedback) model rather than the traditional open loop (broadcast) model. A message must be modified, retransmitted, and remodified on the basis of feedback in a continuous cycle until the emitter is satisfied that the receiver has understood the desired message. The best feedback is in the long term based on patient actions and behaviors; however, the most immediate feedback is the oral and visual cues (body language) of the patient. The physician or educator is responsible not only for the message transmission, but he should also be assured that the communication is received, understood, and acted upon by the patient. Without adequate feedback, fulfillment of that responsibility is improbable if not impossible.

## SUMMARY

Effective diabetic education, training, and treatment should be based on a communication process which can be identified, learned, and readily practiced by members of the health care team. Total communication and education is based on a feedback loop model of communication in which the emitter (speaker) transmits a message, receives feedback (verbal reply or overt cue) from the receiver (listener), and modifies the message for retransmission until clear indication is received that the patient clearly understands the message and will probably modify his behavior or take desired actions. The open loop (broadcast) mode of communication is a monolog with only one person (physician, nurse, educator) attempting to pass a message. This mode is inadequate for the treatment and education of diabetics, because no feedback from the patient is received to confirm that the desired actions have taken or will take place.

## SUGGESTED READING

1. Anastasi, T.E. (1976): Communications training. In: Craig, R.L. (Ed.), *Training & Development Handbook. 2nd ed.* McGraw Hill Book Co., New York.
2. Diekman, J.R. (1979): *Get Your Message Across: How to Improve Communications.* Prentice-Hall, Englewood Cliffs, NJ.
3. Drucker, P.F. (1974): Management. Harper & Row, New York.
4. Hopper, R. and Whitehead, J.L. (1979): *Communications Concepts and Skills.* Harper & Row, New York.
5. Millar, D.P. and Millar, F.E. (1976): *Messages and Myths: Understanding Interpersonal Communication.* Alfred Publ. Co., Port Washington, NY.
6. Shannon, C.E. and Weaver, W. (1959): *The Mathematical Theory of Communication.* University of Illinois Press, Urbana, IL.

## GLOSSARY OF TERMS

*Accommodate* – the modification or fabrication of schemes (mental structures that adapt or change with cognitive development). The application of existing structures to a new situation in the environment.
*Assimilate* – the integration of information into existing mental structures.

*Broadcast model* – a one-way transmission with no feedback or method of indication that a transmitted message has been received.

*Concrete operational level* – a stage of mental development involving the individual performing such logical operations as adding or subtracting.

*Emitter* – the individual who transmits or sends a message.

*Extrinsic motivation* – motivation from outside the organism (such as rewards, punishment, money).

*Feedback* – information received by any means (verbal, visual, taste, smell, body language) which indicates how much of a transmitted message is received and understood.

*Formal operational level* – a stage of mental development involving an individual's hypothetical, propositional and reflexive thinking.

*Holistic* – emphasizing the functional relationships between the parts and the whole.

*Intrinsic motivation* – motivation from within the organism (such as sense of achievement, satisfaction).

*Pedagogical* – pertains to teaching.

*Pedagogy* – the art, science or profession of teaching.

# 19. Patient education: individual, group and mass media medical teaching: advantages and problems

JOHN G. ALIVISATOS

## EDITORIAL

*Physicians, nurses, dieticians, and social workers who have to inform, teach, or train patients and/or the general population, are confronted with the size of the client group: 1 person, a small group of 10 or less, a few dozen people, an audience of hundreds or a population with thousands or even millions of people (as with television).*

*It is not the purpose of this article to analyze the use of audio-visual material either with individuals or in groups, but to demonstrate how the medical message must begin with a clear understanding of what is needed as well as what has to be avoided to reach the optimum quality of the message in relation to the size of the audience. Too frequently the physicians give the same medical information in the same way, whether they speak to an individual person or a large group of people. (The editors.)*

## INTRODUCTION

If the ultimate goal of health education is behavioral change, then the health educator must also be responsible for the translation of the information into personal behavior. The dynamics of this process necessitate a knowledge of communication and the ability to analyze factors that could possibly interfere and interact during the process. These are the essential prerequisites which every health educator should know.

This article outlines advantages and disadvantages of various types of presentations used in medical education. One limiting factor, the number of persons involved in the communication, is considered. Dimou [1] examined the differences among the individual, the group, and the mass media approach in the following way.

## A. THE INDIVIDUAL APPROACH IN PATIENT EDUCATION

According to Fletcher [2], the essential element of medical practice is when a person, in the intimacy of a medical setting, seeks advice about his health from a doctor he trusts. The practice of medicine derives from this functional element. People also seek advice and consult doctors for other reasons including life-stressing events, psychiatric disorders, social isolation, and informational reasons [3]. In these cases, the patient is seeking not so much a cure of symptoms, but rather information, explanation, and knowledge.

The following are advantages of the individual approach (Table 1).

First, it gives the possibility to develop for the listener a multi-feedback system. You talk to the patient; you register his reaction to what you have just said; you give back an answer; you get his second reaction to your comment; you further adjust your answer, etc. This approach is a communication cycle of acquiring, giving information, and adapting one's next reply based on the partner's last statement. This form of exchange of messages is the essential feature of communication. Communication is not a one-way transmission, but a two-way process: an exchange of messages between 2 persons.

The second advantage is the individualization of this communication. One can focus on the individual case or problem. Within this individualization the patient may give you intimate information which he or she may be reluctant to share with others. The individual approach makes it possible to apply the medical knowledge and skill differently to each person every time. The popular saying applies in this situation that health providers and educators may provide 'different strokes for different folks'.

Thirdly, the dynamics of the interactional process of the communication between 2 people include not only words, but also the feelings of concern emitted by the non-verbal language of the medical care provider. The reciprocal process has both an intellectual and emotional dimension. Both dimensions can contribute toward a better health condition [4].

Table 1   *Patient education: the individual approach*

*Advantages*
1.   Multi-feedback system
2.   Individualization
3.   Interactional process (information and empathy)

*Problems*
1.   Number of individuals limited by their participation
2.   Time-consuming process
3.   Communication training needed for doctors and other members of the medical team

Frequently, patients' non-compliance is attributed by physicians only to the patient. In this view, the patient is passive, without desire for action, unmotivated, and lacks the ability to ask questions about the treatment and the disease. The blame is placed classically on the patient. Few have indicated that the physician's attitude and behavior could be significant factors affecting patient compliance and subsequent patient behavior.

A group of researchers from Southern Illinois University investigated 2 aspects of physician behavior during the interaction between patient and physician. One aspect was 'explanations' given to the patient and the other was 'concern' for the patient. There was a statistically significant correlation between these 2 aspects of physician behavior and patient compliance: the better the quality of the relation, the greater the degree of patient compliance [5].

Accordingly, in the individual approach, the physician's skills in communication need to be permanently present and used. The physician must have the ability to recognize individual differences, evaluate patients' needs, and observe the readiness of patients for information and understanding. The physician must be able to deliver information and empathize with the patient.

The problems of the individual type of communication may be as follows:

First, the individual approach is limited to the small number of individuals who actively seek advice. If we are interested in health education of the healthy, asymptomatic public, this is generally not the right approach unless individuals ask for advice.

Second, the individual approach is time-consuming. If we are interested in attaining a high standard in the patient-doctor relationship and a better patient compliance for therapeutic effectiveness, then we must plan more time for our patients. Training and experience are required for the health care providers to know 'how much' time.

The third problem is a frequent difficulty among physicians to really communicate effectively. Physicians are not trained to communicate; they are trained to act. How many medical schools give special courses on the basic principles of communication? Most training is limited to how to take a medical history, which is only one aspect of all the communication skills needed in medical practice.


## B. THE GROUP APPROACH IN PATIENT EDUCATION

The advantages of the group teaching method may be as follows (Table 2).

First, the important value of the group discussion technique [6] is the personal interaction which develops. In this setting the vital interaction process takes place not only with the educator, but mostly among group members. Sharing experiences with others produces the awareness that other people have similar problems. This is a powerful emotional stimulus.

The saying for this experience could be: 'A sorrow shared is a sorrow halved'.

Furthermore, people within the group can teach one another, especially if these people commit themselves. The group approach can be active rather than a passive educational approach. Getting information and hearing viewpoints from others who have had to face the same problems bring about a new evaluation of attitudes which increases the chances of effective behavioral change. The living example of one person telling another of his or her personal experience with the listener truly understanding and reacting to what has been said, is definitely more persuasive and powerful than any abstract lecture.

What would be the role of the physician or any other health educator in the group process? He or she should be the catalyst for the communication reactions; not the essential communicator or the initiator of every action. The group facilitator provides some guidance and direction to the members of the group to increase group interaction. The facilitator's role needs special skills which are based on specific techniques that can be learned.

Since the pioneer work of K. Lewin in 1948 [7] in using the group discussion-decision approach for influencing dietary practices, group techniques have been widely used in medicine. In the field of diabetology, J.J. Groen et al. applied successfully the so called 'joint teaching' technique between doctor and patient or patient and patient, or the 'communicative education' technique in group discussions with diabetic patients. They used not only physicians, but also diabetic patients as group coordinators (see Chapter 28).

The second advantage is the larger number of people reached as compared to the person-to-person method.

The problems of the group approach may be as follows:

First, the doctor and/or other health care providers and educators have to learn the skills for moderating group discussions. To be a good physician

Table 2   *Patient education: the group approach*

*Advantages*
1.  Interactional process among group members;
    actual, first-person examples;
    'joint teaching' between doctor and patients and/or patient and patient
2.  Larger number of patients possible

*Problems*
1.  Moderator must have effective skills
2.  Preparation and prior appraisal of group
3.  Lack of privacy for patients
4.  Possible tensions within the group of patients

does not necessarily mean that one is a good teacher. To be a good teacher does not automatically mean one is a good group moderator.

Secondly, group discussion needs preparation and a prior appraisal of differences and similarities between members of the group. You do not just walk into a group and start teaching. Additionally, selection of the group members may be a factor in the success of a group. The selection process may be time-consuming.

Thirdly, the group approach may lack privacy. However, this may not be a problem for all individuals.

The fourth consideration is that problems which cause anxiety or tension between the group members may arise. These tensions may produce disruption in the educational group process. Further, some group members may display extremes in attitudes. For example, some members may be completely silent. Others may monopolize the conversation and still others may simply chatter irrelevantly. Overcoming these types of problems requires a skilled and trained moderator with sufficient experience in working with diabetic patients.

## C.   THE MASS MEDIA APPROACH FOR PATIENT EDUCATION

The mass media are capable of exerting powerful influences affecting attitudes and behavior. One of the most famous examples of the dramatic effects of a broadcast was Orson Welles' radio production, 'War of the Worlds', in October 1938. This dramatization of the attack of New York City by aliens was taken as real by the population. A general panic occurred in some sections of the United States after the broadcast. This frightened reaction had not been foreseen by anyone. This extreme example illustrates the possible effect of radio or TV programs on behavior.

Are these powerful mass media of television, motion picture, and radio effective for health education? Are the mass media a tool capable of persuading people to adopt health attitudes and to go as far as changing behavior in order to improve their health? According to Budd and McCron [8], the mass media in health education are of limited effectiveness and are not the panacea to be applied in all cases.

Some of the advantages of the mass media approach (Table 3) are listed below:

The first is the mass coverage in which 'so many with the help of so few' can be reached.

The second, generally accepted advantage is that the influence of mass media lies mostly in reinforcing existing opinions or beliefs.

The third advantage is that the mass media may have behavioral effects, but these usually occur when certain levels of motivation pre-exist within the population.

The fourth point is that the mass media, when properly structured, pro-

Table 3   *Patient education: the mass media approach*

*Advantages*
1.   Mass coverage
2.   Reinforcing existing opinions or beliefs
3.   Behavioral effects when motivation pre-exists
4.   Effective in cognitive changes
5.   Trends can be generated

*Problems*
1.   No immediate feedback, no dialog
2.   Communicator impersonal
3.   No individualization of messages
4.   Audience self-selected
5.   Changing behavior difficult
6.   Technically skilled people needed

duce changes of knowledge, not necessarily attitudes. The mass media have a definite role in information transfer and learning. They can give a general background knowledge about health and can help to settle uncertainties, encourage resolutions, or correct some long-held mistaken beliefs about diseases and drugs. It is generally accepted that the mass media have brought about a definite improvement in public opinion for a number of health problems.

Fifthly, mass media can (sometimes) be more persuasive than individuals, because information can be presented more effectively and dramatically. A trend can be generated by influencing many people at the same time.

The limitations and problems of the mass media approach are many. The following includes a partial list of these problems:

First, there is no immediate feedback. This type of communication lacks dialogue.

Second, the communicators are usually unknown and impersonal with no interaction processes developing.

Third, the message is not individualized and, therefore, cannot take into account social and demographic characteristics such as: age, sex, education, ability, religion, social background, nationality etc. The message has to be simple and clear for large groups because it cannot be individualized.

Fourth, the audience is self-selected. People read the newspaper they prefer or switch to the radio or television programs which they prefer. It is an error to view the target audience as passive recipients of media messages. The target audience should be viewed as active participants.

Fifth, changing behavior is difficult especially when the population is indifferent and apathetic or when a commitment to a difficult, consistent course of action is required. In these circumstances the mass media may not be appropriate for health education.

Sixth, the mass media are a most expensive (of course not per capita) and a most difficult means of communication to organize.

A diagrammatic analogy (Fig. 1) is based on the work of B.K. Tones [9]. Figure 1 shows the spectrum of health education methods and the relationship to the degree of the 'Individualized Interaction Process' as related to the number of people involved in the communication.

According to Tones, the spectrum is a methodological continuum. At one end is the interpersonal approach and at the other end is the mass media approach. In the intermediate positions, different group techniques are available. The traditional lecture method often employed in diabetic education is closer to the mass media than the individual approach. The peaks above the spectrum indicate the degree of the intensity of the interaction process. In position A – the interpersonal approach with the one-to-one ratio – the individual interaction process is expressed as a single peak or, for diabetologists, the 'mono-component peak'. The strength of the individual approach comes from its feedback potentiality. In position B, the group approach, there are 2 smaller peaks: $B^1$ the smallest of the 2, which indicates the patient-doctor interaction and $B^2$, which is higher, the group member interacton. This is the double peak interaction component of the group approach. The interaction process fades away in the other educational techniques as the number of people in the audience increases. The doctor-patient joint collaboration (the individual approach) corresponds the closest to the modern concept of self-care.

How do the patients view the different media in patient education? Little attention has been given to this question despite an increasing concern among health professionals over the lack of active patient participation in the decisions concerning their health and disease.

Gadd et al. [10] examined how patients view different media. The patients of the study had rheumatoid arthritis and glaucoma. The authors

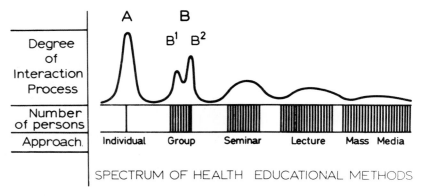

Fig. 1   Spectrum of health education methods and the individualized interaction process (from B.K. Tones).

analyzed the sources from which the patients sought information about their disease and treatment. Outside the health care system they used different media (newspaper, books, TV, friends, and other patients), while within the medical care system, they mainly used information given by physicians. The patients with rheumatoid arthritis did not spontaneously use the same media as those with glaucoma. Therefore, this study might suggest that each medium has a different order of priorities depending on the disease being considered.

## CONCLUSION

This article outlines the advantages and problems of different teaching approaches oriented for various sized audiences from one individual to a general population. All of the methods are useful, but some are more appropriate to solve a specific problem than others.

A mixture of media methods is also effective. In diabetic education, a film on diabetic problems (mass technique) shown to a group of diabetic patients can be followed by a discussion (group technique). The latter could be completed by a doctor-patient consultation if a patient's personal problems need to be discussed.

While the role of communication aids (audio-visual, books, pamphlets, etc.) cannot be emphasized enough and mass media may be useful in reaching large numbers of people, the best attitude, which also can be learned and/or improved, is to communicate with a patient using very 'old fashioned' human interest, concern, warmth, and feeling. The challenge to the health care provider who wants to give medical education is to radiate these essential ingredients of a successful educator-client relationship regardless of which mode of communication – individual, group or mass media – is used.

## SUMMARY

In order to effectively modify the behavior of patients, health educators must select the appropriate mode of communication – by individual, group, or mass media – based on knowledge of the advantages and disadvantages of each mode. This article examines these common modes of information presentation between health educator and client.

The need for effective health education of the public in general, or more specifically of patients in relation to their disease, has become a major theme of interest in recent years. Many believe that this kind of education can have an influence in improving the quality of 'health care' as well as 'disease care'. Education can be of value in preventing disease, facilitating treatment, and lowering medical costs.

The task of the educator is first to provide information and second to assist the individual in utilizing this information for a behavior change to improve health.

The information must be assimilated by the individual to affect personal beliefs and attitudes toward health. A change in attitude is a necessary prelude to a change of behavior. Knowledge alone cannot motivate correct behavior.

## REFERENCES

1. Dimou, N. (1980): Individual, group and mass medical teaching: advantages and problems. In: *A Better Approach to a Diabetic Patient*. 6th EASD-European Postgraduate Course on Diabetes. Laboratoires Servier, Geneva.
2. Fletcher, C.M. (1972): Communication with patients. In: *Communication in Medicine*, Part I, p. 7. The Nuffield Provincial Hospitals Trust.
3. Barsky, A.M. III (1981): Hidden reasons some patients visit doctors. *Ann. Intern. Med.*, *94*, 492.
4. Groen, J.J. (1980): A patient and his doctor: patients are listening better to us if we begin by listening to them. In: *A Better Approach to a Diabetic Patient*. 6th EASD-European Postgraduate Course on Diabetes. Laboratoires Servier, Geneva.
5. Falvo, D., Woehlke, P. and Deichmann, J. (1980): Relationship of physician behavior to patient compliance. *Patient Counsell. Health Educ.*, *4th Quarter*, p. 185.
6. Sutherland, I. (1979): *Health Education – Perspectives and Choices*. George Allen and Unwin.
7. Lewin, K. (1948): Conduct, knowledge and the acceptance of new values. In: G.W. Lewin (Ed.) *Resolving Social Conflicts: Selected Papers on Group Dynamics*, p. 56-68. Harper, New York.
8. Budd, J. and McCron, R. (1981): Health education and the mass media: past, present and potential. In: *Health Education and the Media*, p. 33. Intern. Conf., Edinburgh. Pergamon Press.
9. Tones, B.K. (1981): The use and abuse of mass media in health promotion. In: *Health Education and the Media*, p. 97. Intern. Conf., Edinburgh. Pergamon Press.
10. Gadd, A.S., Norell, S.E., Kvarnstrom, A.C. and Strandler, U. (1981): Different media in patient education. The patients view. In: *Health Education and the Media*, p. 369. Intern. Conf., Edinburgh. Pergamon Press.

# 20. The use of audio-visual media in diabetes education

LUTZ F. HORNKE

## EDITORIAL

*As audio-visual systems are more and more often used in diabetes education centers (mainly to save personnel) a professional description of the potential advantages and pitfalls of this new medium should be of great value. In this context, the following article outlines a number of important features of the audio-visual media to be used for improvement of diabetes education. Thus, audio-visual techniques can be used to present certain information, but they may also be quite helpful for observation of certain behavioral patterns of the patients. Furthermore, they can be instrumental to provide information to the patients' relatives or even to the general public. It seems to be of particular interest that any teaching feature using audio-visual media should be programmed in such a way that the transfer of information can easily be evaluated at the level of the patients. Furthermore, it should be stressed that the restriction of the entire diabetes education to audio-visual programmes for the patients will not serve a good purpose. Only for certain items in the diabetes teaching curricula may audio-visual techniques be used in preference to other educational methods. Professional cooperation with specialists in (adult-) education seems to be necessary to exploit the full potential of the audio-visual media for the goals of diabetes education. (The editors.)*

## EDUCATIONAL APPROACH

Like the work of the Diabetes Education Study Group, this volume is founded on the belief that diabetics do need help to improve their everyday life and thereby prevent future infirmity. Biochemical and physiological causes and mechanisms are necessary parts of a general practitioner's knowledge that enable him/her to diagnose diseases, to conceive of therapeutical programs and to counsel patients accordingly. However, it is the patient who has to live along prescribed guidelines in order to achieve relative health. The practitioner-patient contact thus very much resembles a teaching situation, and this is why educators might be called for assistance.

Therapeutical programs are effective only to the degree that the patient complies to them. From a democratic or partnerlike point of view 'obedience'

139

cannot mean sheer subordination to given prescriptions. It is the patient who has to live actively with his disease. Thus – as the Diabetes Education Study Group considers as a fundamental value – the patient has to aim at emancipated independence from medical personnels' guidance. To achieve this far-reaching end, special training programs are needed that teach the patient to manage his diabetes with as little help as necessary from others but with as much acquired skill as possible.

To 'educate' – or, a little less presumptuously, to 'teach' – patients becomes a challenging enterprise which might want to follow guidelines developed by education specialists. Here cooperation between medical doctors and educational doctors is called for to work together on curricula and to evaluate their effects. By *curriculum* is meant a rationally planned enterprise to bring out changes in diabetics. However, the ultimate goal might be to achieve well-adjusted blood sugar levels under varying life conditions, i.e. to change a patient from others-dependent to self-dependent by equipping him with diabetes-relevant knowledge, insight and actions. To achieve this a joint plan of present day knowledge of diabetes mellitus and proper patient behavior has to be made. This plan will then guide training of teachers as well as patients, since all criteria of effective teaching behavior, useful media and present/future patient activities are deducable. Seen from this point of view, *curriculum* means deciding upon goals, choosing diabetes-relevant information, defining behavioral objectives, training teachers, designing appropriate materials, installing media and evaluating their effects on patient behavior which represents 'independence'.

A well-understood curriculum and its evaluation as an ongoing process directly leads to a circular system of teaching where senders (teachers) interact with receivers. That the patient (receiver) learns from the teacher (sender) is quite an established fact. However, the teacher who adapts to the needs of his patients or who uses their life examples or recognizes feelings expressed by relatives 'receives' himself, too. However, to optimize this circular system of teaching it is necessary to gather information on its outcome and to change teacher and patient.

Behavioral goals/objectives are stressed here since it is through proper behavior that patients maintain or plan their well adjusted glycemia level. It ought to be understood that 'behavior' is not a flourish term but the observable entity so that patients' self-monitoring can be judged objectively by what they are doing. Behavior as stressed here encompasses a broad concept insofar as cognitive, psychomotor and affective dimensions are concerned.

However, to start with the patient in diabetes education would mean to put the cart before the horse. A learner presupposes a teacher, which means that training the medical (teaching) personnel ought to come in the first place and deserves thorough attention, be it medical doctor or teaching nurse. This in turn presupposes an entire curriculum, i.e. contents, objectives and media.

Seen from this educational point of view, diabetes curricula form systematically planned teaching-learning interactions of which media are but one part. So it will not suffice here to describe various audio-visual devices, but it will be stressed that these media are useful tools in many respects, some of which might not occur immediately to laymen.

## DIFFERENT MEANINGS OF 'MEDIA'

'Medium' is a very opaque term, and a closer look reveals that it denotes something that stands between 2 agents, namely the sender and the receiver. The sender is forced to encode messages which the receiver has to decode subsequently. However, for a diabetes education context it is the sender who is charged with the burden of proper encoding so that the receiver, i.e. the diabetes patient, will be able to reliably decode behavioral guidelines in everyday terms and to store and retrieve them accordingly when needed. Here, proper behavior of patients serves as an overall criterion for successful mediation/transmission/teaching. Since it is the sender who has control over different media, it is of interest to consider the latter in detail.

In general, one might want to distinguish between audio and visual media(tors) or a combination of both. As far as audio mediation is concerned spoken words are subsumable here. In any counseling context 'audio media' are used by the practitioner's talk or the nurse's lecture. Taped self reports of former patients or didactical interviews might be used as well. It should be clear that from the perspective taken here the use of 'audio' messages, like any other, will have to follow a systematic set of rules which are trainable as such with medical doctors or nurses. Small talk or casual conversation uses audio media as well but in a more or less unintentional way, since changing a person's behavior seldom comes in the first place. The contrary holds in educational contexts. Audio messages given once or twice have to be remembered and/or transformed so that the patient himself generates proper actions in varying situations. Systematic 'mediation' will help to ensure this end. Systematic 'teacher talk'/'guidance talk' in life lectures or radio transmissions is but one essential step.

Visual media aim at the same goals just mentioned. However, visualization might be identified with a whole gammut reaching from script, still pictures, handouts, diet charts, medication information, instructions and letters to the patient in magazines to formal textbooks for diabetics. Written instructions represent by far the general kernel of this kind of 'media'. But any of the above mentioned aims at representing by a minimal set of words something which, when properly remembered, effectively guides patient behavior. This is quite obvious as far as injection instructions or self control instructions are concerned, but it still holds when dose adaptation or holiday planning is called for. In any case, patients have to retrieve memory codes about what they had read a while ago, which first enables them to relate different information items, then to draw conclusions from them, and finally to behave accordingly. Again, it is believed here that different ways of 'visualization' affect patients' information processing quite differently. So it becomes necessary to investigate diverse effects of different visualization techniques before a subset of them can be used in diabetes education. This does not only pertain to 'visual' media but to all other kinds, too. To identify some of them in short: still-slides, picture books, graphs and the age-old blackboard. From the educational research literature it is not yet possible to rank-order visual media from poor to good, from ineffective to effective. Therefore it is necessary to design and conduct different small-scale studies which investigate the above-mentioned visual media and their effects in different clinical settings. The teaching personnel also has to be trained in the proper use of them. Instead of starting to write in the upper right corner of the blackboard – as many of us will do – training to start in the upper left corner is necessary, for example.

To teach a patient or to get any message across deserves much work. Using the entire gamut of media yields a show but does not guarantee anything. For example a teaching nurse might 'say and demonstrate': 'Take the syringe and put the nozzle slowly into your skin', demonstrating this with an empty syringe and an orange. The problem here is whether the patient will learn from this audio-visual context proper injection techniques. The oral message is cast in everyday language terms but obviously is not valid as instruction to guide injection behavior. Also the visualization lacks essential parts that serve as visual traces in the patients' behavioral memory repertoire. Using visual *and* auditory sensory channels such as lectures, film, slide shows or TV represents forms of audio-visual media.

Again, any audio, visual or audio-visual medium is but a means to achieve an end, namely to install proper patient behavior in varying life contexts. Colorful pictures, fancy TV movies and the like do not accomplish this by their dramatic make. It is necessary to design any mediated instruction according to educational guidelines that more or less ensure evaluable behavioral effects.

## DIFFERENT USES OF AUDIO-VISUAL MEDIA

It was stressed above that the general function of using audio-visual media is to improve patient behavior. To achieve this, teacher behavior has to be improved in the first place. Other target populations are represented by patients' relatives and the general public which deserves training in the third place. In the following paragraphs guidelines for each group are given.

## 1. 'Teacher' training

Knowledge of physiological facts and relations does not guarantee good teaching by itself. The teaching staff has to be equipped with special teaching skills, like how to ask questions of a patient, how to manage a group session, how to evaluate patient progress or the like. They all represent small behavioral skills that are trainable in the first place and have proven to be effective, i.e. to foster patient learning, in the second place. Teaching is considered here less an art than a trainable set of behavior.

To establish a teaching behavior repertoire, audio-visual media are very well suited, not only by presenting good teachers to trainees but also by designing small-scale life training sessions for trainees who actually will have to display and exercise certain chosen skills. The first-mentioned usage emphasizes model learning from some effective teacher model. In previous evaluation studies the model's teaching behavior had to be proven effective as far as patient behavior is concerned. Even multiple models are useful to present for example a doctor's questioning style, a nurse's diet explanation, a patient's verbalization of her emotions, a youngster's expertise in insulin injection, a father's physical activity planning or the like. Models who accompany their own actions – that have to be representatives of behavioral objectives – with their own words will help the learning patient to recognize essential relations and to store relevant information in order to retrieve them later when necessary in order to generate situation-bound proper behavior himself. The above-mentioned model behaviors 'questioning', 'explaining', 'verbalization of emotional states', 'injecting insulin' and 'planning' are but a subset of a far-reaching teaching behavior repertoire, bits and pieces of which are trainable separately, be it by means of model observation, controlled life exercise or a combination of both.

The second use of audio-visual media is far more direct, might be labelled 'learning by doing' and is suitably characterized by small-scale training sessions where each trainee displays a certain skill. He/she is being videotaped in front of a small group of colleagues or patients. Later the videotaped teaching unit is replayed and discussed with a proctor, education specialist or advanced colleagues. Special emphasis is given to analyzing how well videotaped skill behaviors resemble their theoretical descriptions. Several teaching-discussion cycles will approximate the trainees' behavioral repertoire/competence to the level desired. Adding another skill to the training program finally yields a repertoire from which the teacher, medical doctor or nurse in this case will be able to draw deliberately in real life teaching situations. This approach is called microteaching and proved to be effective with teacher students.

Very well-described skills are the kernel of this approach. Especially for counseling situations the following skills are recommended:

1. use of questions
2. reinforcement of client's responses
3. verbal explaining
4. introduction/opening interview
5. closing interview
6. paraphrasing
7. reflection of feelings
8. sustaining.

The 'use of questions' for example will become clearer when open questions, where answers draw upon material not contained in the question asked, versus narrow questions, where often a 'yes' or 'no' response is required, are considered. Both types do have their virtues and place in diabetes education. However, they relate to different levels of objectives. 'Right'/'wrong' differentiations are necessary with basic facts, but 'higher order questions' are useful to test a patient's understanding, i.e. knowledge of and construction of relations between facts or even synthesizing future behavioral actions. However, to ask questions purposely in a teaching situation is to give the learner, i.e. the patient, the chance to put into his own terms what he is to learn. This directly relates to what one might want the patient to remember, i.e. to store in his memory. If the patient is able to encode verbally-presented material, to store it appropriately, to retrieve it from his memory and to put it into action, then one might say that he 'learned' something, i.e. reached the objective intended. Questioning is but one teacher activity that helps the patient to fulfill this. The better the questioning as such, the better will be the learning success of diabetes patients – probably. Teacher behavior is regarded as a fundamental condition for patient progress.

Another important skill is to 'give feedback' or to 'reinforce'. Here teaching behaviors range from nonverbal gestures (e.g. nodding) to open positive verbalizations like 'Your description of the relation between insulin and glycemia level was very clear and comprehensive'. Whereas most 'teacher trainees' regard 'good' or 'so-so' as sufficient feedback in the beginning of a training session, they will finally have access to an entire set of 'reinforcements' that reach the patient individually.

'Very good' or 'ok' as such may be good reinforcers but are hardly sufficient sometimes to indicate to the patient what part of his answer/thinking/planning was considered. Differentiated feedback like 'Dear reader, I do thank you for having read so far and absorbed ideas of model learning and learning by doing' may be considered from 3 perspectives. 'I do thank', for example, emphasizes the relationship domain between reader and writer, 'read so far and absorbed' does represent reader behaviors to be installed, 'model learning and learning by doing' repeats key concepts dealt with. To disrobe 'reinforcement' from playing dirty tricks it is important to recognize that detailed feedback demands immediate evaluation of patient responses and subsequent verbalization/'gesticulation'. This, however, is hardly play-ing tricks but a systematic and objective-oriented cognitive activity on the teacher's side. It is hard labor, especially for beginners with too little under-standing of patient learning processes.

To complete the skill list given above, 'verbal explaining' emphasizes differentiated steps in presenting new material. Here the teacher will have to cast his explanatory comments into patient language, which should not be confused with slang or informal talk. Technical terms and/or Latin shorthand should be avoided, a difficult task for someone who is used to dealing with fine discriminations in medical contexts. To consider but one possible problem: 'diabetes mellitus' might confuse some patients because its two-word character instigates the question which other diabetes might exist. Surely, there is more than one diabetes, but what would their knowl-edge contribute to mellitus patients? Next to nothing, so one ought to skip 'mellitus' for this reason. This was but one example of problems in verbal explaining, and one might want to see imperatives like 'Use short sen-tences!', 'Try to give many examples!', 'Use everyday-like situations as example!', 'Complete ideas within a couple of sentences!'. Each impera-tive, however, will give rise to interesting analyses of teaching behaviors and nearly by itself instigate 'inventions' of good or even better teaching responses which are trainable separately.

'Opening' and 'Closing an interview' are teacher behaviors that make patients ready for or dismiss them from teaching. 'Good morning, ladies and gentlemen, welcome to our today's conversation about diet for diabet-ics' might stop chatting or 'embarrassment', direct attention to the teacher, and inform about forthcoming activities. The reader might want to take the message of above and cast it into a variety of versions. Anyone will discover his own awkward phrases when considered from the patient point of view. 'To come to an end' often evokes a feeling of relief and a closing of memories. As in writing, where the full stop indicates a unit, closing phrases serve as intellectual brackets and help the patient to keep things mentally together.

'Reflections of feelings' and 'Sustaining' underscore emotional domains. For a patient who displays concern about injection a smile might be of some help. But a smile is not always a smile, and all of us have to learn to do it. 'I smiled' may be someone's assertion, but the video replay reveals nothing but a twitch of his lips for one third of a second. The point here is that one has to make sure one smiles when one wants to. All this, however, is re-garded less from the observable teacher behavior but from the effects inten-tional, i.e. teaching, behavior has on patients. For gestures as well as ver-balizations this means that either prolongation, emphasis, or unequivocality are trainable domains.

Training sessions are set up to modify someone's behavior and someone's cognitions of himself and others. To some degree this becomes a 'therapeut-ical' or, less presumptuously, a relearning enterprise. One guideline might be to say that one wants to see how others see one's behavior, but this does not mean to subdue to others' evaluations or modification ideas. Self awareness and restructuring of one's behavioral repertoire is one goal of teacher training, but this is far from indoctrination. This is why such teacher training has to be handled with expertise and tactfulness. Well-trained educators are needed here to insure positive outcomes.

## 2. Patient instruction and behavioral assessment

Since diabetes education emphasizes patient instruction in the first place, the predominant role of audio-visual media will be described here.

Slide shows require but a cheap and light apparatus that is easily installed. Any change in slide sequence, however, as a result of a program evaluation calls for a change in the audio-tape as well, unless one uses a device where sound comes with the slide itself. Try-out versions or the like are easy to design and to fieldtest. Here 2 tape recorders and a set of slides will be sufficient. More recent devices even allow limited speed control by interspersing pauses demanded by patients. This is a crude but in many cases sufficient adaptation to patient learning speed.

Film, like TV, has the major advantages of cutting or editing desired versions of teaching spots. In case smaller teaching spots are cut, audio editing becomes a problem, and audio dubbing will have to be done for the entire program. But a pair of scissors will suffice to yield different try-out versions of a teaching program. The effort seems worthwhile, however, because moving pictures allow to present processes, be it injection techniques, physical exercise, or modelled patient-doctor interaction. The edited film strips yield instructional films that might be used even without medical personnel's assistance. The latter might be planned for a discussion roundtable or individual counseling.

TV – as it is available at present – has one major drawback. It requires very complicated devices to edit a final instructional sequence to obtain dramatic effects like broadcast TV.

Besides technical considerations, educational objectives come in the first place. They guarantee to generate a reasonable textbook and dramatic script. For our own work we started with a set of objectives concerned with 'introduction to diabetes'. Subsequent to their formulation a raw script was written and revised to achieve clear and codeable messages for patients. Several versions of a scene will be videotaped and linked together with others selected to yield 2 or 3 try-out versions. These are fieldtested with patients to get reactions and evaluative information. Here immediate recall of facts and relations represent the different levels of objectives, i.e. knowledge and comprehension. Also we decided for one version to present questions/problems via the TV screen and have the patients work alone and in groups. From a learning theory point of view this will help patients to overcome mere reception, to become active and use materials previously presented. Hereby we want to prevent 'media entertainment'. It is not yet a settled matter whether interspersed activation will foster learning or not. A lot of empirical educational research needs to be done in diabetes education.

The above reflections about audio-visual media and their possible uses are but a short glimpse of the entire set of possibilities. Another area of application is the assessment of patient behavior. This is very much alike the uses in teacher training in that actual problem behavior is videotaped. The difference, however, lies in the way the information obtained is used. Videotaped patient behavior from self control, insulin injection, dose-adaptation, record-keeping or the like is not replayed to the patient but used as a non-volatile behavioral report for the evaluation team. Many replays might reveal to the expert deviations from proper behavior that ought to be trained. So revised trainings will result, be it by instructing teachers, by rewriting instructions or by redesigning instructional films. Formative and summative evaluation of patient learning is possible, too. Correctness of patient behavior will be objectively judged by videotaped activities, which is scarcely possible if the observer participates in the moment the behavior is displayed.

Another application might be to record patient behavior when watching instructional films. Here immediate responses are of interest. Sometimes frowning, yawning or chatting tell that the instructional spot contains unintelligible information which ought to be revised. Laughter, 'clear faces' or murmured problem solutions tell the contrary and thus give rise to analyze the spot such that its 'dramatic make' will be described and used again.

Audio-visual media used in assessment reveal patients' proper or improper reactions and decisions and thus yield far more advanced data about what patients actually can do instead of what they 'will/might do' as is assessed in questionnaires or tests. The problem situation is there and the behavior is recorded in the situational context and not off context as with tests etc. Although *in vivo* recording of patient behavior has advantages, it does not outmode other means like observation or questionnaires but supplements them in a way that real life goal dimensions become observable. For group settings it might even be possible to design videotaped items and to record patient responses accordingly. In the long run many patient behavior 'protocols' might be used themselves to yield instructional spots in that previous patients' behavior serves as model behavior that is analyzed and cast into instructional explanations. What someone did right or wrong becomes obvious to future patients using videotaped reactions of former ones.

It is hoped that the two uses 'instructional' and 'assessment' will stimulate further creative TV applications. We expect widespread installation of TV player sets over the next years. In combination with small computers, even programmed audio-visual instruction might become possible which allows even more individualization of the learning pace according to patients' needs. Later video discs will carry entire instructional programs with many spots, each of which will be retrievable by the touch of a key. Objective oriented instruction becomes possible as well as 'watching/looking up' already forgotten information. However, more advanced techniques do require sound medico-educational research of effects. Technical means don't guarantee effective instruction by themselves. They should not be abused as entertainment-and-advertisement means in GP's waiting areas. The stance taken here is on continuous formative and summative evaluation of any diabetes instructional program.

## 3. Information for relatives and the general public

The above paragraphs approached diabetes education from training medical personnel and instructing patients. Here emphasis will be on informing relatives and the general public about diabetes. These are groups which are affected by diabetes in that they have to live with a patient, which creates problems now and then.

The mother or husband whose child or wife, respectively, has diabetes has to have some information about this disease. There are even many instances when actual emergency help might be needed, but most problems occur in everyday life. Physical activity like dancing, housework, shopping, hiking or the like will have to be planned by the patient, which affects his surroundings as well. Relatives do have to understand this and take an active part in necessary precautions and planning. At least they should know how to prevent and treat hypoglycemia. Psychological help plays an important role, too. 'Affective' objectives might be considered for informational programs designed for relatives and the general public. Here audiovisual media offer great advantages. In waiting areas informational programs are offered that are watched by patients and relatives together. Spots about the nature of diabetes, necessary precautions, dietary schedules and emergency situations will help a lot. One major psychological 'goal' will be to reduce 'sickness gain', i.e. hypochondric or exaggerated demands of the patient due to his experienced restrictions.

However, the latter desiderata are easier to formulate than to realize. Public broadcasts are to be considered here as well. They aim at informing the general public to take steps to prevent diabetes infirmity.

In both cases dealt with above, evaluation seems badly needed because relatives as well as the general public are not supervised closely by medical personnel. Here acquired knowledge, change of attitudes or the like are central points. It is necessary to start with well-designed objectives and design informational programs accordingly.

The distinction made here between relatives and the general public is one of degree. Anyone might meet a diabetic at work or at a party or at a sportsground. For mutual understanding and acceptance some basic information for the stranger seems necessary. Dutch television approaches this by 'Diabetes Voorlichting', a public broadcast. However, it seems that very casual objectives serve as guidelines too often. Here educational thinking might help to improve public information and its subsequent evaluation.

## CLOSING COMMENT

It should have become obvious that 'media' are already used in diabetes education. Be it speech, written material or audio-visual TV, it is necessary to start with properly-defined behavioral objectives and contents of interest. The latter two then guarantee that what is being mediated will be observable/assessable in one way or the other as effects from instructional efforts.

As far as audio-visual media and especially TV are concerned, many uses are identifiable. Instructional and informative functions will help patients, relatives, and the general public. However, a distinguished function is given with training medical (teaching) personnel to install proper teaching behavior and/or to improve their teaching skills. The latter point clearly emphasizes that instructional media are not meant to replace teaching personnel. Quite the contrary is true: teaching personnel receives assistance by instructional media.

The above-mentioned catalog of functions is neither meant to be comprehensive nor exclusive. The good old lecture or individual counseling will have its place as well as modern TV training/instruction/information. However, the stance taken here is in favor of modern media because much thinking and revising has to go into a single and sometimes simple spot. All this labor ought to have a recognizable payoff as far as patient behavior/ health is concerned. It is not denied here that a good counselor has a positive effect, too, but 'good media' instruction always has an effect within a larger group – on the average – and may be transported elsewhere. Repeatability of effects and transferability of teaching enterprises is what is needed if one considers a large number of diabetes patients.

## SUGGESTED READING

Instead of adding numerous titles from the educational literature, only a few are suggested for further reading or information.

1.  Bloom, B.S., Hastings, J.Th. and Madaus, G.F. (1971): *Handbook on Formative and Summative Evaluation of Student Learning*. McGraw Hill, New York.
2.  Green, L.W. and Kansler, C.C. (1980): *The Professional and Scientific Literature on Patient Education*. Gale Research Company, Detroit.

# 21. Problem-oriented participatory project work: an alternative way of education

JOHNNY LUDVIGSSON, ANNE GÖRANSSON AND ULLA RIIS

## EDITORIAL

*The authors decribe a system of problem-oriented education in which the learning process is activated by participatory project work performed by the patients. Similar to the method of interactional learning (as described in Chapter 24), this approach aims at an activation of the patients. A sophisticated attempt is presented to have the patients actively acquire knowledge by collecting, presenting and discussing information – rather than letting them retain the traditionally passive role of a pupil who consumes information. The authors maintain that more active ways of learning and acquiring knowledge will facilitate the emancipatory process of diabetic patients and adolescents in particular. Finally, the authors discuss the results of a study (published elsewhere) in which they have compared the efficacy of conventional group teaching and the problem-oriented participatory project work as educational methods in a clinical setting. In accordance with their theoretical assumptions, the method of active learning proved to be more effective. Finally, practical recommendations are given concerning the planning and use of the problem-oriented participatory project work in diabetes education. (The editors.)*

Diabetes mellitus affects every part of life all day long, year after year. Few if any diseases need such a complicated treatment. It seems self-evident that diabetics need knowledge. Nonetheless, most studies have shown no or a negative relationship between knowledge and degree of metabolic control [1-7]. There may be several possible explanations for such findings. We may have inadequate methods to estimate quality of treatment and degree of metabolic control and also inadequate methods to assess knowledge. Perhaps the relationship between quality of treatment and degree of metabolic control is too weak. It is also known that lack of motivation and compliance make even good knowledge useless and without effect on the treatment [8, 9]. Poor metabolic control may of course lead to repeated information, recommendations, prescriptions and prohibitions which lead to a large body of knowledge, but the metabolic control may remain poor.

150

Knowledge is too often superficial and passive. In this chapter we will discuss some requirements to get a qualitatively deeper knowledge and describe an alternative method to the conventional teaching which can be used in patient education.

## LEARNING IS MORE IMPORTANT THAN TEACHING

Usually education aims at reproduction of knowledge in the pupils. It seems reasonable that those who know, the older generation, convey their knowledge to those who do not know. The consequence of this ambition will be that in the educational process the focus is on the teacher, and 'education' has often been treated as synonymous with 'teaching'. However, the crucial point is of course whether the pupils learn or not. Knowledge about a certain phenomenon can have different meaning and quality for different pupils [10]. The situation and opinion of the pupil should be the basis for the educational method [11]. To render the learning process more effective we know that *an appropriate motivation* is invaluable [12]. Lack of motivation is usually the problem, but too much arousal may also interfere with the ability to learn [13]. Secondly, it is most important to consider the *mental development* and the *intellectual capacity* of the pupil, especially when educating children [14]. Thirdly, the more *active the pupil*, the more effective will he learn [15, 16]. We all know that it is easy to remember knowledge or experience which we have sought for or have been forced to seek to solve a certain tangible problem. However, most educational methods do not take advantage of the potential of the pupils' own activity. We are usually prone to estimate the effectiveness of an educational method as the amount of facts a teacher brings about in a certain amount of time, although it is learning rather than teaching that needs to be emphasized.

## PROBLEM-ORIENTED PARTICIPATORY PROJECT WORK

This educational process [17, 18] can be divided into two parts:

1. *Introduction phase*. The participants get to know each other and the educational method is introduced to them. They make an inventory of their resources and limitations such as the topics to be studied, the time, localities and other frame factors available. Finally, they decide the working forms for their project.

2. *Project work*. First of all the participants have to choose problems within a field given by others (e.g. the doctor who has decided that the patients should be invited to study diabetes mellitus and its treatment).

Problems are stated which can be empirically investigated. After this follows a phase of data collection, e.g. through literature, interviews, questionnaires, hearings with specialists etc. These data are analyzed and should be presented in some kind of report or other concrete product. The participants may choose to present their results as a poster, a paper, a film, an article in a newspaper etc. This product should be criticized and discussed by the specialist and other interested people, so that errors can be corrected and the product as a whole refined before the final presentation.

This educational method requires problem-orientation and participation. A problem is not a problem from the psychological point of view unless the pupil experiences it as such [17]. Participatory project work implicates that those who are supposed to learn also actively take part in the decisions regarding the education, its content and methods, even if these decisions are limited by certain frames, e.g. economical and juridical. In addition to 'problem-orientation' and 'participation' we add 2 other concepts: meaningfulness and extroversion. The problems should be meaningful not only for the pupils but also for the people outside this group. From this follows the expectation that the final product will be presented to persons outside the educational situation. In summary, it should be evident that this educational method is very similar to the common research method.


## BACKGROUND OF OUR OWN STUDY

The majority of diabetic children, even teenagers, have an unsatisfactory knowledge about their disease and its treatment [1-4, 19]. Although the parents may have become well-informed at the onset of the disease, the children themselves too often do not understand. Schoolchildren may follow the prescriptions and recommendations more or less passively. They get most of their information in a negative form: you must not do so, you should do that, etc. At the beginning of puberty the teenager wants to and is also supposed to become independent. If knowledge about diabetes and its treatment is incoherent and incomplete and if its treatment is experienced as oppression, the emancipation may be very difficult. In an effort to prevent such problems we have tried to reeducate diabetic children in prepuberty as if they were newly diagnosed. Group information was chosen, as we hypothesized that, in comparison with the individual information group education would need less resources, give better motivation, make it easier for the patients to accept their disease and perhaps might even give qualitatively better knowledge. As conventional teaching seems to give passive short-term knowledge, we decided to try problem-oriented participatory project work as a promising and more active form of learning.

Table 1   *Comparison between traditional education, problem-oriented participatory project work and actual study on education of diabetic children*

| | Traditional education | Problem-oriented participatory project work | Actual study on education of diabetic children |
|---|---|---|---|
| Learning style | The basis of education is general theories or principles which the pupil should apply on concrete situations (deductive learning). | The basis of the education is tangible problems which are supposed to be expressions for structures of society. The pupil tries to enlargen his conceptions (inductive learning). | The children decide themselves what they experience as problems within the field 'diabetes' and its treatment; by solving this problem they get more and more knowledge about connected facts. |
| Learning implies | To get new knowledge. | To acquire insight into how facts are connected to each other, to understand entities. | For the children: to acquire knowledge about their disease and its treatment and to understand the different treatment components and their interaction. |
| The learning process | The teacher conveys his own knowledge or experience to the pupils. | The pupil chooses his problem, studies, acts and puts the results in relation to society and to other theories. | The children choose a problem of their own and try to solve it. |
| Needs of learning | It is supposed that the pupils need to learn the same things. | The pupils have different needs of learning, depending on problems and developmental state. | The children were divided into 2 age groups, as it was supposed that children before or in the beginning of puberty have different problems and psychological development. The next step was to consider differences in interest. |

Table 1   *Comparison between traditional education, problem-oriented participatory project work and actual study on education of diabetic children (continued)*

| | Traditional education | Problem-oriented participatory project work | Actual study on education of diabetic children |
|---|---|---|---|
| The role of the teacher | The teacher is the expert. He/she gives lectures, recommends literature, demonstrates, etc. | The teacher gives the frames and keeps the pupils aware of the aim of the education. | The group leader and the children have agreed upon the frames for the group activities. The group leader carried the responsibility of actualizing the aim when necessary. |
| The role of the pupil | The pupil receives the facts, reads, etc., and is relatively passive in the education situation. The knowledge is not transformed into action. | The pupil works intentionally and actively to cover new fields, to compare theory and practice, to convey his knowledge to others. He/she works to improve unsatisfactory conditions. | The children tried to get knowledge on diabetes and its management. They got knowledge from each other and by cooperation, and they decided how to report what they had learned. This report (a booklet) aimed at improving the knowledge of classmates, parents, etc., and comprehension of diabetes. |
| Responsibility | The teacher is responsible for the learning process of the children. | The teacher is responsible for the relevance of the problem and for the practical arrangements. The pupil is responsible to himself and to others for the relevant learning to occur. | The group leader took responsibility for ensuring that the problem to be chosen was relevant. She strove for making the children responsible for the learning. |

| | | | |
|---|---|---|---|
| Mistakes | The pupils try to make as few mistakes as possible. | In the educational situation new ways and means may be tested without fear of failure. In the extrovert parts of the work, mistakes should be avoided as they may harm the aim of the project. | The same condition as in the preceding column. However, the group leader had the task of preventing the children from mistakes that would be hazardous to the treatment of their diabetes. |
| Control | The result of the education is controlled by putting questions or problems to the pupils in a test situation. | The result of the education is controlled through the assumption that there is a practical use of the knowledge outside the educational situation. | The result of the education is controlled both by the use of the knowledge outside the educational situation, its impact upon selftreatment and by special knowledge interviews. |
| Evaluation | The teacher evaluates the pupils' knowledge and gives certain marks. | The pupil himself evaluates together with the teacher the use and value of the product for himself and for others. | A doctor scrutinizes the final product and discusses this with the children and with the group leader. |
| Learning results | The knowledge has a relatively intellectual and theoretical character. | The pupil has learned new skills, new ways of solving problems and has got new insights into the conditions of society. | The children have acquired new knowledge, new skills and have also learned a new way of how to get further! |

*J. Ludvigsson, A. Göransson and U. Riis*

## DESIGN OF THE PATIENT EDUCATION

We invited 37 children aged 10-14 years who had had diabetes for 2 years or more to participate in the study. Only 1 family refused to participate, but 3 others had to be excluded because of e.g. complicating disease. The remaining 33 patients and their families were included in the study. We started with a pre-testing period including estimation of knowledge about diabetes and its treatment, responsibility for the treatment, family relationships and mental state of the child [20] and the general health-related motivation according to the Health Belief Model [21, 22]. In addition we evaluated both quality of treatment and degree of metabolic control in several ways. After these pre-tests the patients were divided into 6 groups: 4 groups working under an experimental condition with the problem-oriented participatory project work and 2 groups under a control condition with conventional group information. All groups met every other week from October 1979 to April 1980 for 1½ hour every time. In each group there was 1 adult group leader. Two persons, educationally but not medically trained, served as group leaders. In addition the groups had access to the ordinary staff members of the clinic. The subject to be dealt with was insulin-dependent diabetes and its treatment.

The problem-oriented participatory project work started with an introduction phase. The members of the group learned to know each other and their leader, and the subject matter was introduced to them as well as the rest of the identifiable frame-factors. Then the instructional method was introduced thoroughly. Following this introduction came the project phase. The patients chose a problem to work with as a project. Already during these discussions they ventilated quite a lot of personal experience and ideas before they chose a problem which was both real to them and relevant to the topic 'diabetes and its treatment'. It was important that this problem should be one which could be solved realistically by the patients during the time they had at their disposal. The next step was to start working with the problem by formulating questions and trying to have them answered by studying literature, posing questions to invited experts or older diabetics, etc. The patients could and also did ask the medical staff for short lectures on defined topics. After all information had been gathered, the patients prepared their product. All groups decided to make a booklet from which the classmates and teachers at school would understand the life situation of a diabetic child. When the product was completed it was scrutinized by one of the patients' doctors so that incorrect facts could be revised.

The conventional group information included lectures, films, etc., organized by the teachers (medical staff) in the usual way. No special attempts were made to activate the patients although, of course, they had the possibility to ask questions in connection with the lectures. There was no special group leader.

Below follows a comprehensive comparison between traditional educa-

156

tion, problem-oriented participatory project work and the actual study on education of diabetic children [10, 23].


## RESULT AND DISCUSSION

Two main questions were to be answered by the study:
1.  Can one or both of the two educational settings serve as a functional model for patient education within the clinical work?
2.  Did the patients acquire more knowledge and/or different kinds of knowledge under one of the two educational conditions?

The question of attitudes and responsibility can be considered as parts of the second question above.

Firstly, it can be concluded that on a practical basis the problem-oriented participatory project work exceeded the conventional teaching method. In the latter case, the patients showed less interest and the absence and drop-out rate was higher. This had a negative effect on the enthusiasm of the medical staff engaged in this instruction.

Secondly, it can be concluded that the problem-oriented education was feasible in the clinical situation.

Thirdly, it can also be concluded that in the present study differences in knowledge-increase, attitudes and responsibility were in favor of the problem-oriented education, although the differences were small.

The fact that the differences were small may be interpreted as partly due to the fact that the problem-oriented participatory project work method was not fully carried through. Evidently the patients had too few meetings, as it took quite a long time before they really had defined their problem and started to work. Another important factor is the group leader. The leader must have a clear idea about the theory and the underlying principles of the method. He must also be able to carry through the instruction according to these principles. Otherwise there is the risk of the group leader's choosing either to use his conventional teaching strategy or to refrain from using any strategy at all; both courses make the work ineffective. However, if we suppose that the problem-oriented education method really was carried through in our study, there may be several explanations why the result was only slightly better than in the conventional group information. Maybe some of the young children actually did not experience the treatment of diabetes as their problem but rather as a problem of their parents. Furthermore, our evaluation shortly after the education period shows less differences than might be seen 1 or 2 years later, especially if the problem-oriented education has made the patients more motivated and has also taught them how to get further knowledge.

To investigate whether the problem-oriented education is even more suitable in somewhat older patients, we have continued our studies by using the method in 3 different groups of diabetics aged 16-17 years, 18-20 years and

*J. Ludvigsson, A. Göransson and U. Riis*

21-24 years. In this case only those patients participated who showed interest, which of course is a selection disturbing the evaluation. However, we dare to conclude that in these age groups the method, at least for these patients, seemed to be very useful and stimulating. The activity and motivation was very high among the participants, and all 3 groups produced relevant products bearing indications of coherent, integrated, active knowledge.

## CONCLUSION

There are many reasons why diabetics should have a metabolism as normal as possible. No medical staff can ever reach this goal without an active cooperation with the patient, who is the one realizing their ideas about the treatment. This implies that the patients should have both adequate knowledge and motivation to transfer this knowledge into compliant behavior. Different approaches are suitable in various situations, for individual patients and doctors. We have questioned the conventional group teaching which may result in passive, superficial knowledge without changing attitudes or activities; that is, treatment. Instead, both theory and our practical experience indicate that problem-oriented participatory project work is an educational method that has quite other qualities. An introductory course may initiate interest and teach the patients how to get further skills and knowledge. This can of course be followed by other courses or complemented by other types of education. When the patient can work with questions experienced as his own problems that need solution, then the motivation to learn increases. Such knowledge is stored in the memory and can be used actively outside the education situation. Then education will not only increase self-respect, independence and confidence, but will also contribute to a good treatment, an improved metabolic control and better quality of life for the diabetic patient.

## REFERENCES

1. Collier, B.N. and Etzwiler, D.D. (1971): Comparative study of diabetes knowledge among juvenile diabetics and their patients. *Diabetes, 20*, 51.
2. Karp, M., Manor, M. and Laron, Z. (1970): What do juvenile diabetics and their family know about diabetes? In: Laron, Z., *Habilitation and Rehabilitation of Juvenile Diabetics*, p. 83. Stenfort Kroese, Leiden.
3. Watkins, J.D., Williams, T.F., Martin, D.A. et al. (1967): A study of diabetic patients at home. *Am. J. Public Health, 57*, 452.
4. Williams, T.F., Martin, D.A., Hogan, M.D. et al. (1967): The clinical picture of diabetic control, studied in four settings. *Am. J. Public Health, 57*, 441.
5. Etzwiler, D.D. and Robb, J.R. (1972): Evaluation of programmed education among juvenile diabetics and their families. *Diabetes, 21*, 967.

6. Strauss, M.B. (1969): Diabetic regimens – procrustean beds. *N. Engl. J. Med.*, *281*, 1482.
7. Tietz, W. and Widmar, T. (1972): The impact of coping styles on the control of juvenile diabetes. *Psychiat. Med.*, *3*, 67.
8. Ludvigsson, J. (1976): *Metabolic Control in Juvenile Diabetes Mellitus. The Influence of Some Clinical Biochemical and Socio-psychological Factors.* Linköping University Medical Dissertations, No 42.
9. Ludvigsson, J. (1977): Socio-psychological factors and metabolic control in juvenile diabetes. *Acta Paediat. Scand.*, *66*, 421.
10. Riis, U., Göransson, A. and Ludvigsson, J. (1983): *Knowledge about Diabetes and its Treatment as an Effect of Problem-oriented Participant-controlled Patient Education.* Linköping University, Department of Education Reports. In press.
11. Bruner, J.S. (1968): *Toward a Theory of Instruction.* Norton Co, New York.
12. Ausubel, D.P. (1968): *Educational Psychology. A Cognitive View.* Holt, Rinehard and Winston, New York.
13. Broadhurst, P.L. (1957): Emotionality and the Yerkes-Dodson law. *J. Exp. Psychol.*, *54*, 345.
14. Inhelder, B. and Piaget, J. (1958): *The Growth of Logical Thinking from Childhood to Adolescence.* Basic Books, New York.
15. Skinner, B.F. (1954): The science of learning and the art of teaching. *Harv. Educ. Rev.*, *24*.
16. Bligh, D.A. (1974): What's the Use of Lectures? Penguin Books, Harmondsworth.
17. Illeris, K. (1974): *Problem-Orientation and Participation. Design of Alternative Didactics.* Munksgaard, Copenhagen.
18. Illeris, K., Fibaek Laursen, P. and Simonsen, B. (1978): *Society and the Pedagogy.* Munksgaard, Copenhagen.
19. Etzwiler, D.D. (1962): What the juvenile diabetic knows about his disease. *Pediatrics*, *29*, 135.
20. Ludvigsson, J., Cederblad, M., Göransson, A. et al.: Group information of diabetic children. A multidisciplinary approach. *Pediatr. Adolesc. Endocrinol.*, in press.
21. Ludvigsson, J., Richt, B. and Svensson, P.G. (1980): Compliance and the health belief model – relevance to the treatment of juvenile diabetes mellitus. *Scand. J. Social Med., Suppl. 18*, 57.
22. Svensson, P.G., Ludvigsson, J. and Richt, B. (1983): The health belief model applied to juvenile diabetes. Psychosocial aspects of diabetes in children and adolescents. *Pediatr. Adolesc. Endocrinol.*, in press.
23. Berthelsen, J., Illeris, K. and Poulsen, S.C. (1977): *Project Work. Experience and Practical Guidance.* Borgen, Copenhagen. (Danish.)

159

# 22. Computer-assisted instruction for diabetics

## The DOCEO II system developed at the University of Liège, Belgium*

PIERRE J. LEFEBVRE, MUTIEN-OMER HOUZIAUX, COLETTE GODART, MYRIAM SCHEEN-LAVIGNE, MICHEL BARTHOLOME AND ALFRED S. LUYCKX

### EDITORIAL

*Among the various methods which can be used to transmit knowledge, computer-assisted teaching will certainly play an increasing role in patient education. Home-computers are becoming increasingly available, so it is likely that patients will gradually come to accept this technique more readily.*

*If computer-assisted teaching is a very useful tool for providing knowledge, further development of this technique should also help the student to develop new skills. However, knowledge and skills will only become therapeutic if the patient is able to change his behavior with regard to the treatment of his diabetes. Technical equipment alone will not help people to change their behavior, and therefore a computer-assisted program will be only one, albeit valid, step in a more global approach towards patients. Personal discussions with health-care providers remain essential. The use of technical equipment might help health-care providers save precious time which could then be devoted to patients in the form of greater and improved personal interaction. (The editors.)*

One of the limiting factors in the development of teaching methods for diabetics is the great amount of time required from qualified individuals. In recent years, modern educational techniques such as teaching machines have been used as an aid in this matter [1-5]. Our group at the University of Liège has developed an original audiovisual Computer-Assisted Instruction (CAI) system, and a special programmed course for teaching diabetics has been designed [6].

In its present state, the program consists of 7 lessons dealing with various

---

*Slightly modified version of an original article published in *Diabète et Métabolisme*, 7, 127 (1981), reproduced with permission of the editors and the publisher (Masson Ed., Paris).

aspects of insulin-dependent diabetes. A detailed assessment program (also computerized) has been conducted in order to collect data on a patient's knowledge of diabetes self-care before and after completing the computer-assisted teaching program (and so, to determine the improvement of his score).

The aim of this paper is to describe briefly: (1) the initial conditions and objectives; (2) the adopted methodology; (3) the characteristics of the CAI system; (4) its experimentation; (5) its evaluation and (6) its acceptance by patients.

## 1. INITIAL CONDITIONS AND OBJECTIVES

Insulin-dependent diabetics were initially selected to participate in this educational program because a major part of their successful management involves the greatest degree of knowledge and therapeutic initiative from the patients themselves. Other factors relevant to good care include intellectual ability, age and sociocultural level [3, 7-9]. The course was designed to *individualize* teaching in order to give a minimum of basic information to a maximum of patients. The only prerequisites were the ability to read fluently, knowledge of the usual language and absence of serious mental deficiency.

The main objective in this CAI program has been to supply the patient with *knowledge*, to arouse his desire and to increase his ability to put his knowledge into *practice*. In this perspective, we assumed that the patient would be able not only to repeat something memorized (as a result of a Skinnerian conditioning), but also to use his knowledge to solve most of the problems encountered in his daily life as a diabetic.

The content of the program has been defined in view of its integration into a broader educational context. For this purpose, we have selected questions which both pertain to the theoretical aspects and solicit inductive and deductive skills rather than mere memorization. Topics of the lessons developed so far are: (1) carbohydrate metabolism; (2) pathophysiology of juvenile-type diabetes; (3) insulin: aspects, packaging and use; (4) types of insulin and principles for adapting doses to standard daily situations; (5) hypoglycemia; (6) dietary basic principles; (7) testing urine for glucose and ketone bodies.

## 2. METHODOLOGY

The target population being rather heterogeneous, we adopted a tutorial approach, in which the learner's rhythm and abilities, such as they appear in the conversational process, are taken into account.

161

Functionally, the general structure of the CAI system-learner relationship can be described as shown in Figure 1.

The part played by the system consists in giving the learner information and checking the efficiency of the message by displaying a question (a). Each answer is stored (b) and formally analyzed in contrast with stereotypes (c). The result of this analysis is memorized (c') and applied in the decision process (d). The nature and the content of the program feedback, i.e. comment, remedial sequence and/or selection of the next question (e), is determined either on the basis of the last answer or, in a more sophisticated and adaptive way, by referring to the content of the computer memory. Further details will be found in the description of the software (see 3.c.).

In this teaching method, it appears that making an error is considered, just as in daily life, as a natural occurrence (playing the role of a vaccine), provided it is immediately recognized as such by the learner [10].

In the same way, the lessons arouse the subject's observation and reasoning as much as possible in order to enable him, after a certain time, to reconstruct mentally vanishing notions and to increase his transfer of learning aptitudes, which the process of solving problems inevitably entails.

The matter has been thoroughly analyzed: with the help of relational matrices, it has been possible to bring out its various topics and their relationship.

Most items make use of the multiple choice technique, which is easier for the patients than the constructed response and turns out to be satisfactory as far as the diagnosis of mistakes and the determination of the appropriate remedial sequences are concerned.

The flexibility we intended to reach led us to adopt a great variety of programming structures. Yet, in the process of writing lessons, a certain number of standard algorithms emerged and, owing to their efficiency, have been repeatedly used in the course.

An example is given in Figure 2 in which the diagram shows the structure of one of the last sequences of the first lesson devoted to the role of insulin.

After a theoretical teaching sequence, the patient is asked to answer the following question:

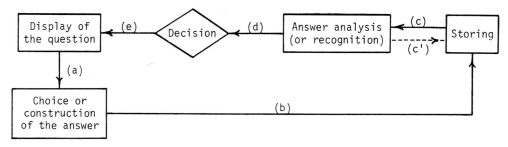

Fig. 1 General structure of the CAI system-learner relationship.

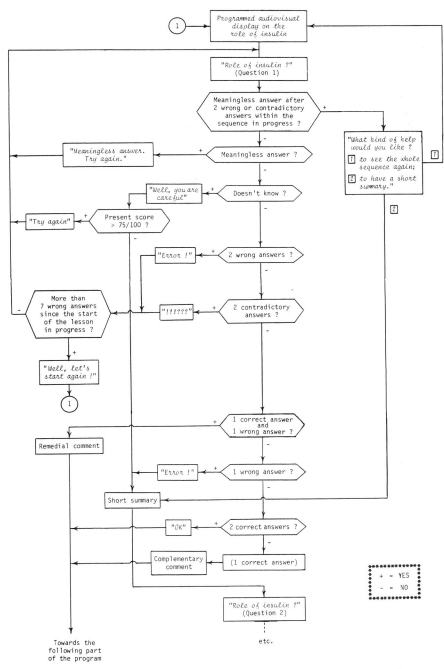

Fig. 2    Flow-diagram of a sequence about the role of insulin.

163

Insulin produces:  a rise in blood glucose                          1
                   an increase of glucose penetration into cells    2
                   a reduction of glucose penetration into cells    3
                   a reduction of blood glucose                     4
                   I don't know                                     5

From the beginning, the patient had been told that the correct answer was included in the list of the proposed answers and also that it could consist of one or several of the propositions (*e.g.* 1; or 1 and 3; or 1, 2 and 4, etc.).

The diagram shows how specifically the system reacts according, not only to the given answer, but also to information gathered during the lesson about the 'pupil's' performances since the beginning of the lesson.

For practical reasons, the wording of the comments and other messages in the flow-diagram depicted in Figure 2 has been considerably condensed: it is actually far more explicit and occasionally rests on illustrations (Figure 3).

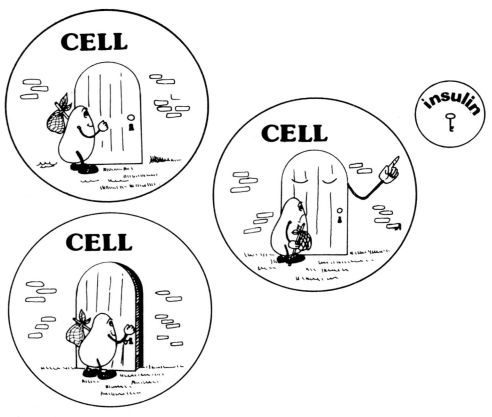

Fig. 3  Illustration used to explain that insulin plays the role of a key allowing glucose to enter the cell.

Question 2 is the same as question 1 except for the last answer (I don't know), which has been withdrawn. The treatment of the answers is also similar, but if the patient, in spite of the help he has received, is still unable to provide the right answers (in this example, answers 2 and 4), the system gives them to him as explicitly as possible.

## 3. FEATURES OF THE SYSTEM

The system has been named SIAM-DOCEO II: SIAM for 'Système Informatique d'Anamnèse Multilingue', DOCEO from the Latin *doceo*, I teach, and 'II' since the system presently used is derived from the original DOCEO I system developed in 1965-1966 by one of us [11].

It consists of a central unit and a series of terminals for the hardware, and of specially designed software.

### a.  The central unit

The central unit consists of a DEC PDP-8E mini-computer* with a 32K (12 bits-words) core memory, 2 disks of 32K, 3 disks of 1600K and 2 DECtapes (196K each). This configuration is capable of managing up to 10 terminals in time-sharing.

### b.  The terminals

Each specially-designed terminal (Figure 4) includes: an alphanumerical cathode-ray tube with an associated alphanumerical keyboard, a random-access Kodak® slide projector with a rear projection screen, a Uher® tape-recorder modified for randomly selecting audio-items from a hybrid (analog-digital) tape, earphones and interface circuits.

### c.  The software

A special-purpose software has been elaborated which does not require a large central memory but allows great flexibility in programming lessons.

One of the main functions of the operating system, called RTS-LPC (Real-Time-Sharing in Language for Programming Conversational processes), is the interpretation of author's programs (A.P., i.e. courseware) written in a symbolic language, the LPC. To avoid the description necessary to account for all the possibilities of this language, we shall merely point out

---

*The transfer of our system onto a DEC PDP-11/44 is currently in progress (November 1981). For further technical information, please contact M. Bartholomé and M.-O. Houziaux, co-directors of the project (SMATI, Bât. B19, Université de Liège au Sart-Tilman, B-4000 Liège, Belgium).

its main functional features. Users' answers can be chosen *or* constructed. In the first case, the user responds to a series of items by selecting one or more of the proposed answers, or by rejecting all of them. If, in the other case, the answer is constructed, the technique of keywords is applied: as a matter of fact, the program is able to test their presence or their absence, the order in which they appear in the given answer, their number and their associations. Common misspellings are detected by simple algorithms.

At each step of the dialog, the system may be programmed to modify its

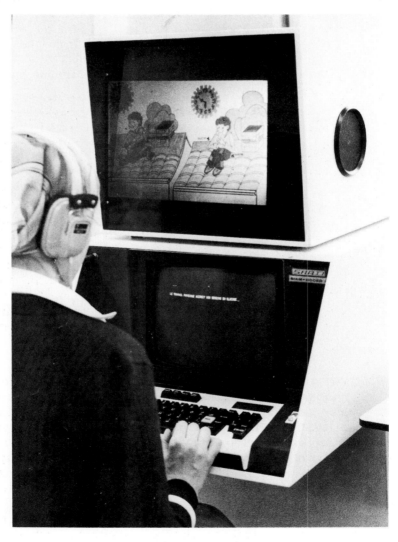

Fig. 4   Audiovisual terminal of the DOCEO II-system.

166

responses according to various criteria: whole or part of the previous pathway (including prior sessions), psycho-pedagogical profile of the user, latency of his answers, and so on. All these criteria may be combined in Boolean expressions. A number of routine control operations are automatically executed by means of permanent instructions included in the monitor program. The capacity of the system is considerably increased thanks to the availability of a set of auxiliary programs (written in Assembler), which may be activated from the A.P. Each lesson concludes with the storage of the different files (for the purpose of subsequent statistical analysis), and, if requested, with the printing of detailed reports for the users (patient, educational nurse, physician etc.).

## 4. EXPERIMENTATION

So far, 218 patients have participated in the experiment, which was supervised by two nurses specialized in teaching diabetics. Most patients were in-patients. All were individually informed about the twofold aim of the course: (1) to give them the opportunity to become more knowledgeable about their disease, and (2) to improve the efficiency of the methods and the lessons designed for them.

Our first program-trials soon revealed a number of methodological shortcomings we immediately corrected. For example, we soon realized that, in one of the sequences, we had failed to respect one of the principles we had decided to adopt when defining the methodology: patients should not be considered as pupils in the usual sense (i.e. their self-respect should not be affected); it was, therefore, decided to forgo a rule which is generally followed in programmed instruction or computer-assisted instruction: learners should not be allowed to progress until they have mastered the notions taught so far. When really needed (e.g. to prevent a patient to become disheartened), the correct answer with an appropriate and explicit comment is provided.

## 5. EVALUATION

Rather than comparing results gathered in very dissimilar conditions, it was decided, at this stage of the experiment, to limit the evaluation to the elements of the experiment which were sufficiently homogeneous to be statistically analyzed. The present evaluation, therefore, deals only with the first 4 lessons attended by 50 in-patients during a period of 1 or 2 weeks.

All were insulin-dependent diabetics and were hospitalized either for initiation to insulin therapy or for changing insulin regimen. All were mentally alert, not confined to bed, and aware of the diagnosis of diabetes. There were 26 males and 24 females. The mean age ($\pm$ S.D.) was $36 \pm 15$ years (range 13-74).

The efficiency of the teaching program was evaluated by submitting the patients to a 19-item questionnaire before (pre-test) and after (post-test) completing the first 4 lessons. The content was the same in the pre- and post-tests, but the formulation of the questions was not identical.

The pre-test was performed immediately before the first lesson and the post-test 24-48 hours after completion of the fourth lesson.

As shown in Table 1, the mean ± S.D. of the simple scores (SS) was 10.95 ± 3.95 before the course (pre-test) and 17.68 ± 1.76 after the course (post-test). When the scores were corrected for guessing (SG), they were 9.59 ± 4.43 and 17.04 ± 2.26 respectively (paired *t* test: $p < 0.001$). Those figures indicate not only that the average score has improved markedly, but also that the dispersion of the individual scores has been considerably reduced, as shown by the values of the standard deviations.

Figure 5 shows an analysis of the distribution of the learners' improvement rate. The generally-recommended formula for tabulating relative gain (absolute gain/possible gain) did not satisfy us since, with this formula, apparently equal relative gain might have very different meanings.* That is the reason why we adopted the formula established by P. Lambert (IR, Improvement Rate) to eliminate this effect of homogenization by taking into account relative gain *and* absolute gain.** The figure clearly shows a bimodality in the distribution of the improvement rates. The gain was quite impressive (IR = 6 to 10) as for the 43 patients whose improvement rates in score corrected for guessing constitute the main peak on the right of the figure. The smaller group of 7 individuals whose IR ranged from 2 to 5 corresponds to patients whose scores were either high in the pre-test (14.7, 15.1, 15.8 and 17.2) and moderately increased in the post-test (respectively 17.5, 16.1, 17.8 and 18.6), or mediocre but above the mean in the pre-test (10.9, 11.6 and 13.3), with relatively little improvement in the post-test (respectively 13.3, 14.4 and 15.8).

Figure 6 shows the cumulative frequency curves of the scores corrected for guessing in the pre- and post-tests. One is favorably impressed by the highly-reduced dispersion of the scores on the right of the mean in the post-test. So the initial aim of giving a minimum of knowledge to a maximum of patients was attained: the scores (corrected for guessing) were 20/20 for 8 patients out of 50 (16%), 18.5/20 for 13 patients (26%) and 17-17.5/20 for 12 patients (24%). It should also be noted that the 3 lowest post-test scores (11.5/20) were, indeed, higher than the mean score of all patients in the pre-test (9.6/20).

---

*For example, the relative gain will be of 100% in these 2 cases:
1)  pre-test score: 10/20; post-test score: 20/20;
2)  pre-test score: 18/20; post-test score: 20/20.
**The mathematics involved are too complex to be detailed here. For further information, consult M.-O. Houziaux et al. [6].

Table 1   *Results of testing before and after the first 4 lessons*

|  | WA | OM | RA | SS ± S.D. | SG ± S.D. |
|---|---|---|---|---|---|
| Pre-test | 194 | 236 | 520 | 10.95 ± 3.95 | 9.59 ± 4.43 |
| Post-test | 92 | 18 | 840 | 17.68 ± 1.76 | 17.04 ± 2.26 |

WA:   wrong answers
OM:   omissions
RA:   right answers
SS:    mean of simple scores (out of 20)
SG:    mean of scores corrected for guessing (out of 20)
S.D.:  standard deviation

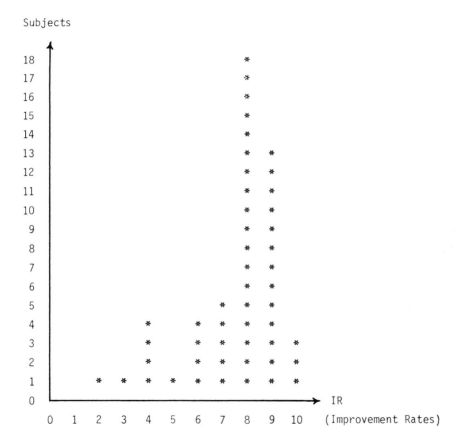

Fig. 5   Distribution of improvement rates in 50 patients after the first 4 lessons of the course.
(From Houziaux, M.-O. et al. [6], with courtesy of Scientia Paedagogica Experimentalis.)

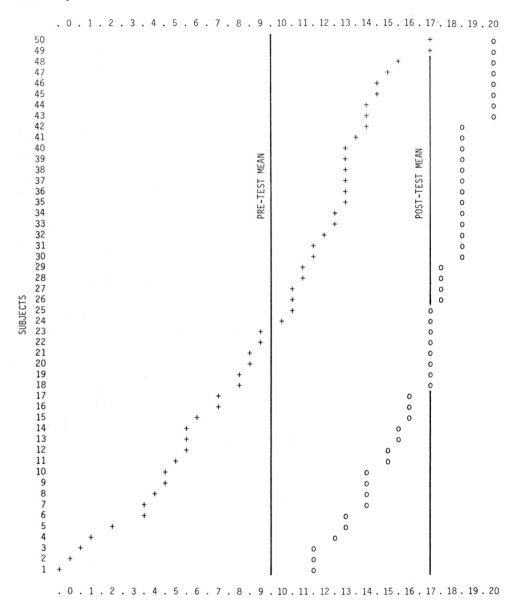

Fig. 6   Cumulative frequency curves for the pre- and the post-tests.
(From Houziaux, M.-O. et al. [6], with courtesy of Scientia Paedagogica Experimentalis.)

## 6.   ACCEPTANCE BY THE PATIENTS

Because of the flexibility of the teaching procedure in the present system, the time spent by the patients for a given lesson varied greatly from individual to individual. A mean of 30 minutes was needed for each of the first, second and fourth lessons with a range of 18 to 43 minutes. The third lesson lasted an average of 19 minutes (range 12-25 min.).

Each lesson ended with a multiple choice question allowing the patient to give his opinion on the method and the content of the lesson. Table 2 illustrates the answers given. A totally positive opinion was given by a vast majority of patients (from 88 to 100% of the opinions); we cannot exclude the possibility that this high percentage of positive opinions may have been inspired by the wish to please the personnel involved. With regards to the specific opinions, only the presence of a comment (positive or negative) was to be considered, since patients were quite free to answer the questions or not. So, omitting 'good understanding' does not mean 'difficult understanding'. As evidenced in Table 2, the first lesson has been found 'difficult' by 8% of the patients; its presentation will be slightly modified in accordance. Many patients expressed their opinion orally and emphasized the usefulness of the lessons, their interest in such a modern way of teaching and, often, their gratitude for what had been specially planned for them.

Table 2   *Patients' opinions on the CAI course*

| SUBJECTS | Lesson 1 % | Lesson 2 % | Lesson 3 % | Lesson 4 % | Mean % |
|---|---|---|---|---|---|
| Totally negative opinion | 12 | 6 | – | 2 | 5 |
| Totally positive opinion | 88 | 94 | 100 | 98 | 95 |
| **SPECIFIC OPINIONS** | | | | | |
| Respect of personal learning rhythm | 38 | 32 | 46 | 64 | 45 |
| Good understanding | 38 | 42 | 64 | 70 | 53.5 |
| Relaxed atmosphere | 52 | 52 | 58 | 64 | 56.5 |
| Alertness maintained | 60 | 84 | 80 | 84 | 77 |
| Too rapid a rhythm | 2 | 2 | – | 2 | 1.5 |
| Difficult comprehension | 8 | 2 | – | – | 2.5 |
| Difficult handling | – | 2 | – | – | 0.5 |
| Weariness | – | 2 | – | 2 | 1 |

## 7. CONCLUSIONS AND PROSPECTIVE

Convinced that teaching diabetics is a cornerstone in their management and faced with the difficulties of providing every diabetic with the individualized education he/she may require, we have attempted to develop an original computer-assisted instruction course. This course has been designed to provide individualized teaching and to give a minimum of basic information to a maximum of patients. Our opinion is that such method is not to replace other more conventional ways of teaching (e.g. private conversations with qualified professionals, formal lectures or seminars, publications, movies, etc.) but should rather be incorporated into a general multimedia teaching policy which, of course, will vary from place to place, depending on the human, technical and financial possibilities available.

The evaluation of our system on 50 insulin-requiring diabetics having completed the first 4 lessons of the course is rather promising, considering the impressive gain in knowledge and the 88 to 100% enthusiastic acceptance by the patients. At the time of writing, a total of 218 patients have been involved so far, and the method is used routinely in our Institution. Such evaluation has been performed on the basis of a pre- and post-test paired comparison. Given the positive results obtained and the positive impact on our population of insulin-dependent diabetics, we have decided to pursue the experiment. Further long-term studies are in progress to determine whether increased knowledge leads to better self-care [12], improved control and, ultimately, reduced incidence of diabetic complications.

## SUMMARY

An experiment conducted at the University of Liège, Belgium, in the computer-assisted teaching of juvenile-type insulin-dependent diabetics is reported here. The course was designed to individualize teaching in order to give a minimum of basic information to a maximum of patients. The original computer-assisted instruction system DOCEO II is described; methods and programming techniques are summarized. The course was evaluated on 50 patients who attended the first 4 lessons. The improvement in knowledge was impressive: scores corrected for guessing were $9.59 \pm 4.43$ out of 20 before the course and $17.04 \pm 2.26$ out of 20 after the course (paired $t$ test: $p < 0.001$). The system was enthusiastically accepted by the patients and is now routinely used in our Institution. Long-term studies are in progress to determine whether increased knowledge leads to better self-care, improved control and, ultimately, reduced incidence of diabetic complications.

## ACKNOWLEDGEMENTS

We acknowledge with thanks the help of D. Leclerq, Ph.D., and P. Lambert, Ing., in the analysis of our data. We also thank Mrs. N. Mawet for her daily assistance in the project and Miss F. Jamart for her help in the preparation of this manuscript. The secretarial help of Mrs. M.B. Counet is gratefully acknowledged.

# REFERENCES

1. Graber, A.L., Christman, B.G., Alogna, M.T. and Davidson, J.K. (1977): Evaluation of diabetes patient-education programs. *Diabetes, 26*, 61.
2. Etzwiler, D.D. and Robb, J.R. (1972): Evaluation of programmed education among juvenile diabetics and their families. *Diabetes, 21*, 967.
3. Hassel, J. and Medved, E. (1975): Group/audiovisual instruction for patients with diabetes. *J. Am. Diet. Assoc., 66*, 465.
4. Etzwiler, D.D., Cohen, E.B., Verstraete, D. et. al. (1970): Diabetes detection and education center. *Minn. Med., 63*, 1035.
5. Miller, L.V., Goldstein, J. and Nicolaisen, G. (1978): Evaluation of patients' knowledge of diabetes self-care. *Diabetes Care, 1*, 275.
6. Houziaux, M.-O., Godart, C., Scheen-Lavigne, M. et al. (1978): Une expérience d'enseignement assisté par ordinateur chez des patients diabétiques insulinodépendants. *Sci. Paedagog. Exp., 15*, 214.
7. Etzwiler, D.D. and Sines, L.K. (1962): Juvenile diabetes and its management: family, social and academic implications. *J. Am. Med. Assoc., 181*, 304.
8. Etzwiler, D.D. (1962): What the juvenile diabetic knows about his disease. *Pediatrics, 29*, 135.
9. Miller, L.V., Goldstein, J. and Nicolaisen, G. (1978): Computerized assessment of diabetes patient education. *J. Med. Syst., 2*, 233.
10. Houziaux, M.-O. (1972): *Vers l'Enseignement Assisté par Odinateur*, p. 93. Presses Universitaires de France, Paris.
11. Houziaux, M.-O. (1965): Les fonctions didactiques de Doceo. In: *Compte Rendu du XIIe Colloque International de l'Association Internationale de Pédagogie Expérimentale de Langue Française*, 47.
12. Watts, F.N. (1980): Behavioural aspects of the management of diabetes mellitus: Education, self-care and metabolic control. *Behav. Res. Ther., 13*, 171.

# 23.  Active diet learning

FRANÇOISE DOURVER AND JEAN-PHILIPPE ASSAL

## EDITORIAL

*In this article the authors stress that the learning of a diet should be an active procedure if we hope to achieve lasting effects on the part of the patient.*

*Various forms of diet prescription exist; some demand more participation by the patient than others, but all of them can be active to a certain extent.*

*The article does not offer 'ready-made solutions' but might suggest new ways of training patients for more efficient meal planning. (The editors.)*

## I.   GENERAL CONSIDERATIONS CONCERNING DIETARY PRESCRIPTIONS

### Diet and/or meal planning?

The term 'diet', with its connotations of restriction or deprivation, is gradually being replaced by the more neutral 'meal planning'. This term is particularly appropriate for non-obese insulin-dependent diabetics who require a carbohydrate and caloric ration equivalent to that of the general population. Nevertheless, the proposed 'meal planning' does not eliminate all constraints: quantitative restrictions, a requirement for identical carbohydrate rations each day, as well as the requirement for regularity of meals. Many diabetics find it difficult to schedule their meals exactly in relation to both the timing of their insulin and the variables of daily living.

The term 'diet' is applied principally for caloric restriction in the overweight diabetic. Low-calorie nutritional programs are difficult to follow, and the term 'diet' correctly reflects the constraints imposed. Diet or meal planning? Whatever the designation used, special diets will continue to be considered as a constraint.

### Information, teaching or training of the diabetic patient?

The general objective of the person prescribing the diet is that the patient acquire an understanding of his dietary requirements, along with the know-how necessary for application and integration into everyday life.

*Dietary information*. By 'information' we refer to the one-directional transfer of knowledge where the person doing the teaching does not verify that the information has actually been understood. This is the situation when diabetics read books or the various documents supplied by diabetic associations, or watch television programs.

The 'annual' conference on nutrition and diabetes, organized by the various diabetic associations, can also be considered to be aimed much more at providing information than at teaching. Despite the fact that these programs can lead to the formulation of specific questions by the patient, it is a mistake to expect too much from the presentation of general information. Overall, this approach can provide a non-negligible aid to the initial orientation of the diabetic patient.

*Dietary training*. Training involves a second dimension in which the patient is an active participant: e.g. with the preparation of meals or the choice of foods from a buffet. This type of active response is essential in the learning process, for it helps the patient apply theoretical notions to practical needs.

Learning can only occur in an active manner in which the patient should be guided, observed and corrected by the dietician. Correction of errors plays a primordial role in the acquisition of proper habits and is best done during training at the time of a buffet.

*Teaching the diabetic*. This type of transmission of information requires more active participation by the teacher who must verify that the information has been properly understood by the patient. It is thus the *evaluation* of the information transfer which allows differentiation between information and training.

A dietician addressing a group of patients is engaged in teaching only when he or she seeks to make certain that the message has been fully understood by members of the group. To achieve this goal it would seem essential that medical personnel be assisted by teaching specialists.

## The role of the dietician in the medical system

The dietician is a member of a 'paramedical' profession. The term itself reflects the ambiguity of the position of the dietician in the medical world. In the hospital the dietician is too often excluded from the medical team.

The dietician frequently runs into problems with the medical hierarchy which is particularly preeminent in the hospital setting. The physician describes the diet, the nurse transmits the orders. Whenever a problem arises, discussion takes place through at least one, if not several, intermediaries. The dietician does not have ready access to the physician. The patient is generally not informed on the diet he or she is being prescribed.

In urban, out-patient care the dietician runs into a different problem. Frequently working alone and having no contact with the physician, the dietician has very little medical information available concerning the individual patient. Physicians frequently do not know what services to request from the dietician because of lack of practical knowledge in nutrition and unawareness of possibilities offered.

The dietician faces other specific problems. One of these is the difficulty of *evaluating the results of a diet*. While the effects of a diet can be followed in obese patients on the basis of body-weight curves, the situation for insulin-treated diabetics is more difficult. Despite the occasional exception, dieticians are generally not informed on the blood-glucose levels and indeed, if they do enquire, nurses and physicians frequently react as if the dietician was getting involved in other people's business. The tailoring of the diet to therapeutic requirements is rendered difficult by this lack of information and cooperation.

## The dietician and the individual with diabetes

One of the major responsibilities of the dietician is the training of the patient. However, dieticians frequently have a tendency to overlook the fact that individuals initially show a great reticence towards the acquisition of new dietary information, especially when forced upon them. This dietary learning is particularly difficult since it requires that the patient abandon his usual habits of eating and ways of thinking. This is especially difficult in nutrition. In prescribing a new diet, the dietician or physician runs the risk of disturbing emotional, social and even cultural factors which may provoke a great deal of resistance. To maintain a proper diet, the diabetic must acquire a new set of eating habits and this may be disturbing, even threatening.

When addressing the patient it is essential that dieticians only bring about the minimum change in eating habits, regardless of how uncommon or even strange the patient's habits may seem. In man, eating is integrated into the entire social framework. Food has a considerable symbolic content (whether conscious or not) and occupies an important place in all cultures in terms of rituals of friendship, hospitality and celebration.

In hospital many diabetics deny that they have consulted a dietician. Thus they pretend to forget the diet itself, the restrictions, their attempts at compliance, difficulties and failures. When requesting changes in their diet, patients more readily address themselves to the nurse, even in the presence of the dietician! The dietician becomes the symbol of all of the dietary constraints they have come up against over the years. For many, the dietician is a 'painful' symbol.

In order to overcome these difficulties, it is essential that, from the first interview onwards, the dietician becomes the patient's advocate, and the patient's tastes, habits and desires should be seriously considered before the diet is prescribed. Only after having acquired knowledge on the latter points can the dietician deal with the practical aspects of the diet. The discussion of dietary habits must not proceed like a police interrogation. *Open questions* will facilitate a wide range of patient replies, allowing a better perception of the psychological and sociological context. If an obese diabetic is asked the question: 'How many kilos have you lost?', the only answer we will obtain will be a fixed number. However, an open question will permit the patient's underlying problems to surface. 'How would you explain your weight loss?' would be another way to approach the patient. It is through such an open question that I learnt that one of my patients had lost 10 kilos during a period of mourning, rather than this being due to a low-calorie diet. (The patient's wife had died 2 months previously.) With an obese woman, who was unable to lose weight, open questions led to the discovery that she panicked at the first signs of weight loss as her husband had died of cancer in a state of severe cachexia.

**The physician and applied, practical dietetics**

Physicians ordinarily have an adequate theoretical understanding of nutrition and meal planning. However, problems arise in the application of this knowledge since their medical training neglects the practical aspects of dietetics.

In a recent study by our group, we found that practical knowledge concerning diet was not significantly better for physicians than for patients. Both were requested to fill out an identical multiple-choice questionnaire concerning the practice of a diabetic diet. Out of a total of 40 questions, the average number of incorrect responses by patients was 19, while physicians made an average of 14 mistakes. As a result of these findings, we now organize a training program for our residents during the weekly activities of our Diabetes Treatment and Teaching Unit. This training of residents goes through 3 stages: 1) practical training at the daily buffet (Figure 1); 2) practical dietary exercise at a 1-hour workshop held weekly, and 3) the obligation for the residents to explain the diet to one of their patients every week, supervised by the dietician.

## II.  THE 3 DIMENSIONS WHICH CONSTITUTE THE HUMAN DIET

Food and eating habits seen in the most general sense should fulfil 3 basic needs (Table 1). One eats in order to be nourished = survive, one eats because food is enjoyable and one eats because it favors social contacts.

### 1.  Nutritional factors

In the case of diabetes mellitus, carbohydrate and caloric intake must be adapted to the degree of insulin lack. Metabolic function in such patients requires the diet to be adapted in terms of quantity, quality and distribution

Table 1   *The three dimensions of a proper balance in eating*

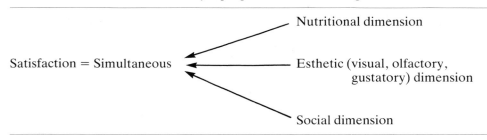

Satisfaction = Simultaneous

Nutritional dimension

Esthetic (visual, olfactory, gustatory) dimension

Social dimension

over a 24-hour cycle. The patient must acquire an understanding of these complex requirements and must learn to choose the necessary quantity of carbohydrates and calories among a virtually infinite range of foods.

## 2.   Gustatory, olfactory and visual characteristics of food

These factors, called 'sensory', 'aesthetic' or 'emotional' are of particular importance when survival is not jeopardized by lack of food. Sight, smell and taste contribute to the pleasures of eating. Even though these factors are not essential metabolically, one can clearly differentiate between agreeable foods and those which do not satisfy the senses.

## 3.   Social factors

People usually do not like to eat alone. What celebration takes place without a meal? It is hard to imagine a baptism, a marriage or a funeral without the ritual of eating. The family is united at meal-times, while in business a good meal is well known to facilitate discussion between participants.

The feeling of satisfaction and well-being which follows a meal is the result of a balance between the nutritional, aesthetic, emotional and social factors. All 3 of these factors must be present in order to provide a sense of physical, psychological and social satisfaction.

## 4.   Prescription of a diet requires integration of the 3 dimensions: nutritional, aesthetic and social

The metabolic exigencies of a special diet are nutritional (Table 2). While this factor is essential for the correction of metabolic disorders, the long-term success of the diet depends on the other 2 dimensions – aesthetic, ( or emotional) and social. Very poor compliance, usually seen with low-calorie diets, is probably due to the relative neglect of the latter 2 factors.

In the light of current knowledge concerning the preparation of meals, the wide range of foods available and the wide multiplicity of techniques for cooking, it should be possible to meet aesthetic requirements, even for

Table 2   *The problems of a diet prescription*

Loss of the *integration* of the three dimensions in the proper balance of eating

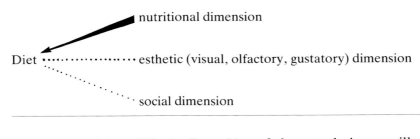

patients requiring difficult diets. Use of these techniques will require the participation of the dietician.

## III.   DIETARY PRESCRIPTIONS REQUIRING AN INCREASING DEGREE OF PARTICIPATION OF THE PATIENT AND THE DIETICIAN

Compliance with a diet requires constant effort and discipline on the part of the patient. Temptation to eat non-prescribed foods must be resisted although the difficulty of this is understandable in view of the gustatory, aesthetic and social factors involved with eating.

A whole world separates the prescription of a drug and that of a diet. Trained to prescribe drugs, physicians tend to prescribe diet in an excessively vertical and theoretical fashion. Diet is learned by practice. Errors which may arise can be corrected by the patient if he or she is assisted in his/her learning by the dietician who can intervene at the appropriate moment.

Specialists in education have shown that acquisition of a concept or a technique is more effective where there is a phase of practical application both by the subject and by the instructor. Teaching of meal planning with the buffet system is probably the optimal means of training for diet.

There is no hope of long-term success for a meal-planning program if the patient to whom the diet is prescribed does not understand the nature of diabetes, how and why a person becomes diabetic and which types of treatment can be planned. It is essential that the patient understands the role of his diet in the treatment of diabetes. This lack of information about diabetes is often seen in outpatient practice and in the hospital. How many times have we seen patients who have neglected their diet simply because they had no reason to follow it – because nobody had explained why it was necessary?

The following is a presentation of 6 various methods of providing a diet prescription to diabetic patients. These methods are listed in increasing order of the patient's participation and, therefore, of learning efficiency.

## 1. The passive prescription: the prepared meal-tray provided at the hospital

Upon hospitalization, the diabetic initially receives a precisely measured diet made up of 3 daily meals, sometimes interspaced with 2 or 3 snacks. Total rations correspond to those prescribed by the physician. Nevertheless, even this obligatory diet may be less passive than imagined. With an increasing duration of hospitalization, the patient receives a large number of standard meals, and perhaps acquires the habit of eating a given quantity of carbohydrates and calories.

Indeed, the hospital meal may be a fairly primitive sort of teaching method. The meal-tray is a highly concrete example of an appropriate diet, and, with a variety of menus, diabetics undergoing long-term hospitalization should acquire an idea of what constitutes their diet. More than one diabetic has picked up the habit of eating light snacks between meals when in hospital, while elderly patients who take only a very light meal in the evening (a cup of coffee with milk and a few biscuits) realise that this very simple meal is entirely compatible with proper diabetic meal planning. On occasion, a patient may even become active to the point of copying down the menu, attempting to estimate the quantity of carbohydrates and/or noting the information shown on a meal card. Unfortunately, this is an exception. The medical team does not encourage this approach which would optimize the 'meal-tray effect', so patients usually accept their diet passively.

## 2. The 'starch-free diet' (without potatoes, pasta and pastries, rice and bread etc.)

This overall prescription is frequently used by the busy physician in order to give some idea of dietetic requirements to the patients. A very succinct list of prohibited foods is delivered orally to the patient: no pasta, no bread, no potatoes, no pastries, no fruit, no rice, no sugars or sweets. Whenever it is observed at the consultation that the patient has high blood sugar, the list is simply repeated by the physician. With this type of prescription, the diabetic listens to the list and tries to memorize the 'forbidden' foods. This memorization is possible only within an extremely simple framework, and after several consultations and numerous repetitions, memorization is achieved and dietary results may at times be good.

Another form of qualitative diet is to provide the patient with a written list of the 'forbidden' foods. Learning is enhanced by reading the list aloud with the patient, since if this is not done, the patients usually set the list aside without bothering to read it. Usually, the physician does not solicit the participation of the patient and never knows whether the written message has been understood.

The drawback of this approach is the prohibition of the carbohydrate-rich foods, while leaving the others available in unlimited quantities. This method also leads to a considerable drop in carbohydrate consumption and often at the same time to a drop in the caloric intake, which results in weight loss at the beginning of the program. Patients rapidly grow tired of this diet which excludes bread, pasta, rice or potatoes and generally is experienced as being monotonous. This kind of diet constitutes a major constraint when patients eat in restaurants or cafetarias, where meals are generally based on starches rather than on green vegetables or meat. Patients undergoing such restrictions frequently feel guilt or anguish when they don't comply with the restrictions.

Finally, the majority of diabetics require a minimal daily carbohydrate ration of 120-200 g, and an over-zealous restriction of carbohydrate may not always improve diabetes. We have observed hyperglycemic states with patients receiving no more than 40-50 g carbohydrates per day and improvements in their blood glucose when we have raised the carbohydrate intake to 120-150 g/day.

## 3. The 'standard' printed diet

This printed diet includes lists of food which are allowed, restricted or 'forbidden'. Such lists are far more precise than the rather contrived lists discussed above. The patient can re-read them whenever necessary. The general practitioner usually has 2 or 3 'standardized' diet lists: usually 1400 calories – 140 g carbohydrates, 1600 calories – 160 g carbohydrates and 2000 calories – 200 g carbohydrates. Each diet is printed on a sheet for distribution to the patient. Most of the time the list is given with little or no explanation, although, at times, it may be read and discussed with the physician or dietician. This diet has the advantage of being precise, clear and is usually easily understood by the patient.

With this 'printed' diet the choice of foodstuffs is limited and from the patient's point of view, prescription may be poorly adapted to eating habits, tastes, budgetary restrictions and occupational schedules. No active participation can be asked of a patient who is given a 'printed' diet without explanation. In the best of cases, active participation will take place later when the patient reads the diet sheet at home and tries to apply what he has read.

## 4. The individualized diet

This type of prescription is the first in our list where the physician or dietician must take a diet history where the patient's personal habits and lifestyle are taken into account. This approach requires that the dietician or the physician spend sufficient time with the patient in order to fully discuss his eating habits. Unlike a medical history, a complete diet history is often not made by physicians since this requires special skills.

The individualized prescription is frequently supplemented with a carbohydrate-exchange list. Unfortunately, while they are reasonably simple for the physician, the available systems of food equivalents generally include somewhat abstract notions which do not fit in with the ordinary dietary practices of the patient. It is not self-evident, for instance, that a given carbohydrate equivalent of 25 g glucose is found in 50 g bread or 120 g potatoes. Patients often tend to simplify matters by replacing 50 g bread with 50 g rice or 50 g potatoes. The carbohydrate equivalent tables require that the physician or the dietician provide clear, logical and especially repeated explanations; time for questions should always be allocated. Physicians or dieticians should realize that the prescription of a diet constitutes a therapeutic programme which cannot be constituted in a single consultation. When dietary explanations are given during several consultations, the experience of the patient can then be used and can significantly contribute to improve the adherence to, and practice of, the diet.

The gradual improvement in the control of diabetes should increase dietary motivation. Since efficacy of diet can be evaluated only through blood and urinary glucose or body weight, it is essential that the dietician be aware of these parameters. Too frequently the dietician is not informed about the metabolic control of the patient and therefore the prescription tends to be both too general and uncoordinated with the rest of the treatment.

## 5.  Practical training: the buffet supervised by the dietician

The buffet is one of the best ways we have found for the diabetic to be more active in the learning process. At the buffet the diabetic can serve himself according to the dietary prescription and according to his/her taste. The choice of food can be observed and corrected by the dietician. This type of learning experience must be well planned (Fig. 1).

Since 1974 this system has been used at all evening meals in our Unit, and allows patients to choose from a wide range of carbohydrates. 2 or 3 types of starches prepared in various forms are available at each meal (rice, pasta, potatoes). The preference for one food over another is not only an intellectual decision based upon knowledge of carbohydrate and caloric values, but is also bound to subjective preferences. The simultaneous presence of both the emotional and the nutritional factors increases the usefulness of this teaching experience. This approach can only be effective if the dietician participates in the learning process and helps the patient by leading him to find out how he should select his food. Corrections concerning the amount taken should not be imposed on the patient by the dietician. Discovery should be stimulated by open discussion and the patient should then adjust the amount of food taken according to the results of the discussion.

Learning is enhanced when an active approach is used, and this type of approach requires discovery, repetition and even error. Errors contribute

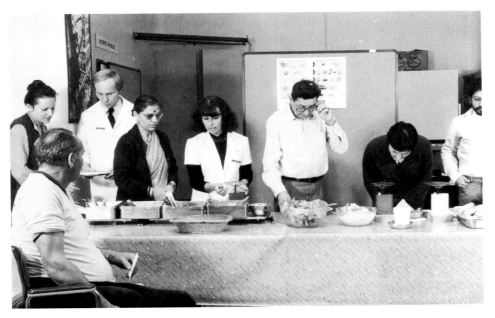

Fig. 1   Diet training of medical residents: one resident (3rd from the left) eating with diabetics at the daily buffet supervised by the dietician (5th from the left).

to learning when they are corrected and this occurs when the involvement of the medical team is mandatory, both for educational and for therapeutic reasons. In the classical 'classroom' approach, the patient is forced to follow the logic of the instructor. At the buffet, the diabetic is encouraged to use his own reasoning and this tends to promote learning.

## 6.   Preparation of a meal with the dietician

This is another useful procedure to encourage active patient participation in the learning of meal planning. Since this system requires a great deal of time, it is hard to carry out on a large scale.

Experimental sessions have shown that diabetics are very interested in this approach and a steady dialog is established between the patient and the dietician during preparation of the meal. Visiting nurses, physicians and dieticians should consider this approach whenever possible since supervised preparation of meals brings to light numerous personal questions which would not otherwise have arisen.

## IV.   ORGANIZATION OF DIETARY PRACTICE IN OUR DIABETES UNIT

### Organization of the Unit

The Diabetes Treatment and Teaching Unit was opened in 1974. Patients are hospitalized in the Unit for control of their diabetes. They undergo a complete medical examination aimed primarily at early detection and treatment of complications. Along with the classical therapeutic measures such as diet and drugs, there is the obligation to follow a complete educational program. Patients are hospitalized for either 5 or 10 days, starting on Monday morning and returning home Friday evening.

The teaching program includes 3 group classes daily which have a duration of 45 minutes each, as well as an individual interview lasting approximately 1 hour. Each group of patients goes through the progressive program together. This progressive approach is important: the risk of confusion, due to the presentation of complex information to patients who have not yet fully assimilated the basic principles (hyperglycemia, glycosuria, the role of insulin etc.), is decreased by refusing to include new patients during the weekly session. In cases where it is urgent to begin training a diabetic who is not integrated into the group, the teaching program is presented individually and the patient is included in the group the following week.

### Dietary approach

In our Unit the dietary program is run by the same dietician who takes the diet history for each patient and who gives the final diet program upon release. The dietician works together with the medical personnel: nurses, nursing aides and physicians.

There are *4 educational objectives* to be attained with diabetic patients during this week of training.
1.  To teach and evaluate the patient comprehension on food exchange lists of carbohydrates.
2.  To teach and evaluate comprehension of specific problems, such as prevention of hypoglycemia, adjustment in cases of increased physical activity and intermittent diseases as well as the imbalance of diabetes.
3.  To increase the independence of the patient as much as possible for those individuals undergoing a 5-day period of hospitalization twice, so that they may continue training during the weekend spent at home between the 2 periods of hospitalization.
4.  To promote discussion and exchange of personal experiences both among the patients themselves and between patients and the medical personnel during the round-table discussion 'What does a meal mean for me?'.

The dietary program for each patient is as follows.

*A diet history* (approximately 1 hour) is taken to gain the best possible overview of dietary habits.

*3 hours of group instruction* (1 hour daily) with active discussion (Fig. 2) of the following subjects: carbohydrate content of foods; carbohydrate exchange lists; calories; the role of alcohol; animal, vegetable fats and cholesterol; dietary products for diabetics; prevention and treatment of hypoglycemia; dietary measures in case of increased physical activity; dietary measures in case of intercurrent disease.

*A round-table discussion: 'What does a meal mean for me?'*

The group discussion is moderated by a dietician, with the participation of a physician. Diabetics and their entourage are encouraged to express their feelings during these group sessions which are designed to help them learn how to participate in meals in family, social or occupational settings. During the approximate 1-hour session, the dietician provides guidance and technical information as required. Patients who have never participated in a group discussion are frequently apprehensive, as they see the dietician or physician as the representative of the strictly medical approach. At the beginning of the meeting, when asked what a meal means to them, the answers usually are something like: 'A meal is properly controlling my

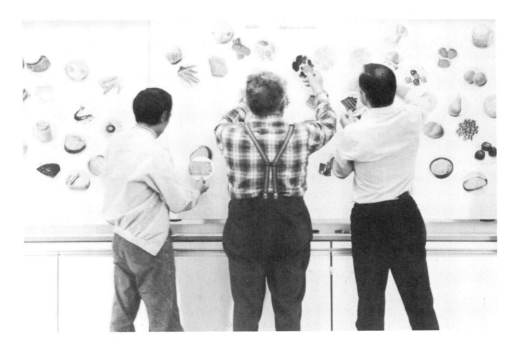

Fig. 2   Active training of patients: organizing food groups using pictures displayed on a magnetic board.

carbohydrate intake', or 'To consume a quantity of calories corresponding to my needs' etc. Progressively the scope of the discussion broadens and only later the pleasure of consuming pleasant food in good company is discussed.

The round-table discussion serves as a catalyst for the theoretical courses and the practical exercises at the buffet. Learning is facilitated by the fact that the patients realize that the medical staff is fully aware of the social and emotional importance represented by food in their daily routine.

## The daily buffet

The buffet (Fig. 1) constitutes both the optimal means for training the patients in practical dietetics and the ideal situation for observation and evaluation of their skills. The practical set-up of the buffet is as follows: the buffet is carried out in the dining area and the 10-15 patients serve themselves under the supervision of the dietician assisted by an aide. It is laid out on a table 3 metres long and 80 cm wide. Each patient serves himself, and the platter is then checked together with the dietician who discusses with the patient any corrections which might be necessary. Since the food is weighed on kitchen scales which have small calibration units, the table is illuminated with spotlights. Warmed plates are stacked in the vicinity of the hotplates, with hot dishes placed on one side of the table and cold dishes (cold cuts, salad, fruits) on the other. Patients serve themselves trying to meet the requirements shown on a postcard-sized diet card (Fig. 3), which they keep with them. The kitchen scales and 200 ml graduated cups are available for measuring food. Patients can choose between a light or heavier meal, depending upon how hungry they are. They can, for example, choose soup, meat, vegetables, starches and a dessert; or simply coffee with milk and bread. All of these choices are possible thanks to the system of equivalents, the weighing of foods and supervision by the dietician. Wives and husbands are invited to participate in the choice of foods during the buffet hour.

The preparation of a buffet for 10-15 persons requires a great deal of cooperation with the central kitchen facilities of a 2000-bed hospital. Furthermore, the time of the buffet – 6.00-7.00 p.m. – makes it more difficult to find specialized personnel prepared to work at this time of the day. This schedule has been set for therapeutic reasons: it is not acceptable for diabetic patients to have their evening meal at 5.00 p.m., as is frequently the case in hospitals.

## Individual interviews

At the individual interview which is held at the end of the patient's stay (after the group classes, buffets and the round-table), a general review of dietetics, along with a prescription of the final diet upon release from hos-

# Unité de Diabétologie. HÔPITAL CANTONAL UNIVERSITAIRE DE GENÈVE

| Nom: .......................................... | K calories / ........ | Glucides ........... ...g |
| .......................... **date:** .......... | / Jour | Protides. ............. g |
| (g = grammes. Eq = Equivalent.) | | Lipides ........ g |

| **PETIT—DEJEUNER** g | .......... **H. MIDI** g | ........ **H. SOIR** g |
|---|---|---|
| Fromage.............. | Viande................ | Viande ........... |
| Margarine........... | Graisses.............. | Graisses ........... |
| | Légumes.............. | Légumes ........... |
| FARINEUX.......| Eq | FARINEUX.........| Eq | FARINEUX ......| Eq |
| LAIT ............. | FRUIT............. | FRUIT........... |

### COLLATIONS

| ........ **Heure** | Eq | g | ........ **Heure** | Eq | g | ........ **Heure** | Eq | g |

1000 6.80 IFRA

Fig. 3   Diet-card (postcard size) used by patients during the buffet.

pital, are discussed. It is particularly important that the diabetic's entourage be present at this meeting.

The individual meeting should be very carefully structured. In outpatient practice, it is unacceptable that the patient be seen merely once or twice by the dietician. Diet prescription and proper control of a meal-planning program require a substantial body of knowledge. It is therefore necessary that a series of short interviews (10 to 15 minutes each), rather than a single long one, be held. Such a procedure is generally unfamiliar to the dietician. The only document usually available to the dietician is the prescription sheet. Optimal care would require that the entire medical record be available to the dietician so that the patient could be followed over a period of months. There is a fundamental need to follow the patient for a long period of time if we want to favor a lasting change in attitude. This approach can be compared to that in physiotherapy in which one cannot hope to treat a patient efficiently in one single session.

## CONCLUSIONS

Numerous explanations can be offered as to why results of prescribed diets are usually disappointing. One of these is that physicians and dieticians rarely take into account the complexity of such a prescription. A diet cannot be injected like a dose of insulin; of all the constraints imposed by therapy for diabetes, dietary prescription produces the greatest interference with the patient's social, professional and family life. While the formulation of the diet itself (calories, grams of carbohydrates, etc.) is a function of objective nutritional factors, the 'sale' of the prescription to the patient and his subsequent compliance all depend upon a complex balance of personal, subjective and social factors.

For the patient to maintain good compliance with his diet, a change in attitude is essential. Such a change will only be brought about by a regular dialog between the physician, the dietician and the patient himself. Only repeated dietary consultations allow for proper coordination and development of a diet which will be followed by the patient. To fulfil its essential therapeutic role in the treatment of diabetes, the diet must be properly coordinated and developed through repeated consultations which provide time for action feed-back and learning between the patient and the medical team.

Does the teaching of dietetics to the patient free him from constraints or, on the contrary, does it actually increase such constraints? Physicians and nurses are perhaps overly optimistic that proper teaching will invariably tend to make the patient independent. Although a balanced and healthy diet without major restrictions is proposed and the system of food exchange allows for the widest possible variety of diet, it must be borne in mind that a low-calorie diet or a meal-planning system for insulin-treated diabetics does impose significant limitations. Some patients are faced with a desperate avoidance of calories, while others are required to eat at rigidly scheduled meal-times. Indeed, a proper system of training will both liberate and limit the patient at the same time. The limitations will be better accepted when their importance is clearly understood, thanks to appropriate explanations, and when the patient experiences changes in his state of health.

## SUMMARY

While it is well established that an adequate dietary program is the basis for therapeutics in diabetes and that without appropriate diet no form of diabetes can be controlled, most diabetics still show inadequate compliance with diet. There are numerous possible explanations for these failures, including both inadequate instruction by the prescriber and the difficulty of the patient in terms of adherence to prescription.

This paper deals with the dietary treatment of diabetes, with special reference to a dietary education system requiring an increasing degree of participation by the patient with practical training in the proper choice of food. This approach to dietary education provides more opportunities for 'true learning', to use the definition of Jean Piaget, as opposed to the 'false learning' of memory work. 'True learning' is based on the adaptation of the learning situation to the individual's intellectual stage of development, interest and language, and in the learner's interactions with concrete objects in the presentation of all-new concepts.

## SUGGESTED READING

1. Assal, J.-Ph. and Mousset, F. (1979): Psychological problems in nutrition. In: *Pediatric and Adolescent Endocrinology, Vol. VII*, p. 128. Karger, Basel.
2. Bierman, E.L., Aalbrink, M.J., Arky, R.A. et al. (1971): Principles of nutrition and dietary recommendations for patients with diabetes mellitus. *Diabetes, 20*, 633.
3. Christakis, G. and Miridjanian, A. (1970): In: Ellenberg, M. (Ed.), *The Nutritional Aspects of Diabetes in Diabetes Mellitus: Theory and Practice*, p. 594. McGraw-Hill, New York.
4. Davidson, J.K., Delcher, H.K. and Englund, A. (1979): Spin-off/cost-benefits of expanded nutritional care. *J. Am. Diet. Assoc., 75*, 250.
5. Davidson, J.K. (1975): Educating diabetic patients about diet therapy. *Int. Diabetes Fed. Bull., 20*, 1.
6. Etzwiler, D.D. (1967): Who's teaching the diabetic? *Diabetes, 16*, 111.
7. Etzwiler, D.D. and Hess, K. (1973): *Education and Management of the Patient with Diabetes Mellitus*, p. 27. Ames Company Division of Miles Laboratories.
8. Hinkle, L. (1962): Customs, emotions and behavior in the dietary treatment of diabetes. *J. Am. Diet. Assoc., 41*, 341.
9. Kaufman, M. (1965): The many dimensions of diet counselling for diabetes. *Am. J. Clin. Nutr., 15*, 45.
10. Ley, P. and Spelman, M.S. (1966): *Communicating with the Patient*. Staple Press, London.
11. MacRae, N.M. (1967): The dietician in private practice. *J. Am. Diet. Assoc., 51*, 52.
12. Maguire, R. and Rutter, D. (1976): Training medical students to communicate. In: Bennett AE (Ed.), *Communication between Doctors and Patients*. Oxford University Press, for Nuffield Provincial Hospital Trust.
13. Miller, L. and Goldstein, J. (1978): Evaluation of patient's knowledge of diabetes self-care. *Diabetes Care, 1*, 275.
14. Ohlson, M. (1968): Suggestion for research to strengthen learning by patients. *J. Am. Diet. Assoc., 52*, 401.
15. Phillips, M.G. (1971): The nutrition knowledge of medical students. *J. Med. Educ., 46*, 86.
16. Sansum, W.D. and Blatherwick, N.R. (1926): The use of high carbohydrate diets in the treatment of diabetes mellitus. *J. Am. Med. Assoc., 86*, 178.
17. Stone, D.B. (1965): A rational approach to diet and diabetes. *J. Am. Diet. Assoc., 46*, 30.
18. Sund, R.B. (1976): *Piaget for Educators*. C.E. Merrill, Colombus, Ohio.
19. Weinsier, R.L. and Seeman, A. (1974): Diet therapy of diabetes. Description of a successful methodologic approach to gaining diet adherence. *Diabetes, 23*, 669.
20. West, K.M. (1973): Diet therapy of diabetes: an analysis of failure. *Ann. Intern. Med., 79*, 425.

21. William, T.F. and Anderson, E. (1967): Dietary errors made at home by patients with diabetes. *J. Am. Diet. Assoc.*, *51*, 19.
22. Young, M.A.C. (1968): Review of research and studies related to health education practice (1961-1966). In: *Patient Education, Vol. 26*, p. 49. Health Education Monographs.

# 24. Interactional training and learning: the Metaplan method

W. SCHNELLE

## EDITORIAL

*The learning experience is most of the time a difficult one, characterized by an active teacher and passive students. Patient education is often dispensed this way. The Interactional Training Technique offers ways to activate the learner. In the first symposium of the Diabetes Education Study Group (DESG) W. Schnelle, a communications' specialist, utilized this technique among physicians who were responsive to the activation. At the request of the editors, Schnelle describes his personal reactions and observations in this paper. He generally thought that, in a learning experience, the Interactional Training Technique was particularly beneficial for demonstrating to the doctors a stimulating method for sharing experiences and ideas. Furthermore, with this technique the learners can express themselves, which may be particularly useful in patient education because the patient's personal experience with the disease plays such an important role. (The editors).*

The following example of Interactional Training is taken from a preparatory workshop where participants convened to organize the first European Symposium of the DESG in 1979. Fourteen physicians from different European countries participated in the meeting.

In the 1979 Interactional Workshop the Metaplan moderator stood in front of a tackboard or pinboard which was completely covered with brown paper. On this brown paper there was the statement: 'Educating diabetics – the physician's nimbus helps!' Underneath this statement were 4 boxes which represented a scale of evaluation from 2 minuses to 2 plusses (Fig. 1).

The moderator asked the participants to indicate whether they agreed completely (++) with the statement, agreed more than disagreed (+), rejected it more than they accepted it (–), or fully rejected it (– –). Each participant received a little self-adhesive dot and, after having decided where to place the dot according to their answers to the questions presented, each participant came to the tackboard to place the dot in the appropriate box corresponding to his answer.

When all the participants had finished placing their dots on the tackboard, the results were as follows: 7 dots for 1 or 2 plusses (acceptance), 5 for 1 or 2 minuses (rejection) and 2 on the center line (undecided). The

191

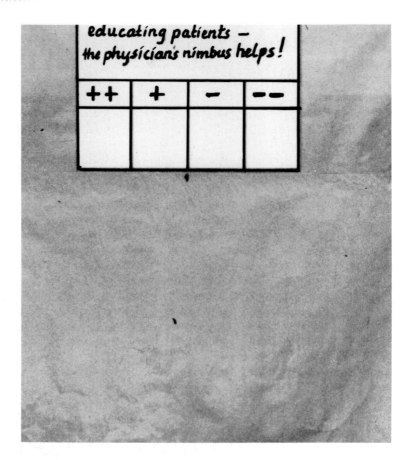

Fig. 1    Interactional Learning: Exposure of the question.

physicians were suprised at the amount of differing opinions among themselves about this statement. The moderator first asked those who rejected
the statement to give some arguments for their viewpoints. He wrote down
these arguments on little cards with a felt pen and attached the cards under
the corresponding minus boxes (Fig. 2). The same procedure was followed
for the 'plus' side of the answers.

   As soon as one of the participants said, 'It provides a good start', another
physician contradicted by adding, 'but a bad end'. The moderator drew a
mark in the form of a flash of lightning ( ⚡ ) on the attached card with the
argument which had been contested. He also wrote the counter-argument
on an oval card and pinned this oval card next to the previous card (see
lower left of Fig. 3).

   Finally the moderator asked to hear the arguments behind the dots on
the center line. 'The statement is too vague', was the typical response from

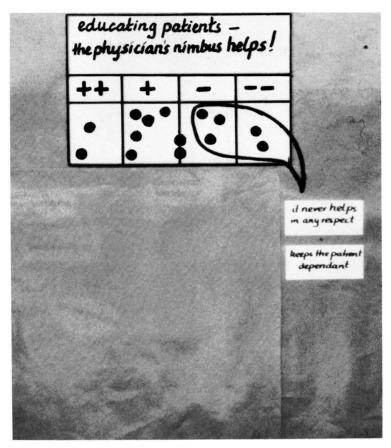

Fig. 2   Interactional Learning: Answers of participants.

scientists who have been educated only to accept well-defined statements.

This example illustrates some steps used in Interactional Training. These techniques stimulated active participation and allowed clear statements to be made by participants with responding opposition also heard. The discussion was mediated by a moderator with the use of pin- or tackboards, cards, dots, etc.

In 1979, as an expert in communications preparing and organizing the First DESG Symposium on Diabetes Education, I had to learn almost everything about diabetes, diabetic patients, and especially about diabetologists. These physicians discussed a lot about patient education. The more I listened to their debates about this subject, the more I began to doubt whether they really grasped the idea and concept of educating patients. While the following may be exaggerated assertions, they describe the physicians' problems in patient education:

193

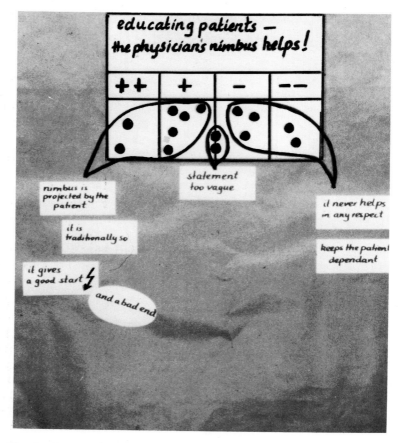

Fig. 3   Interactional Learning: Further discussion of the question.

1.   Physicians cannot distinguish between educating and consulting patients and, therefore, cannot understand that they need specific teaching skills.

2.   Physicians think of education as the process of imparting information about the disease and its treatment. They seem to be unaware that educating is not only teaching, but also building a suitable patient mentality and attitude.

3.   Physicians think of education as an appendage to medication that, if necessary, can be left to the nurse or dietician.

4.   Physicians are not aware that their nimbus may hinder the educational process. Physicians are the paternal figures to whom the patients very often hand over the responsibility for the treatment of their disease. Patients want to stay under the doctor's protection and might be inwardly disturbed when the same 'demi-gods' teach them self-care and self-control.

Perhaps physicians have such difficulty in learning how to educate patients because it is so foreign to their usual way of thinking. Professionals of any kind typically have specific difficulties in learning to adapt approaches demanding skills which are outside their accustomed field of vision and, therefore, strange to them. In such cases, it is more or less useless trying to teach and convince physicians what they should learn.

Interactional Training and Learning presented an opportunity for the physicians to explore, for themselves, possible solutions for their own problems.

Interactional Learning or Training by Interaction is based on the following didactic principles:

1.   What has to be learned should be correlated to the learners' own experiences; better still, it should be drawn out of their experience.
2.   The learners should really become involved during the process of learning. Statements and questions should 'hit them'. Learners must experience personal discrepancies to be able to detect that there is something 'between heaven and earth' that they have not yet noticed.
3.   The learners should have the opportunity to observe whether their peers or colleagues reject or accept what should be learned. Professionals do not want to be either the first or the last to accept something new.

The following is an example of a Metaplan learning experience (Fig. 4). The question, placed on the tack- or pinboard in front of the physicians is: 'As for your own learning habits and abilities, what is different now when you compare with your childhood?' The moderator suggests that the physicians should think of recent learning situations to be able to answer this question correctly. Examples of such learning situations for these physicians might be something new about immunology or how to do autogenous training.

Having presented the question, the moderator provides the participants with little cards and felt pens asking for 2 or 3 answers to be written legibly on separate cards. After a while he collects the cards; reads them aloud; and, following the advice of the group, arranges them in clusters on the pinboard according to clusters of the same meaning. The moderator draws a circle around the cards with similar meanings. He then writes a title on round cards for each cluster. As soon as a participant wants to contradict an argument seen on the board, the relevant card will be marked with a flash of lightning symbol ( ⚡ ). The counter argument is written down on an oval card and pinned next to the card being contradicted.

At this stage, the moderator summarizes all the clusters on the board. The reflection is continued by asking the participants the following question: 'If these are the typical learning attitudes and habits of physicians, which of them are also valid for educating diabetics and which are not?' He provides everybody with 2 black dots for 'valid' and 2 white dots for 'not relevant'. Then the physicians go to the pinboard and put their dots where they want them. The moderator points to the clusters on which both types of dots are located and starts a discussion between the proponents

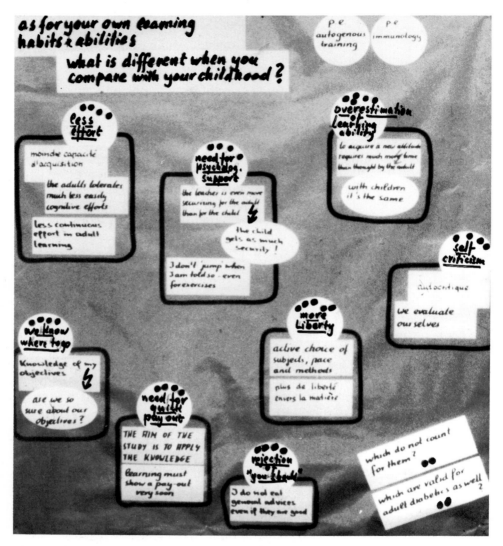

Fig. 4 Interactional Learning: Answers to questions on small cards, grouping of answers and 'votation' on answers.

and opponents of the learning habits proposed as suitable for the education of diabetic individuals. This is the way that the Interactional Experience allows the participants to discover, for themselves, the process of true learning: how it actually occurs.

The core of Interactional Training and Learning by the Metaplan Method is as follows:

The moderator stimulates interaction among group members.
The moderator triggers simultaneous and visible answers with a question or statement.
These answers will be given on cards or by dots that will be displayed on pin- or tackboards covered with brown paper.
Suspense and curiosity arise among the participants to see if their own view-point is confirmed or disputed.

Although this method has been used successfully in many DESG workshops, there remain 2 critical questions:
1. Is it necessary or at least beneficial to the performance of learning to know, consciously, that learning is taking place during these Interactional Workshops? Very often participants in Interactional Workshops are not aware that they are attending a learning session.
2. Will physicians, in particular, need to be taught by reputable experts in any field other than medicine, especially the various disciplines of human sciences, if they are really to accept and adopt new things? In Interactional Training and Learning the moderator might not be taken to be such an authority.

## CONCLUSIONS

The outlook for Interactional Training and Learning in diabetes education is positive. The Metaplan Method is – in the context of the DESG – an almost accepted way of training the medical team. Interactional Learning can become a good means of educating diabetics as well as physicians. Will the doctors then be able to take over the moderator's role? One would hope so.

## SUMMARY

Interactional Training, using the Metaplan Method, is a technique in which learning takes place through discovery and discussion among the participants. The moderator acts only as a facilitator and not as a lecturer or dispenser of information. The technique is an 'oral and written' discussion where participants express themselves on small cards of paper which then are pinned on a tackboard, grouped according to common subjects, and discussed by the participants. This technique appears to be a strong activator in learning and training experiences and could be used in several fields of medicine and patient education.

*W. Schnelle*

## SUGGESTED READING

1.  Schnelle, W. and Stolz, I. (1977): *Interactional Learning. A Guide to Moderating Groups of Learners*. Metaplan GmbH, 2085 Quickborn, Western Germany.
2.  Schnelle, E. (1979): *The Metaplan Method. Communicaton Tools for Planning and Learning Groups*. Metaplan Series no. 7, Metaplan GmbH, 2085 Quickborn, Western Germany.

# 25. The emotional and social aspects of eating

GYUALA CEY-BERT

EDITORIAL

*Adherence to a diet is usually difficult for each patient and lack of compliance often leads to frustration for both the diabetic and the physician and/or dietician. Meal planning is almost always nutritionally oriented with only discussions of carbohydrates and calories, while the social and emotional aspects of eating are too often ignored. This article tries to strengthen the links among the nutritional, emotional, and social aspects of food and eating. Failure to approach the concept of diet from this global perspective can negatively affect the success of the prescription. (The editors.)*

Food has always been one of man's fundamental preoccupations throughout the ages and in all societies. For a long time his preoccupation was a quantitative one: he wanted to eat as much as possible in order to survive. But now the emphasis has changed. His preoccupation has become a qualitative one.

Today, in our industrialized countries the main consideration is what to eat to keep fit and well, to recover a slim and attractive appearance, to enjoy oneself more, or to better convey expressions of friendship to others. People are becoming more interested in nutrition and are vaguely realizing that its global concept includes the physiological, psychological, and social dimensions of eating which combine to make the foundation for achieving a satisfying and balanced quality of life.

Food is a fundamental, symbolic form of expressing desires, hopes, and expectations, as well as deep-seated anxieties and fears. Food reflects an essential relationship between the quality of life with its leisure enjoyments and the need to eat. This essential relationship between life and food is what determines the motivational background of feeding behavior composed of the following 2 main categories of motivation:

1. *Eating for survival and security* is associated with a desire to gain a sense of security through food, both quantitatively and qualitatively. This means eating to live, to maintain good health, and/or to preserve an esthetic and attractive physical appearance.
2. *Eating for freedom and pleasure* is associated with a desire to gain a sense of freedom through food, to escape from everyday constraints,

to relax, and to enjoy oneself. Eating becomes a pleasurable pastime to feel comfortable and free.

These 2 motivational categories, which are codified in the pattern of eating habits, simultaneously express the 2 fundamental needs of life itself: the need for a sense of security and the need for a sense of freedom and enjoyment. This motivational polarity – the desire for freedom and the desire for security – can be discerned in any choice of food and diet. Certain eating patterns are more strongly influenced by the desire for security, while others show a greater desire for freedom. The choice of milk or vegetables, for instance, reveals a stronger desire to feel secure. A bottle of champagne or a portion of *foie gras* express the desire for freedom combined with pleasure. The 2 motivational categories of security and freedom determine the physiological, emotional, and social development of food habits.

There are, in fact, 3 distinct aspects of eating: the physiological aspect, the psychological aspect, and the social aspect. However, the physiological aspect of eating is considered by several branches of science as its only essential function because it is easier to measure and quantify. Modern dietary research is making a big mistake in solely trying to ascertain the physiological determinants of nutrition: only its measurable and quantifiable aspects.

Both dietetics and medicine are being increasingly conditioned by this one-sided approach and it is the fundamental cause of failure in a great many cases of unsuccessful medical treatment. This limited attitude results in the unhappy, depressive attitude of people who have lost the pleasure of eating because they only consider food in terms of the number of calories or grams of carbohydrates absorbed. Each meal, with its anxious calculation of the calorie content, becomes a source of fear and tension. Even in the most extreme circumstances, the pleasure of eating combined with the emotional aspect of food mixes the physiological with the psychological aspect.

The physiological factors are very impo.    .t, of course, but any analysis of their influence in the diet must also consider their close interaction with the emotional and social factors. In fact, the physiological factors of appetite are rarely displayed directly. Their influence is indirect because they are integrated into general behavior. A feeling of hunger might not be triggered by hypoglycemia if the emotional state or social context is not conducive to eating. The diabetic individual may desperately need some quick carbohydrates, but may be so absorbed in an activity that he or she is totally unaware of low blood glucose. This means that the emotional and the social aspects are essential functions in determining feeding behavior.

The physiological, emotional, and social aspects of behavior should not necessarily be considered as independent factors or motivations separate from one another. Dietary motivation, i.e. the desire to eat a specific food, is determined by the close interaction among the physiological, emotional, and social factors. Consequently a motivation initiated by an emotional stimulus will only become a genuine motivation depending on the physiological state of the body and the symbolic and social value attributed to the food. The motivation of feeding behavior is a combined result of these 3 factors.

Eating is a ritual behavior. It is precisely this ritual aspect of eating which forms the indispensable links among the emotional, social, and physiological functions of feeding. The rites involved are a crystallization of social regulations transposed into symbolic actions. When I raise my glass and say 'Cheers' to my neighbor at the dinner table, it is a ritual act conveying an emotive message which creates a greater sense of security both for her and for me. Similarly when a bottle of champagne is ordered in a 3-star restaurant, it is a significant ritual act indicating a high level of esteem, affection or appreciation for the person invited. Thus the ritual of food and drink is a symbolic act of communication. These symbolic acts serve to convey a sense of security concerning the correct treatment of food in the physiological, the emotional, and the social context.

In the ancient societies without written traditions, knowledge essential for the survival of the community concerning the production, processing, and preparation of food was passed on from generation to generation through the ritual language of dietary laws and customs. Discoveries of the physiological properties of certain foods were translated into ritual customs. The ritual consumption of fermented mare's milk by the ancient peoples of Central Asia is a very significant example. Being breeders of horses and cattle, they were condemned to endless struggles to preserve the pastures vitally needed for their existence and livelihood. Above all, these Central Asian people were big meat-eaters. Their diet included very few fruit and vegetables, an indispensable source of vitamin C. A deficiency of vitamin C would have resulted in dangerous dietary disorders. It would have been a mortal threat to their survival by sapping their physical strength and ability to fight.

For a long time no one could understand how these people compensated for the lack of vitamin C in their diet. It is known that the consumption of fermented mare's milk (koumiss) was a strictly enforced institution among the peoples of Central Asia. According to a Baskir legend it was 'Tengri', the supreme deity of the community, who ordered that 'koumiss' should be regularly and ritually consumed so that 'the Baskir fighters would be swifter, stronger and more powerful in battle ...'. Similarly the regular consumption of certain fruits, herbs and plants mixed with certain dairy products was prescribed by ritual dietary customs.

Thanks to the link established between the physiological needs and the symbolic ritual connotation, the ancient peoples of Central Asia largely managed to solve the problem of insufficient vitamin C in their diet. This link was established in 3 successive phases according to the 3 fundamental aspects of eating:

201

1. *Physiological aspect:* first the physiological needs emerged, a deficiency of vitamin C;
2. *Psychological aspect:* once the physiological solution had been discovered in the form of fermented mare's milk or 'koumiss', emotive and sensory properties were attributed to the milk and it became desirable, good, and appetizing;
3. *Social aspects:* finally the discovery was institutionalized on a social level, enhanced with symbolic meaning, and the consumption of 'koumiss' became a highly recommendable social obligation.

This process of linking the physiological, psychological, and social aspects of eating by imbuing them with a symbolic, ritual significance, likewise explains the beneficial effects of more ritualized, traditional eating habits in the prevention of certain serious illnesses. In a recent survey conducted in Hawaii, being able to read and write Japanese proved to be one of the best indicators of cardiovascular health for more than 8,000 men of Japanese extraction, born between 1900 and 1919. These were the Japanese men in Hawaii who had escaped becoming westernized. Those men who had retained or learned their ancestral language had also continued certain traditional ways of living including ritual eating habits. The traditional Japanese food customs, with a diet rich in complex carbohydrates and fish, seem to be in inverse proportion to the danger of heart disease.

This ethnographical example of the Japanese food customs is a perfect demonstration of the importance of the dietary ritual in creating links among the physiological, emotional, and social aspects of eating. The whole purpose of this coordination is to attain the *physiological equilibrium* which is indispensable for physical health; the *emotional equilibrium*, indispensable for psychological health; and the *social equilibrium*, indispensable for a sense of social happiness and well-being.

The following examples illustrate the present day emotional and social aspects of eating. It is important to consider the constant underlying interaction of the emotional and social aspects of eating for a correct interpretation of these examples.

THE EMOTIONAL ASPECT

The emotional aspect of eating is determined by the search and desire for oral and affective pleasures. Oral pleasures are determined by perception of the visual, affective, gustatory, and tactile aspects of food. Affective pleasures are determined mainly by memories of previous pleasurable experiences which prompt an emotional response in our state of mind. The memory of a Peking duck enjoyed during a dinner in the company of a particularly charming and attractive Chinese woman can emotively determine a preference for Pekinese cooking.

On an emotional level, the pleasures of sight, taste, and smell mainly determine the development of food preferences and the gastronomic evolution of distinctive national cuisines. Thus some national cuisines seek above all to enhance the visual and esthetic pleasures of food, whereas others attach greater importance to the pleasures of fragrance and flavor.

Japanese cuisine, for instance, is primarily a gastronomic art designed to give visual pleasure. The exquisite presentation of food is a true work of art. French cuisine is a most harmonious and comprehensive combination of the oral pleasures of gastronomy. It seeks to blend the pleasures of fragrance and flavor with the visual and tactile pleasures (the consistency of food).

In the New French Cuisine described by Gault and Millau, the traditional cooking style with its attention to flavors and fragrance, accentuating above all the merits of natural products, is simultaneously combined with the visual dimension in the esthetic presentation of Japanese food and the quest for the complete harmony of oral pleasures found in Chinese cuisine. On the emotional level, however, the originality of the New French Cuisine lies in another even more important aspect. It is the first attempt by a national cuisine in Europe to consciously restore contact among the physiological, emotional, and social aspects of food.

This contact has been broken among the physiological, emotional, and social aspects of eating in the living conditions of modern society because of the destruction of traditional dietary values. These values were traditionally based on the interaction of these 3 factors, whereas modern values are based either on overestimated emotional and social factors or, to a lesser extent, on the quantitative aspects of overestimated physiological factors (the anxious counting of calories).

Why was this contact broken? For modern affluent mankind, the problem of hunger does not exist. On the contrary, he is overfed and has weight problems. Quantitatively, the problems of food have been solved and nutrition has become a question of qualitative selection. Following new eating habits largely based on only the emotional and social aspects of meals, people eat for enjoyment, relaxation, and a feeling of freedom.

## THE SOCIAL ASPECT

An analysis of the ritual significance of the dinner to celebrate an urban marriage in modern society is an excellent illustration of the growing importance attributed to the emotional and social aspects of food. The emotional influence of food shared together plays an important part in forming and consolidating the union of the young couple to be married. We conducted a survey interviewing 600 young, newlywed couples and our analyses of the results revealed the following main points:
- all the couples belonging to the sample group had met privately several times for meals or rendezvous at various restaurants or in their respec-

tive homes. They were unanimous in considering that eating together had played a considerable part in developing and strengthening the bonds of affection between them;

– in 33% of the cases the couple's decision to get married was taken during a *tête-à-tête* meal;
– in 54% of the cases, the young couple had a meal together the same day that they decided to get married or the day after their decision to 'celebrate the decision to get married' or 'to discuss the details'.

This means that in 87% of the cases, the meal together played an important emotive part in the decision to get married. This is a perfect example of how very important the emotional and social aspects of eating are as a means of human communication.

At the same time, we are experiencing a decline in the influence of the physiological consideration of eating, an important factor of dietary equilibrium. One of the principal causes of the modern dietary problems of overfeeding and unbalanced nutrition is the great difficulty of maintaining contact among the physiological, emotional and social aspects of eating. The development of fast food restaurants is a significant example of this problem, as well as the modern tendency of overestimating the social aspect. The main customers of these American styled, fast food restaurants such as MacDonalds are young people and adolescents seeking a social atmosphere and environment different from that of traditional restaurants. In this new social environment, where general behavior is more relaxed and easy-going, the eating ritual has been socially modified:

– the food offered is finger food which re-establishes the direct emotive contact with the food;
– the ritual is freer: one can eat standing up, sitting down, or wandering around; and items ordered can be taken away;
– the atmosphere is young and tolerant with unconventional behavior and clothing being accepted.

Surveys that have been conducted clearly show that the majority of customers at fast food restaurants are attracted not only by considerations of time and money, but also by the social aspect of the younger, more relaxed, and easy-going style of eating. But the surveys also show that the hamburgers and other items sold in fast food restaurants are physiologically and nutritionally unbalanced. The fast food catering, characteristic of today, clearly illustrates the declining importance attributed to the physiological aspect of food and the parallel overestimation of the social and emotional aspect.

In the earlier ethnographic example of the consumption of fermented mare's milk, the purpose of the ritual was to establish the indispensable linkage among the physiological, emotional, and social aspects of food. The fundamental physiological need was vested with the emotional and social connotations of its ritual consumption.

In the example of modern fast food catering the sequence is reversed: there is a basic social need which is given an emotive significance. The physiological need is secondary. The result is the nutritional one-sidedness of the fast food restaurants which simultaneously reflects the generally unbalanced attitudes toward food and the eating habits of our time. In order to restore the necessary equilibrium, it is essential to restore contact among the 3 main aspects of eating – the physiological, emotional, and social aspects.

## CONCLUSION

The following points should be emphasized:
*1.* The physical, psychological, and social equilibrium of man is closely connected with his feeding behavior. Only by establishing and maintaining the indispensable links among the physiological, emotional, and social factors in eating habits and attitudes can equilibrium and well-being be assured.
*2.* The overestimation of the quantitative aspects of the physiological factor by certain branches of science and the medical world creates anxiety and psychological stress.
*3.* At the same time, the overestimation of the emotional and social aspects of eating by much of the population results in a lack of nutritional equilibrium with all its harmful effects.

Let us not forget the indispensable combination of these 3 factors either when we are prescribing a diet to someone who is ill or when we raise a glass of champagne to say 'Cheers' to a friend.

## SUMMARY

This article presents a 2-part analysis of the emotional and social aspects of eating. The first analysis defines the underlying significance of feeding behavior by distinguishing between the 2 most important motivational categories which determine eating habits. The second analysis outlines the significance of the emotional and social aspects of eating which are closely related with the physiological aspect. A number of ethnographical examples and instances of modern life are cited.

## SUGGESTED READING

1. Gault, H. and Millau, Ch. (1977): *Gault et Millau se Mettent à Table.* Plon, Paris.
2. Castaneda, C. (1971): *Voir.* Gallimard, Paris.
3. Cey-Bert, G. *Le langage des préférences.* Alimentories. Manuscript.
4. Dioszegi, V. (1978): *Az Osi Magyar Hitvilage.* Gondolat, Budapest.
5. Hemardinquer, J.J. (1970): *Pour une Histoire de l'Alimentation.* Arman Colin, Paris.

6. Mayer, J. (1974): *Human Nutrition*. Charles Thames, Springfield.
7. Revel, J.F. (1979): *Un Festin en Paroles*. Pauvert, Paris.
8. Tannahill, R. (1973): *Food in History*. Eyre Methuen, London.
9. Tremolières, J. (1973): *Nutrition*. Dunod, Paris.

## BIBLIOGRAPHY

1. Cattel, R.B. and Radcliffe, J.A. (1963): The nature and measurement of components of motivation. *Genet. Psychol. Monogr., 68*, 49.
2. Scarr, S. (1969): Genetic factors in activity motivation. *Child Dev., 40*, 823.
3. Minder, M. (1947): Didactique fonctionnelle. In: Dessain, H. and Diel, P. (Eds), *Psychologie de la Motivation*. Presse Universitaire de France.
4. Frisse, P., and Piaget, J. (1963): *Traité de Psychologie Expérimentale*. Presse Universitaire de France.
5. Giraud, J. (1964): *Clefs pour la Pédagogie*. Editions Seghens.
6. Gfeller, R. and Assal, J.-Ph. (1980): The diabetic's subjective experience. *Folia Psychopractica*. Hoffman-La Roche, Basel.
7. Hameline, D. (1980): *Les Objectifs Pedagogiques en Formation Initiale et en Formation Continue, 2e Ed*. Editions ESF, Paris.
8. Ford, D.H. and Urban, H.B. (1963): Freud's Psychoanalysis. In: *Systems of Psychotherapy*. Ch. 5, p. 109. John Wiley & Sons, New York.

# 26. Developmental stages of patient acceptance in diabetes

R. GFELLER AND J.-PH. ASSAL

## EDITORIAL

*The chances of success in the treatment of a chronic disease depend on several factors: some are related to the approach of the physician, others depend on the patient. In chronic diseases, patients' active collaboration in the treatment is mandatory, particularly when the disease has new symptoms. Active collaboration of the diabetic patient requires acceptance of the disease. Coping with the disease is the positive result of an individual's progression through a developmental sequence of difficult adaptations which occur when a person has lost good health.*

*These psychological adjustments of the patients to their disease are fundamental and need to be recognized by the physician/nurse/dietician. Only by listening to the patient's subjective experiences can the medical team adapt their therapeutical approach to the patient's real needs from a global, comprehensive perspective of that individual. (The editors.)*

In a synthetic and comprehensive or global approach to medicine, each and every illness has a psychological and social, as well as an anatomical and physiological dimension. The physician treats a case of diabetes in the classical sense of diagnosis and treatment of the metabolic disorder. In the sense of *global* diagnosis and treatment, however, the physician has to treat both the metabolic imbalance *and* its bearer, the diabetic patient. This approach broadens the therapeutic relationship which is no longer one between doctor and illness (glycemia), but between doctor and patient (glycemia and its bearer, the patient with diabetes).

This relation between the health care worker and the patient is decisive in obtaining the optimum therapeutic effect, particularly in chronic diseases. The treatment can only be successful if the physician/nurse/dietician know and take into account the subjective experience of the patient. Neglecting the bearer of diabetes and his experience as a diabetic amounts to practicing all alone without a patient. Such a therapeutic relationship is only one of doctor-disease, rather than doctor-patient. The reciprocal doctor-patient relationship can only exist when the doctor takes into account the diabetic's experience. The doctor and patient dialog is a decisive factor in the successful treatment of chronic diseases.

*R. Gfeller and J.-Ph. Assal*

The psychological understanding of a patient with a chronic illness can be analyzed according to 2 periods: (1) before the occurrence of the disease and (2) after discovery of the disease. In the first situation the psychological profile of the patient can sometimes be part of risk factors directly or indirectly influencing the outbreak of a disease. The following sequence is an example: a person having psychological problems which lead to overeating and then obesity followed by peripheral resistance to insulin and, finally, diabetes mellitus. The second situation is a question of a patient's psychological reactions to the discovery of the disease. This article will discuss the various adaptations of the patient to the disease.

Thanks to weekly discussion groups, which were recorded on audio tape, it has been possible to listen to the observations of more than 1,500 patients on how they live with their illness. These Round Table discussions revealed to what extent diabetes was poorly accepted from all points of view: metabolic, psycho-social, professional and familial. A large number of diabetics, even those who were quite well-balanced, had not yet accepted the limits imposed by their state of health and the obligations which had to be met by a treatment that is complex.

## THE ROUND TABLE WITH PATIENTS AND ITS POSITION IN A GLOBAL HEALTH CARE PROGRAM

In our Diabetes Treatment and Teaching Unit the patient is structured in 3 dimensions:
1.   A medical, organic check-up and treatment which is determined by the biological feedback from the laboratory results.
2.   A teaching and training program for patients including 13 hours of group lectures and 3 hours of individualized teaching a week. The feedback of this pedagogical dimension is in the demonstrated skills of the patients, i.e. selecting their diet from a buffet or performing a blood glucose self-monitoring test, etc.
3.   The third dimension is centered on the patients' subjective experience. Thanks to open questions asked by the moderator, topics such as the following are discussed: 'How do you live with diabetes?'; 'What are the best strategies for adapting to the disease?' etc. Although patients can express themselves during personal interviews, it is at the time of the weekly Round Table that they seem to feel free to express themselves the best. The discussion and, therefore, the feedback to the medical personnel present is centered on the patient's personal experience with the disease.

## THE CHARACTERISTICS OF THE ROUND TABLE DISCUSSIONS

The weekly Round Table Discussions with the patients of the Unit, which include 15 to 20 patients and other people significant in the patients' lives, last for 1½ hour. All patients as well as physicians, nurses and dieticians of the Unit have to participate. The Round Table Discussion is moderated by a specialist in psychosomatic medicine (R. Gfeller). Since the opening of the Unit in 1975 this Round Table Discussion has been held systematically every week.

This Round Table Discussion is preceded by a meeting between the moderator and the medical team. In this meeting the doctors, nurses and dieticians try to define the personalities of their patients and the way these patients adapt to diabetes. Immediately after this group discussion, the medical team participates in a staff meeting which allows them to discover ways to provide the patients better psychological support.

The topic of the Round Table Discussion, 'What does diabetes mean for me?' goes to the heart of each diabetic's experience. The discussion group has the role of a *catalyst of relationships* in the Unit. It provides a good atmosphere for patients to verbalize emotions about their acceptance of diabetes while also allowing the medical team to discover the patients' subjective experiences and their own counter attitudes as physicians, nurses and dieticians. These counter attitudes of the medical team are discussed with the moderator at the post-table which immediately follows the group discussion with patients.

For the functioning of a diabetic unit as a whole, the discussion group provides feedback which enables the medical team to become attuned to the individual needs of the patient. Observation of patients and consideration of their diabetic experiences and feelings have led to the greatest improvements in the organization of the Unit, patient education and training.


## THE NOTION OF FEEDBACK

Feedback can be conceptualized by a theoretical reference system, the cybernetic model, which plays a fundamental role in communications theory [1]. It is during the discussion group that the personal feedback of patients is best verbalized and quite apparent.

During their stay in the Unit, and according to the classical medical scheme, the patients are the *receivers* of the medical care and knowledge about diabetes. The members of the medical team are *transmitters* of the care and the diabetic message. This model only allows for one-way information between the doctor/nurse/dietician and the patient. In the group discussion with patients (providing the medical team is present) the roles are reversed: the patients are the transmitters and the medical team is the receiver. Since personal experience varies from one patient to another, the doctor/nurse/dietician must try to listen actively to each patient. The feedback from patients is particularly valid because it is first-hand experience. This experience cannot be found and learned in any textbook on diabetes!

This feedback, verbalized in the discussion group, has brought about profound changes in the global approach to the diabetic; in the short term, a change of attitudes to certain patients; in the medium term, a modification of pedagogical methods; and in the long term, an alteration of the structure of the unit. Feedback is an essential element in any relationship between adults which is characterized by reciprocity and dialog between the two individuals.

The utilization of feedback is an important influence in patient education and training. Learning is a process in which the receiver (the diabetic) tries to assimilate an information bank from the transmitter (the medical team). Feedback, for its part, is the information which comes from the receiver (the diabetic). The feedback then enables the transmitter (the doctor/nurse/dietician) to adjust his or her information to the understanding of the receiver (the diabetic). By consciously seeking to use the feedback and to maintain its stability, the medical team will rapidly be on the same 'wavelength' as the patient and continually improve the dialog.

## THE DIABETIC'S SUBJECTIVE EXPERIENCE

Although there are as many personal experiences with diabetes as there are diabetic individuals, several common attitudes in the various adaptations to accept diabetes can be observed. The acceptance of a chronic disease like diabetes means nothing less than the acceptance of the loss of one's biological normality and psychological integrity. In other words, acceptation of a disease is the mourning of health.

Freud [2] described the 3 stages of normal mourning: (1) denial of reality, (2) depression and (3) adaptation to the new reality. In *On Death and Dying*, Kübler-Ross [3] went into even greater detail by describing the phases of revolt. She distinguished 5 stages of mourning: (1) shock and denial ('No, not me ...'), (2) revolt ('Why me?'), (3) bargaining ('Yes, but ...'), (4) depression with hope, and (5) acceptance. Analysis of tape recordings of 150 Round Table Discussions [4, 5] with patients showed that acceptance of diabetes was a continuous dynamic process in which certain stages could be identified that were very close to what Freud and Kübler-Ross had described.

These stages are artificial steps in the sense that they are 'man-made' labels to help understand the dynamic process which normally occurs as an individual process in the difficult period of disease acceptance. This is evident in the case reports which are included later in this article. The reader must always remember that the developmental stages of mourning are never entered into in isolation, one at a time, but rather in relationship to the stage before and after. For example, a person in the stage of 'revolt' might, at the same time, be partially in the stage of 'shock and denial' while also exhibiting characteristics of the stage after 'revolt' which is 'bargaining'.

The speed at which one passes from one stage to another varies greatly from one individual to another depending on the individual, his or her personal surroundings, and the medical relationships he or she has experienced. Therefore, there are many factors which favor the acceptance or inhibit the evolution.

To accept one's own disease is an eminently dynamic process. One moves both backward and forward. The general movement goes forward towards active acceptance with intermittent backward moves when there are setbacks. A chronic illness always presents a series of painful situations which one must surmount or to which one must adapt. In the beginning, the diagnosis of diabetes must be accepted, but afterwards come constraints from the treatment and, later, complications which must again be faced and accepted. *The difficult phases in the process of acceptance are absolutely normal*. What is abnormal is to remain for months or years at one or two of the intermediary stages. The dialog with the patient should positively activate the patient's movement towards the evolution to acceptance.

The next section is a closer examination of the 5 evolutionary phases towards acceptance. Case reports recorded during the weekly Round Table Discussions and followed by a short commentary will illustrate the patients' personal experiences with diabetes.

*First Phase*: SHOCK AND DENIAL OF REALITY: 'This can't be happening to me …, I'm not a diabetic!'

The *denial* stage in the evolution to acceptance is the period in which the person is the most negligent. The refusal to face reality induces negligence of medical control and treatment. This denial of the illness, in addition to negligence, is often realized retrospectively after the period has been passed. The denial is often easier to maintain if there are no overt signs of the illness, particularly when it is asymptomatic.

At the stage of *denial* it is an illusion to think that teaching will be really effective when the disease is not real to the patient. A good attitude which is possible for the doctor/nurse/dietician is not to force the issue, but to create a receptive climate by waiting and active listening.

The following is an example of denial of reality recorded during a Round Table Discussion with patients.

*Case Report*: DENIAL OF REALITY
Dr. G.: 'As we do every Thursday, we are going to discuss the topics 'What does diabetes mean to me?, What is the best possible way to live with diabetes?' and 'How well do I accept this chronic illness?' Who would like to speak first?'

Mr. A. (55 years old, farmer, non-insulin-dependent diabetic for 10 years, admitted to hospital with hyperglycemic coma with severe dehydration):

'My diabetes has never bothered me. I've been living with it for ever so long. Here in the hospital I was given insulin at first, but I haven't needed it now for some days. I've almost been cured of my diabetes because I'm not being treated any more'.

211

Dr. G.: 'It's interesting that you say you once had diabetes, but don't have it any longer. Are the classes you are taking on diabetes really of any use if, as you say, you no longer have diabetes?'

Mr. A.: 'Oh yes, they're very important. If I had had a better idea about my diet, I wouldn't have had this accident with my diabetes. So if I know the illness a little better, I'll be able to deal with any problem if the disease comes back. I think it's very important to be in the care of a doctor who has a good knowledge of diabetes'.

*Commentary*

Denial of reality. During the Round Table Discussion, Mr. A. went from denying his illness ('I don't have diabetes') to claiming he didn't have it any longer. He considers the courses useful because he might have diabetes again some day. He does, however, feel the need to be in the care of a doctor interested in diabetes.

*Second Phase*: REVOLT AND AGGRESSIVENESS: 'Why is this happening to me ... My diabetes is due to my problems at work ... (or) ... to my divorce ...'

The stage of *revolt* and *aggressiveness* of the patient follows, in general, that of denial and negligence. This stage represents progress and should be utilized, for it is only an active attitude which can lead the patient towards the acceptance of his diabetes. During the stage of revolt, the aggressiveness of the patient prevents him from listening and following the medical guidelines correctly. It is very difficult for him to deny that he is ill. A number of situations, usually exterior to his illness, permit the patient to express internal revolt. At this stage the patient is often considered to have a difficult personality by the people surrounding him (the medical team, family and friends).

*Case Report*: REVOLT AND LONELINESS

Mr. B. (65 years of age; male nurse; became diabetic suddenly, 8 years previously with loss of weight; glycosuria and ketonuria; insulin treatment; wife is an invalid with valvular heart disease):

'It was a real shock for me when I was told that I had diabetes. From my training I knew right away that I was faced with an irreversible and chronic disease, often having very serious complications. I felt I was alone with my problems. I couldn't burden my wife with my worries because she herself has a severe illness and is under a lot of physical and mental stress. I only saw limitations wherever I looked: a daily discipline which meant that I had to break with so many old habits! I revolted at the idea of my diabetes. Why did I have to have yet another such trial in my life? Why, just when I had adjusted to my wife's illness, did I have to adjust to this new blow? Would I be strong enough to stand this new test? I felt really alone and misused'.

Dr. G.: 'Did you tell your doctor about this feeling of revolt?'

Mr. B.: 'No, my doctor was always in a great rush, but he gave me good treatment. He took a lot of blood glucose tests and analyzed my urine. In any case, I wouldn't have wanted to tell him my problems; I don't like to gripe. You know, it's a disease you don't see from outside. Other people don't realize it. Everything seemed to be crumbling around me, and there was nothing to hold on to. In the streets too, I am alone with my diabetes, cut off from the rest of the world. No sharing. I felt despair and an inner revolt. How could I manage to meet my professional obligations? How could I work as actively as before? Would I be able to finish my career or would I have to change jobs once again? This revolt inside me was an awful strain and I wondered whether I had enough faith to overcome this obstacle. And all alone, I found the answer in the very core of my being: Dear God, have pity on me in my misery. Many people have already made this appeal and tomorrow others will make it. But it was this cry which enabled me to overcome the revolt and feeling of injustice'.

*Commentary*
Revolt and loneliness. Mr. B. has described his revolt against fate. 'Why does this illness happen to me? Life has burdened me enough already'. Moreover, Mr. B. illustrates the feeling of loneliness which almost invariably accompanies the stage of revolt. The loneliness was fostered by the revolt against illness and fate and also by the fact that the illness cannot be seen.

*Third Phase*: BARGAINING: During bargaining, the patient can tolerate certain limited aspects of his illness, but not all of them. One encounters such remarks as: 'If I have to be ill, then I agree to only part of the treatment, but, for the rest, I'll do what I want'.

The ideas in the Bargaining stage are nearer to acceptance than in Revolt. The treatment, in general, is accepted, but not totally. As far as teaching is concerned, the patient appears often very interested in the courses. He or she asks a lot of questions, although they are often the same questions to different members of the medical team. This is done with the undeclared aim of seeking different replies to the same question. When the information given by different members of the medical teaching team is not always exactly the same, the patient will state that some sections of the treatment are impossible to learn, to put into practice, or to accept because the medical personnel's answers differ.

There is a great danger, during this stage of *bargaining*, that the information given to the patient will be distorted. When there is bargaining, one already accepts *part* of reality, so the hope of a solution appears closer than in the previous phases.

*Case Report*: BARGAINING (with some REVOLT)
Mr. H.: (44 years old; diabetic since age 16; automobile dealer; 1 injection of Lente a day; severe hypoglycemic episodes in the afternoon; severe background retinopathy for which laser therapy is proposed; visual acuity 10/10 in both eyes):
'I just came to your diabetic unit to see how to get rid of these "hypos" (hypoglycemia episodes) in the afternoon. You know they often took me for an alcoholic in my office, but I do not drink! I agree to do what I can to avoid these hypos, but I refuse to be treated with 2 insulin injections a day. One in the morn-

ing is enough. How can I believe you when the ideas of the physicians are so different about treatment! One says that with the second injection in the evening, I will have less reactions in the afternoon; another doctor says that it is mainly to protect my eyesight that the second injection is so important. I came here to get rid of these hypos in the afternoon and not to discuss about eye problems. In fact the ophthalmologist told me that my vision was good. I would agree to change my diet. In my profession you will not see me eating at 4 o'clock in the afternoon, but I certainly will eat more at lunch!'

Dr. G.: 'Don't you think that both doctors meant basically the same thing? They both wanted to improve your diabetes control'.

Mr. H.: 'You know, I know physicians who think exactly like me'.

*Commentary*
Bargaining with revolt. Mr. H. has had diabetes for 28 years. Despite the long duration of the disease, acceptance of diabetes is far from being reached. Serious hypoglycemia episodes have forced the patient to come to the diabetic unit. Mr. H. wants to improve, but at the same time he refuses ways to reach better control. He refuses the second injection as well as the necessity of taking, systematically, a mid-afternoon snack.

Mr. H. tries to explain his decisions. He says that the physicians of the unit have apparently no common medical reason for the second injection; even more, he knows physicians who would continue to advise 1 daily insulin injection. He states that the dietician does not understand that his professional obligations make the mid-afternoon snack impossible. But still, this patient was ready to try to prevent the 'hypos' by eating more at lunch. As for the eye problem, the attitude of the patient is denial because he does not accept that control of diabetes might improve his retinopathy.

This case illustrates how the emotional turmoil of a patient who is revolting against his disease can seriously interfere with the improvement of control. There is still hope to help this patient. The entry point is offered by the patient. One might, in a very first step, modify his lunch program because he suggested it.

This phase of bargaining with revolt is probably one of the most difficult times that the patient and the medical team have to face. The ingredients needed for success in helping such a diabetic patient towards a more active phase of acceptance are active listening to the patient without judgement, more patience towards the patient and emotional support of the diabetic individual.

*Fourth Phase*: DEPRESSION-INNER QUESTIONING
Arriving at this psychological point, the diabetic individual might say: 'With everything that I have to do, can I really cope with this?'

In this phase the diabetic individual is overwhelmed by all the information that he or she must assimilate and utilize in daily life. The person honestly wonders if he or she is equal to the task of living with so many restrictions and requirements.

The stage of Depression-Inner Questioning occurs when the illness can no longer be ignored, but must be integrated into daily life. This sort of depression does not manifest itself in a very acute form, but is more insidious and often goes unnoticed. The doctor must identify this phase in the patient.

This phase almost always follows the phases of *revolt* and *bargaining* which are visible and explosive. In the Depression-Inner Questioning phase when the patient is finally more peaceful, the medical team starts to relax and tends to ignore this patient. This attitude is unfortunate because it is in this phase that the patient is more open to the influences of education and training. Teaching at this stage not only improves knowledge, but is an *important psychological support*. The more the patient knows about his illness, the less he will fear it and the better he will be able to live and cope with it.

The phase of Depression-Inner Questioning in the movement toward acceptance has nothing to do with the clinical psychiatric depression manifested by sadness, anxiety, loss of interest, loss of appetite, insomnia and suicidal tendencies. This pathological depression must be immediately treated by psychotropic drugs. Psychiatric depression is not found any more frequently in the diabetic than in the non-diabetic population. Out of 2,000 diabetics in our consultation, there were no more cases of psychiatric depressions than in the control group population. The phases of Denial, Revolt and Bargaining, which are experienced before Depression-Inner Questioning, are the fundamental defense mechanisms used by patients to avoid a collapse into a psychiatric depression without hope.

The Depression which follows the Bargaining phase and precedes Active Acceptance is a reaction fundamentally different from and not as destructive as the psychiatric depression. The inner-questioning is creative and contains hope. Self-respect is preserved.

*Fifth Phase*: ACTIVE ACCEPTANCE
'Even with this problem, I can continue to live life successfully'. Diabetes is no longer viewed, in the Active Acceptance Stage, as an element foreign to the diabetic's personal being, but as an integrated part of it. Limitations from the disease are the same as before, but the diabetic individual has learned to live with them without resenting them.

This acceptance can be characterized as the best possible health condition ('restitutio ad optimum') rather than return to perfect health ('restitutio ad integrum') as before diabetes was diagnosed. The acceptance of not returning to the ideal health condition, but of attaining the best possible health, given the individual's own type of diabetes, will allow the diabetic to live in peace with his disease. This means to integrate it into his daily activities and to be conscious, without frustration and anger, of what can and cannot be possible.

The person in the phase of Active Acceptance has experienced some successes in controlling his or her diabetes and, therefore, has developed some self-confidence in his or her ability to live with the disease. However, the individual's level of acceptance must be maintained, as in the daily training of a person who is attempting to maintain good physical condition. Keeping up a good level of acceptance is a dynamic, ongoing activity for the diabetic individual which requires the person to participate actively in the understanding and application of his or her personal treatment.

*Case Report*: ACCEPTANCE OF DIABETES MUST CONSTANTLY BE ACTIVATED

Mr. D. (55 years old, bank accountant; insulin-dependent diabetic for 25 years):

'I think of myself as an old hand at diabetes. My diabetes was discovered while I was in the Army. I very well remember how I was treated 25 years ago. There was very little time to give us any information. I was taught to give myself insulin injections and to understand the urine tests and the diet, but it was all extremely difficult'.

'Finally, the day of my release from hospital came; a day I well remember. I was frightened out of my wits at having to leave the hospital and manage on my own. Nothing could happen to me in hospital; I was safe there. Then my doctor took over and, although he was very kind to me, he was a very busy man. What helped me in the end to get a better understanding of the problems of diabetics was the *Diabetic's Journal*. I learned a lot from the *Journal* and would go so far as to say that it helped me accept my illness'.

'I was getting along not too badly until the day that I started vomiting after a great physical exertion. My diabetes had become seriously destabilized and I was admitted to hospital with ketoacidosis'.

'Then everything was allright again and I was doing not too badly when my doctor referred me to the Diabetic Unit. I thought I didn't need it because I was an old diabetic hand, but while in the Unit I realized that there are lots of little things, which make life easier, that I didn't know. Looking back, it seems that there have been a number of occasions where better knowledge of diabetes would have prevented many awkward situations. I feel more self-confident and more my own master. I think I have everything I need to take care of myself efficiently without always being directly dependent on a doctor'.

*Commentary*

Acceptance is never final. Several elements in what Mr. D. just said demonstrate that acceptance of diabetes is never final. It goes through positive and negative phases and several factors combine to create acceptance.

Right at the beginning of his illness, improvement of his physical state by treatment in the hospital enabled him to accept his disease at first. The doctor-patient relationship also helped, but was inadequate because the doctor had so little time. The information which he obtained from the *Diabetic's Journal*, increased his understanding; however, when his condition was destabilized, acceptance was in retreat. When the problems of diabetes were approached in the diabetic unit from a global perspective, a positive development (in terms of physical condition and relevant knowledge) is again seen.

216

*Pseudo-Acceptance*: RESIGNATION
'Now that I have diabetes, I'll just have to do what they say. There is nothing else I can do'.

Acceptance for the diabetic means that he or she must live dynamically with the disease rather than passively. This acceptance should not be confused with RESIGNATION. The resigned patients are apparently calm with the disease and seem to follow their medical prescription. It is because of this appearance that Resignation is often mistaken for Acceptance. Resignation appears at times to be Acceptance: 'I might just as well accept this'.

Resignation is failure to progress forward in the movement towards acceptance. The process of resignation commences at the stage of denial. When denial can no longer be maintained, the diabetic individual submits to a passive attitude and destiny instead of mobilizing his active aggressiveness as is done in the phases of Revolt, Bargaining, Internal Questioning/Depression, and Active Acceptance.

## CONCLUSIONS

Coping with a disease is a highly dynamic process. It goes through several difficult phases which are all protective mechanisms against the dramatic resentment of the individual who realizes the loss of his or her organic and psycho-social well-being. To learn about the stages of acceptance requires the physician to listen actively to the patient, because only the patient can explain his or her subjective inner turmoil. The integration of the stages of acceptance by the diabetic must be an essential goal of the therapeutic approach of the medical team. The success of patient education training therapy is highly dependent on how much of the chronic disease is accepted by the patient. A global approach, both biological and psychosocial, to the diabetic by the medical team requires the recognition of these dynamic stages of acceptance by the medical team.

Each stage requires another open attitude and support from the doctor/nurse/dietician whose therapeutic role is also to provide the stimulation which encourages the patient into a movement towards acceptance of the disease. Acceptance of the disease is the optimal stage in which the disease is integrated into the patient's daily life and the patient actively participates in the treatment of his or her diabetes.

## SUMMARY

The diabetic's personal experience with diabetes has to be considered by the medical team for a more efficient treatment of each patient who is learning to live with the daily demands of the disease. This feedback information from the patient can be obtained by listening during the medical consultation. However, an even better opportunity to get this feedback is during Round Table discussions among doctors/ nurses/dieticians and patients. These informal conversations allow the medical team to learn more systematically how patients live with their disease.

In studying tape-recorded Round Table discussions with patients, a sequence of developmental stages towards acceptance of the disease has been observed. 5 phases could arbitrarily be described in the process of accepting the disease after diagnosis of diabetes. The following sequence of phases has been identified:

1.  Denial: 'Why me, I do not understand'.
2.  Revolt: 'No, I do not have diabetes'.
3.  Bargaining: 'OK, I've got the disease, but I refuse to do all of this'.
4.  Depression-Inner Questioning: 'Will I be able to cope with it?'
5.  Active Acceptance: 'Even with this disease I can live an active life'.

Active Acceptance of a disease is a situation in which the disease is integrated into daily life in the best possible way. Thoughts of returning to the former state of perfect health are abandoned for a new intention of obtaining the best possible state of health with diabetes. The diabetic individual is then an active participant in the understanding and application of the treatment.

## REFERENCES

1.  Von Bertalanffy, L. (1968): *General System Therapy*, p. 428. Brazille, New York.
2.  Freud, S. (1917): Trauer und Melancholie. *Gesammelte Werke, Vol. 10.*
3.  Kübler-Ross, E. (1969): *On Death and Dying.* Macmillan, New York.
4.  Gfeller, R. and Assal, J.-Ph. (1980): The diabetic's subjective experience. In: *Folia Psychopractica.* Hoffman-La Roche, Basel.
5.  Assal, J.-Ph., Gfeller, R., Kreinhofer, M. (1981): Stades de l'acceptation du diabète. Leur interférence avec le traitement. Leur influence sur l'attitude de l'équipe soignante. In: *Journées de Diabétologie, de l'Hôtel Dieu*, p. 223.

## SUGGESTED READING

Balint, M. (1964): *The Doctor, his Patient and the Illness.* Pitman Medical, London.
Balint, M. and Balint, E. (1961): *Psychotherapeutic Techniques in Medicine.* Tavistock, London.
Groen, J.J. (1976): Die Psychosomatik der Diabetiker. In: Jores, A. (Ed.), *Praktische Psychosomatik*, p. 286. Huber, Bern, Stuttgart, Vienna.
Hollender, M. and Hollender, H. (1958): *The Psychology of Medical Practice.* Saunders, Philadelphia.
Watzlawick, P., Helmick-Beavin, J. and Jackson, D. (1967): *Pragmatics of Human Communication. A Study of International Problems, Pathologies and Paradoxes.* Norton, New York.

# 27. Psychological support and careful information at onset – the basis for future success in the self-management of diabetes

SVEN GUNNAR KARLANDER AND JOHNNY LUDVIGSSON

## EDITORIAL

*This paper stresses an extremely important point: although patient education and training are fundamental to efficient therapy, they are not always as effective as they could be for any given patient. Immediately following diagnosis, the psychological turmoil is often such that patients have little energy left to listen correctly and learn efficiently about their diabetes. It is important that the physician/nurse/dietician take this psychological 'background noise' into account and refrain from over-zealous educational programs, especially in newly diagnosed diabetics.*

*This paper also stresses the importance of careful selection of the appropriate time to inform and educate a patient. Just as insulin should be administered cautiously to a patient with high blood glucose and low potassium, so education should be administered with great skill, particularly to patients who are experiencing the personal difficulties accompanying the discovery of their diabetes or new complications which have arisen. (The editors.)*

## INTRODUCTION

Despite increasing interest in diabetes education, problems with education of newly-diagnosed diabetics have attracted only slight attention. This paper will be limited to general considerations based on our own experience and follow-up interviews with patients and parents during the first 2 years after onset [1]. We shall discuss the psychological implications of the diagnosis of diabetes and, in the light of this discussion, some aspects on reasonable goals for the initial education. Finally, we shall also touch briefly on the importance of an organized follow-up on the newly-diagnosed diabetic patients.

Let us first, however, look at a fictitious 'case report' in order to illustrate the difficulties from both the patient's and the physician's points of view.

219

'The doctor is ambitious. He has learnt that information is crucial. Within a day facts pour over the patient. The etiology and pathophysiology are explained in words that are simple and clear for the doctor, but unfortunately not for the patient. The nurse teaches how to give injections and a dietician gives the first lessons in what is forbidden, when to eat and what to eat. In a pause the social worker asks in what way the patient needs help with his job, economy, family, future. After a few days the patient is supposed to know. Soon he leaves the hospital expected to manage the most complicated treatment known in medicine. He is confused, afraid, thankful and disappointed, hopeful and depressed, totally dependent on help from the medical specialists. After some time he has stopped doing self-control at home as he thinks it is boring, reminding him of a disease he anyhow cannot get rid of or do anything about. The doctor does not get angry. This is the usual course for his patients. They never understand. They do not follow the prescriptions. They even cheat. For some peculiar reason these diabetics do not seem to understand what is best for them. But the doctor is extremely patient and helpful. He takes over the management, gives prescriptions which the patient follows now and then. The acute complications are cured. The patient believes that the doctor has saved his life, and the doctor gets almost the same feeling. He is satisfied. Some years later there are new hospital staffs and new ideas. The patient is revealed as ignorant and dependent. Re-education is necessary. The patient accepts unwillingly to satisfy the hospital staff. He listens with his ears but not with his brain. He has already heard this at the onset but his experience has shown something else. After re-education the patient gets better results when tested with a multiple-choice questionnaire. Everybody is happy, but the management of the patient's disease does not really change. The metabolic balance is bad. Finally the complications appear, exactly as he always knew they would. And everything is his own fault. The doctor and the medical staff have done everything they could, they believe. Unfortunately they could not do better'.

## PSYCHOLOGICAL IMPLICATIONS FOR THE DIAGNOSIS OF DIABETES

First, it must be borne in mind that diabetes may start in diverse ways in different patients. Especially from the medical point of view, there is a huge difference between the severely ill, ketoacidotic, often young patient with a sudden and dramatic onset and the subjectively healthy person in whom a slight glucosuria is discovered accidentally during a routine health control.

Nevertheless, there may be psychological similarities. It is considered that the diagnosis of diabetes gives rise to more anxiety than diagnosis of any other serious chronic illness [2]. Generally speaking, previously healthy persons may regard this diagnosis as the first clear evidence of their mortality [3]. In addition, there may be more specific problems, especially fear of the notorious, well-known complications: blindness, kidney failure and amputations in the lower extremities. To this will be added the burden of day-to-day management requiring, among other things, 'interminable diet restriction, which virtually eliminates many highly gratifying foods' [2].

Against this background it is not suprising that the diagnosis of diabetes may result in a state of psychological crisis [3]. During such a crisis, 4 different stages may be discerned. During the initial stage of shock, the patient denies what has happened. Life seems chaotic, and the patient is not receptive to information, although he may look calm superficially. This stage may continue for hours to days. Then there follows a stage of recognition. This is often characterized by feelings of guilt. This prepares for a third stage of objectivity where the patient gradually accepts and adapts to the new situation, and, eventually, a fourth stage or reintegration. Needless to say, in a given patient the development of stages may not be so distinct as described here. Relapses into previous stages are not uncommon. Nevertheless, it may be useful to recognize that a patient is not receptive to any form of education during the first stage. Rather, he should have an opportunity to express his fears and anxieties. It is not until the patient enters the third stage that he becomes accessible to instruction.

What has been said above about the grown-up patient is also true for the parents when a child gets diabetes, and we must not forget that even the adult is rarely quite alone, but has family members who may react in similar ways.

Ideally, initial approach to the newly-diagnosed diabetic must not be limited to the acute state of shock but should take into consideration 2 important later problems: the psychopathological development and patient noncompliance.

During the course of disease it is not unusual for diabetic patients to develop certain psychopathological traits. As summarized by Hauser and Pollets [2] it has been shown in several studies throughout the years that feelings of fear, specialness, inadequacy and depression are more common among diabetics than non-diabetics.

Finally, while patient noncompliance is a serious problem in any chronic illness [4], it is even more important in diabetic patients, who must assume the responsibility for their own management [5, 6]. According to studies using the Health Belief Model, compliance is dependent on patients' beliefs about their susceptibility to their disease and its perceived severity [7-10]. The complexity of the therapeutical regimen must also be considered, more complexity being associated with less compliance [4].

## INITIAL EDUCATION OF NEWLY-DIAGNOSED DIABETIC PATIENTS

In a discussion of educational goals one must distinguish between long-term and short-term objectives. In diabetes education the long-term objective is both an improved degree of diabetes control, brought about by increased knowledge, and an independent, motivated and confident patient [11]. Ultimately, this should result in a reduced risk of complications as well as in a high quality of life. On the other hand, the short-term objective is to teach the patients practical knowledge necessary for their daily management and subjective well-being. It is clear that the short-term objectives have to be reached in order to make the long-term goals possible. From what has been said above on the psychological aspects of the diagnosis of diabetes, it seems reasonable that initial education of the newly-diagnosed diabetic should mainly be concerned with short-term objectives.

From the psychological-emotional point of view the goal should be to relieve fear and anxiety rather than to teach a large amount of facts. The start of education should be unhurried. As mentioned above, the receptivity of the patient may be severely decreased, due to both metabolic derangement and psychological shock. It may be wise to start by listening to the patient instead of briskly imposing 'education'. When the patient has left the early stages of shock, the opportunity should be taken to reassure him. Without going into any details on pathogenesis or the development of late complications it is important at this stage to tell him that good metabolic control will reduce the risk of complications and that diabetes is compatible with a (near) normal life. Remembering the determinants of compliance, this is not to say that the difficulties of being a diabetic should be underestimated, but rather that in this early phase of disease the emphasis should be on reassurance. It is undoubtedly of great value to the newly-diagnosed patient to have an opportunity to meet fellow-diabetics with a few years' duration. This would reduce feelings of fear and uniqueness and enable the newly-diagnosed patients to profit from the experience of the older patients.

As for practical matters, the goal should be limited to making the patient able to manage his own treatment during the first weeks of disease [12]. The need for instruction will depend on factors like type of diabetes, age of the patient, etc. Generally speaking, education should be very simple and down-to-earth. Insulin-requiring patients must be able, psychologically as well as practically, to handle the syringe and to recognize symptoms of hyper- and hypoglycemia. In addition, they should know how to perform tests for blood and for urinary glucose and how to interpret the results.

For overweight type II diabetic patients the paramount importance of weight reduction should probably be emphasized from the beginning, even if a detailed dietary counselling is less advisable during the initial phase.

In summary, we suggest that, apart from the fundamental instruction mentioned above, initial education should rather be a question of psychological approach than education proper. This can always be postponed until the patient had adapted to his disease and is ready to enter a conventional teaching programme. It may be suitable to start on such a programme either during the last days of the first hospital period or shortly thereafter to take advantage of the early motivation. This brings us to the question of follow-up. Because of the great differences in conditions, traditions and practice that exist between various clinics, we shall limit ourselves to some general considerations.

Our warnings against over-zealous education of the newly-diagnosed diabetics presuppose that the patients can be included into an education programme in due time after diagnosis. Education itself should be integrated not only into medical care but also go hand-in-hand with social measures, possibilities to have telephone counselling, etc. [13, 14]. As with all chronic illness, it is important to have continuity among the personnel caring for the patients. Since diabetic patients are prone to have psychological problems and even may relapse into their initial state of crisis [3], it is of great value for them to get acquainted to a certain physician, nurse, etc. Among other things, this will also tend to reduce the number of ambiguous prescriptions as well as the complexity of the regimen and thus work towards better patient compliance.

# REFERENCES

1. Ludvigsson, J., Richt, B. and Svensson, P.G.: The family's experience of the initial care when their child got diabetes. In preparation.
2. Hauser, S.T. and Pollets, S. (1979): Psychological aspects of diabetes mellitus: a critical review. *Diabetes Care*, 2, 227.
3. Kimball, P.C. (1971): Emotional and psychosocial aspects of diabetes mellitus. *Med. Clin. North Am.*, 55, 1007.
4. Gillum, R.F. and Barsky, A.J. (1974): Diagnosis and management of patient noncompliance. *J. Am. Med. Assoc.*, 228, 1563.
5. Koski, M.L. (1969): The coping processes in childhood diabetes. *Acta Paediatr. Scand., Suppl. 198*.
6. Partridge, J.W., Garner, A.M., Thompson, C.W. and Cherry, T. (1972): Attitudes of adolescents towards their diabetes. *Am. J. Dis. Child.*, 124, 226.
7. Kirscht, J.P. and Rosenstock, I.M. (1977): Patient adherence to antihypertensive medical regimens. *J. Commun. Health*, 3, 115.
8. Alogna, M. (1980): Perception of severity of disease and health locus of control in compliant and noncompliant diabetic patients. *Diabetes Care*, 3, 533.
9. Bloom Cerkoney, K.A. and Hart, L.K. (1980): The relationship between the health belief model and compliance of persons with diabetes mellitus. *Diabetes Care*, 3, 594.
10. Ludvigsson, J., Richt, B. and Svensson, P.G. (1980): Compliance and the Health Belief Model – relevance to the treatment of juvenile diabetes mellitus. *Scand. J. Soc. Med., Suppl. 18*, 57.
11. Kelman, H.C. (1958): Compliance, identification and internalization. *J. Conflict Resolution*, 2, 51.
12. Freedman, J.L. and Fraser, S.C. (1966): Compliance without pressure: the foot-in-the-door technique. *J. Pers. Soc. Psychol.*, 4, 195.
13. Miller, L.V. and Goldstein, J. (1972): More efficient care of diabetic patients in a county-hospital setting. *N. Engl. J. Med.*, 26, 1388.
14. Graber, A.L., Christman, B.G., Alogna, M.T. and Davidson, J.K. (1977): Evaluation of diabetes patient-education programs. *Diabetes*, 26, 61.

# 28. How to listen better to patients

H.E.PELSER AND J.J. GROEN

## EDITORIAL

*In long-standing diseases the patient has as much a role to play with his physician in the control of his disease, as his physician has with another member of the medical team. This doctor-patient cooperation in the treatment of the disease requires certain strategies and skills. Group dynamics is one way in which a real dialogue can be introduced between the health care personnel and the patient. The patients also might play an important role among themselves and for themselves. The experience of Doctor Pelser and Professor Groen show that internists, not usually trained in this dimension, can develop a system which can be of great importance in the efficiency of treatment and the well-being of the patient. (The editors.)*

## INTRODUCTION

Many doctors underestimate the emotional burden placed not only on the diabetic patient, but also on his entourage, each of whom has to come to terms with the restrictions of freedom necessary for the effective treatment of his diabetes. These doctors seldom seem to appreciate what it means to have to eat the same amount of food at fixed hours each day; to keep up a constant expenditure of energy from day to day; and to self-administer insulin injections once or twice daily, and sometimes more frequently. And all this for the rest of one's life! They do not seem to comprehend how frightening it is to slip into hypoglycemia, or to live in constant fear of late complications with the dreadful consequences of endless suffering, the possibility of becoming a cripple, or having one's children develop diabetes, too. The patient might equally be concerned about the possibility of losing his job or being rejected for another one because of his disease. These are just a few of the multitude of difficulties with which most diabetic patients are likely to be confronted and have to learn to cope.

## THE DOCTOR'S ATTITUDE

Some physicians argue that these problems are not their concern. The doctor's task is to diagnose the disease correctly and prescribe the proper treatment. It is the patient's responsibility to follow the advice given. Is it really fair for a doctor to hold his patient responsible for the results of his treatment? Since evidence is accumulating that late complications of diabetes can be delayed, if not prevented, by maintaining the blood sugar level within physiological limits, no physician should be satisfied any longer with the kind of diabetic control that the majority of patients have. Good diabetic control cannot be accomplished by the doctor himself; full and active cooperation is therefore mandatory. To this end the doctor must establish a working alliance with his patient which, for best results, has to be based on the *mutual* exchange of information, understanding, and respect.

## THE PATIENT'S EDUCATION

In the teaching process, doctors, nurses, and dieticians usually tell a patient what he or she may or may not do. This approach is currently described as 'the education of the patient'. At first, the rules for the treatment of diabetes do not seem difficult to learn and to follow. Yet one is increasingly alarmed by the many patients, intelligent enough to understand, who still fail to follow these rules. For some reason the patients don't realize that in doing so they expose themselves unnecessarily to the risk of developing late complications. Some diabetologists attribute the poor results of the patients' 'education' to a 'lack of compliance', which again suggests that the doctor holds the patient responsible if the cooperation between the two does not function properly.

The scientific study of education, as a form of human communication, has recently contributed to a better comprehension of the *psychodynamic aspects of the teaching-learning process*. What goes on between educator and pupil, or similarly between doctor and patient, actually is a form of cooperative communication in which *both* partners, be it in different ways, are active. Each of them fulfils his own function which stimulates the other to behave in a certain way. It is only when both fulfil their functions in an optimum way that the learning process can proceed step by step towards results which meet their mutual expectations. In this form of human relationship, the two partners form a unity of cooperation towards a common goal (*identification*) and, in their communication, each fulfils his own role which complements the function of the other (*mutual differentiation*). As the process of education and development proceeds, the pupil becomes more 'independent', the degree and type of leadership and dominance of the educator and doctor in the process decreases and the initiative, responsibility, and self-reliance of the pupil (or patient) increases. In this way a situation can be achieved in which doctor and patient are two experts, working together in the treatment of the latter.

Another important aspect of the teacher-pupil or *doctor-patient educational communication is that it involves both intellectual and emotional fea-*

*tures*. Education and teaching are not only concerned with the transfer of knowledge or the acquisition of skills, but also with the establishment of certain emotional attitudes between the two partners in their cooperation. There is a need for mutual confidence in that both are pursuing the very same goal, and there is the gratification of the educator (or doctor/nurse/ dietician) when the pupil (or patient) responds to the teaching by unexpected behavior and vice versa. These are essential elements in the teacher-learner relationship. The establishment of this intellectual and emotional relationship is furthermore encouraged by the consistency, regularity, and predictability of their mutual behavior and by the observance of certain optimum conditions of time, frequency, and spatial distance in their educational communication. Also, since every student or patient has his own personality, the best results are achieved by an educator who is capable of adapting his or her approach to the individual wishes, requirements, and circumstances of each student or patient.

If we now return to our 'non-compliant' patients, we may recognize that they have been taught (if at all) the rules of their treatment by the usual one-sided intellectual, formal method. This may be why many of these patients do not appear able to use their knowledge of diabetes for the control of their disease. The limitations of the unidirectional teaching method might help us to understand the connection between the 'so-called' intractability of patients with 'brittle' diabetes and their emotional instability inducing them to alternate between overeating and inadequate doses of insulin. Glycosylated hemoglobin determinations confirm that many patients only control themselves carefully during the week or few days prior to their appointment with the diabetologist, but live in more or less severe states of maladjustment the rest of the time.

Due to this therapeutically alarming situation and the threat of late complications, the time has come to ask ourselves critically in what way the methods we commonly use for the education of diabetic patients can be improved. What may be needed for better results are new attitudes by both patients and students. Just as in the modern methods of teaching pupils and students, the newer forms of education of patients have to take into account both the intellectual and emotional aspects of what it means to have diabetes and to lead a diabetic life.

## THE GROUP APPROACH

In searching for better forms of education, it is worth noting that in every culture an important part of the development of attitudes, motivations, skills, and behavior, especially those which prepare the individual for later social communication, takes place in groups. Therefore a group, and by that we mean a *limited number of people in close proximity who are sharing one or more goals*, seems to provide the most 'natural' setting for an educational communication in which intellectual and emotional aspects receive equal attention. Actually, in recent years several methods have been developed to make use of group processes for the regulation and the modification of attitudes and behavior of the participants.

In 1974 we started a pilot project on group discussions with diabetic patients. The main experiences and observations relevant to the patients' behavior and motivation with regard to the control and acceptance of their disease can be summarized as follows:

1.   In each group the subjects, which were discussed spontaneously, were remarkably similar and dealt equally with technical knowledge of diabetes, its complications, and treatment and with the emotional problems of the participants. Most of these problems were concerned with *ambivalent, interhuman relationships between the patients and key-figures*, i.e. parents (especially in the case of young patients, their mothers), marriage partners, and, in many cases, the treating physician. Many patients complained that their doctors were mainly interested in their urine and blood sugar levels and apparently had no time to consider the difficulties of living with diabetes. Almost all patients had gone through far more periods of depression, despair, inner protest, episodes of 'cheating' and non-cooperation than they had discussed with anyone, least of all their doctors.

2.   Several juvenile diabetics, feeling misunderstood as they were unable to discuss their emotional problems within the family, developed *different forms of protest behavior*, e.g. refusing to test their urine or refusing to adhere to their diet. Others felt lonely or depressed and sometimes 'forgot' to eat after having injected insulin. The result was that they went into severe hypoglycemia. At other times they indulged in bouts of eating sweets in order to 'feel better'.

3.   Sooner or later the *fear of late complications*, especially retinopathy, came up in the discussions and then inevitably the question was raised as to whether they could or could not be prevented. The affirmative response from the medical group leader repeatedly provoked very emotional discussions and opposition, especially from the younger group members. In their view the requirement of maintaining the blood sugar level within physiological limits based on a regular diet, the adjusted use of insulin, exercise, and emotional stability would impose a heavy burden on them and only inflict guilt feelings as late complications would occur anyhow no matter how hard they tried. They blamed the group leader for his lack of understanding both in their efforts to regulate themselves as well as possible and in their despair when they did not succeed. In short, it became obvious that many patients, as long as they felt unhappy and inwardly hated their disease, could not possibly attain the equilibrium and motivated concentration necessary to learn how to handle and control their disability.

4.   The group discussions with fellow-patients gave the participants the opportunity to *exteriorize their feelings and talk freely* and at the same time deal with technical problems of diabetes, its complications, and treatment.

By discussing both the nature of these complications and the anxiety surrounding them with the safe and supporting 'togetherness' of the group, the patients were able to help each other to develop more rational attitudes than when these conditions and associated emotions had been either avoided or insufficiently expressed in the previous talks they had had with their physicians. In addition, the patients learned to talk more freely about their emotions in general as well as with their doctors and spouses which, in a number of cases, contributed to an improved relationship both within the family and with physicians. It seemed as if this group education also contributed to the patients' conscious acceptance of the disease and the rules for keeping it under control because it applied the combined discussion of the cognitive aspects with the emotional approach of the problems of the disease, and provided mutual understanding and support.

## FURTHER DEVELOPMENTS OF THE GROUP APPROACH

After 15 to 18 months of weekly group sessions with a remarkable high attendance rate, the participants unanimously expressed their opinion that the group discussions were more valuable than any form of instruction or guidance they had known before with respect to the increase in knowledge about diabetes and the emotional support they had derived from these sessions. They also unanimously agreed that this group approach was a superior form of education and should become available to all diabetic patients. When they realized that this would require a considerable number of group leaders with both sufficient knowledge of diabetes and experience in conducting group discussions and that this combination of capacities is seldom found, most of them agreed to the suggestion from their former group leaders that they themselves could be trained to conduct group discussion with fellow patients.

Coincidentally, a small number of general practitioners and students in medicine and psychology had expressed their interest in becoming involved in a training course for conducting group discussions like ours. We then suggested setting up a joint training course for doctors, students, and patients; all prospective participants readily agreed. Three groups were formed, each consisting of 6 patients, 2-3 doctors and 1 or 2 students, who met weekly. Each group was led by the same instructor (J.J. Groen, H.E. Pelser and H. van Dis) during 7 consecutive sessions, which were followed by a meeting of the 3 groups. The instructors then switched groups for another 7 consecutive sessions whereafter the procedure was repeated. Each session lasted for about 2 hours: the first was taken up by a regular group discussion followed by a discussion of its psychodynamic aspects using the 'Metaplan method' (see Chapter 24). In later stages, the participants took turns in fulfilling the roles of group leader or observer in the discussions.

In the general meetings the participants exchanged their experiences of the previous training period and together evaluated what they had learned. Two additional general meetings were inserted for formal lectures; one on the technical aspects of diabetes and one on group dynamics. Thus, the training course consisted of 24 weekly sessions. During the last session the participants discussed the question of who felt confident enough to act as group leader or observer in a new discussion group with diabetic patients. It appeared that those patients who trusted themselves to fulfil one or the other of these roles were also considered capable to do so both by their fellow group members and by the 3 instructors.

In the next phase of this project these newly trained participants formed 'duos' consisting of a group leader and an observer who started new discussion groups with diabetic patients. Nine groups were formed, comprising 73 diabetic patients. Four 'duos' were diabetic patients, 3 duos consisted of a doctor and a patient, one 'duo' consisted of 2 students, and one couple was formed by one of the instructors (H. van Dis) and a student of psychology.

Once a month these group leaders and their observers met with one of the instructors for a supervision session to discuss their experiences and the problems raised in their respective groups. In this way continuity and consistency are secured and the motivation of the patients maintained.


## RECOMMENDATIONS

Group discussions are now widely used for a great variety of problems and purposes, but also in various ways of the set-up, frequency, duration, and method of conduct. This makes it difficult to evaluate or compare the results of discussion groups whose working conditions are different or ill-defined. Moreover, it appears that the working conditions of every discussion group, in order to achieve optimum results, have to be adapted to the specific problems and goals of the participants. On the basis of our experiences in long-term group discussions with medical patients, we suggest the following guidelines for starting a discussion group with diabetic patients:

1. *Setting the goal for the group*
Every prospective participant should be able to subscribe to the goal of the group. If this goal is formulated too specifically or too ambitiously, it is liable to restrict the number of candidates for participation. The following formula appears to be both suitable for the functioning of the group and acceptable to most diabetic patients: 'To offer diabetic patients the opportunity to meet, under the guidance of experts, in order to discuss not only difficulties associated with having diabetes, but also general problems of life'.

## 2. *The number of participants*

In order for small discussion groups to function effectively the number of participants should not be more than 10 and not be less than about 6, excluding the group leader and observer. Within these limits the group leader can not only give every participant the opportunity to express his views or feelings, but he can also deal with a variety of (sometimes conflicting) opinions to ensure purposeful group interactions.

## 3. *The homogeneity of the group*

Participants in a discussion group should have one or more problems in common, in order to be able to identify with each other. Variety of age, sex, social class, marital status and duration of diabetes among the participants, however, allows for a greater range of the different aspects of diabetes to be discussed. Although non-insulin dependent patients tend to feel left out when insulin dependent participants are involved in lengthy discussions on insulin injections or hypoglycemia, a mixed group of participants usually learn more about diabetes, and are stimulated to maintain a better control of their condition.

## 4. *The frequency of group discussions*

Group cohesion is fostered through weekly sessions. An important feature of a discussion group with diabetic patients is the favorable setting it provides for interactional learning through furthering the exchange of both cognitive information and emotional experience among participants. The development of this essential group interaction is again furthered by the regularity and frequency with which the participants meet for discussions. Because of other commitments, however, most prospective participants are usually unable to attend group sessions more than once a week, except perhaps for in-patients in a hospital or in a diabetes education centre.

## 5. *The duration of a group session*

Group discussions in which equal attention is devoted to the cognitive and emotional aspects of having diabetes and its consequences require at least 90 minutes. However, the group session usually calls for about 2 hours because most groups seem to appreciate having a social chat together over coffee either before they actually start with their discussions or during a prearranged break.

## 6. *The number of group sessions*

It usually takes a discussion group about 7 sessions to develop sufficient cohesion and sense of security to allow participants to disclose their personal life situations and to feel free to share their feelings. With some participants, however, this development of interaction creates ambivalent feelings and they have doubts on whether to continue to attend the group sessions. In order to ensure an uninterrupted group evolution it is important that these feelings are duly recognized by the group leader and are discussed openly within the group. It then often appears that the ambivalent feelings are partly due to environmental reactions in response to the group member's change in attitude or behavior induced by his or her participation in the group discussions. Furthermore, it appears in most groups to take about 20 to 25 sessions before participants begin to develop a more rational attitude towards having diabetes and the consequences thereof. This is a prerequisite for working seriously to improve their diabetic control.

### 7. *How to structure the first group session*

The aim of the first meeting of the group leader and the prospective participants is to agree on the establishment of the group and its procedures. The following structure has shown to be effective:

a. after introducing himself and the observer, the group leader invites the participants one by one to state what their expectations are for this first meeting;

b. after summarizing these expectations, the group leader outlines his objectives for the group;

c. he then invites the participants *as a group* to give their comments on his suggestions, thereby initiating naturally the first group discussion, in which the personal problems of several participants are likely to be touched;

d. after summing up this discussion, the group leader points out to the participants that they have just been engaged in a group activity and that this kind of discussion obviously calls for the observance of a few rules, i.e. regular attendance, sincerity between each other, and discretion towards non-group members about personal disclosures made within the group.

This schedule can be completed within 90 minutes and its result is quite predictable if the group leader keeps strictly to the above sequence. He should however emphasize at the end that this will be the only session in which the structure of the discussion will have been imposed on the group by the leader.

### 8. *Prerequisites for the group leader*

In order to be able to moderate successfully a discussion group with diabetic patients, the group leader should have both sufficient knowledge of diabetes and its treatment as well as sufficient training in the skill of animating group discussions.

### 9. *The goal of the group leader*

In an effort to improve cognitive understanding of the disease and its treatment and to assist the diabetic in the process leading to acceptance, group dynamics are used by the group leader. His aim is *to motivate the participants so that they maintain optimum metabolic control* of their diabetes.

Ultimately the hope is that the participants will learn to cope with all the difficulties inherent to their diabetes.

10. *The functions of the group leader*
They are numerous. The most important are:
a. *to leave the group freedom* in order to determine its own course of action and evolution, both in the choice of subjects and the pace at which topics are dealt with in their discussion, and to ensure that every member is given the opportunity to fully express himself;
b. *to speak as little as possible* and, above all, to avoid interrupting the participants when they are communicating themselves as a group;
c. *not to respond immediately* when questioned by an individual member, but to look around the group asking – 'What do you think of this?'. This should enable as many participants as possible to formulate their own ideas and express them freely, thereby maximizing stimulation of the group's activity. Only when the entire group wants an answer from the group leader should he give his opinion frankly and honestly, taking care to speak as briefly as possible and to avoid a monolog;
d. to emphasize, on appropriate occasions, that *each member is free to express his or her views* on any subject frankly and honestly and that these views will be discussed, accepted, or contradicted. Furthermore, it is functional to point out that the freedom to discuss personal views and personal life situations is best guaranteed if what is being discussed within the group is regarded by all members as confidential and not something to be divulged outside the group;
e. to use opportunities to express that he *appreciates criticism directed against himself* as a token of confidence and will regard it as inspired only by the intention to achieve the common goal, i.e. improvement of the quality of life of the diabetic. In the same vein, the group leader should accept any criticism by the group of physicians, hospitals, the government etc., as well as emotional expressions of self-pity, self-accusation or, occasionally, a crying spell.
f. to pay as much attention to those group members who primarily want technical or scientific information about diabetes as to those who want to speak and hear more about the emotional problems of having to live with diabetes. Thus the group leader will try to guide the group towards *shared awareness of the equal importance of both these biological and emotional aspects* of the disease.
g. to *exercise tolerance*, rather than to resort to intervention, when the group spends a lot of time on seemingly irrelevant subjects. Sooner or later an initiative towards further evolution will come from the group itself. Occasionally certain symbolic expressions, defence mechanisms, silent periods in the discussions, or transference situations call for a cautious intervention, preferably in the later stages of the group's development.

## 11.  *The function of the observer*

Animating a discussion group is a demanding effort, both mentally and emotionally, as it requires unremitting attentiveness and empathy towards various aspects of the discussion and interaction among the group members, as well as between the group and oneself. In this complex task an observer can be of great help by watching the group's activity, making notes and assisting the group leader in evaluating both the group's dynamical evolution and the functioning and attitude of the moderator.

## 12.  *The dissolution of the group*

For most participants the long-term discussion group becomes a special environment where they learn more about diabetes and themselves. It is very likely that they will become attached to the group because of the mutual understanding and support with which it provides them. Therefore the group members should have the opportunity to prepare themselves emotionally for the separation experience through 'goodbye discussions' in the last few sessions before the dissolution of the group. In these sessions the discussion is usually centred around an evaluation of what the group discussions have meant to the participants, e.g. contributing to their knowledge of diabetes and providing emotional and moral support for the problems they face in having to live with their diabetes. Feelings of sadness about the approaching end of the group are usually expressed and, most of the time, the group members spontaneously arrange amongst themselves to have reunions in the future.

## CONCLUSIONS

1.   Long-term group discussions with diabetic patients were considered by all participants as a valuable form of education. It enabled them to learn more about both diabetes and its treatment than any other form of instruction or guidance. It also helped the participants to cope better with the difficulties involved in living with diabetes by developing a more rational attitude towards the illness and consciously accepting the restrictions necessary for its optimal control.

2.   These group experiences apparently motivated many participants to engage themselves actively in an endeavour to make the group approach in diabetes education available to their fellow-patients. Together with doctors and a number of students in medicine and psychology, they undertook a training course in order to become group leaders and observers themselves and started new discussion groups with diabetic patients under the supervision of their professional instructors.

3.   In these 'tertiary' groups, which were conducted by 2 diabetic patients or by a 'duo' of a doctor and a patient (who had himself experienced the same training), the same subjects were spontaneously discussed as in the

'primary' groups and a high attendance rate was maintained. The participants expressed the same satisfaction with this form of diabetes education at the end of the group sessions. These sessions were usually continued for a year's time on a weekly basis. Several of the participants in the tertiary groups also applied for a training course in order to become group leaders and observers themselves for the new discussion groups with diabetic patients.

4.   The joint discussion group experiences of family doctors and patients encouraged doctors, on the one hand, to increase their knowledge of diabetes and its treatment and to undertake themselves the management of their insulin-dependent patients, rather than refer them to diabetologists as had been their normal practice. They also noted that they developed a more understanding attitude towards their patients in general. The patients, on the other hand, learned to appreciate that doctors find it difficult to deal with patients to whom they can offer no cure, especially when these patients do not take the initiative to talk about their emotional problems. Some patients noted that this training group experience enabled them to improve the relationship with their own doctors.

## SUMMARY

Increasing evidence is accumulating to show that consistent maintenance of blood sugar levels within physiological limits contributes to the prevention, on the one hand, of late complications in diabetic patients and, on the other, the recognition that this can only be achieved with the active cooperation of an adequately informed and motivated patient. In consequence, more emphasis is now being placed on the importance of patient education. The growing awareness amongst diabetologists is, however, that of these insulin dependent patients who are precisely most liable to develop late complications, only a minority appear able to adhere to the rules of their treatment, even if they have sufficient knowledge of diabetes. This calls for critical reflections on the effectiveness of the methods commonly used in the education of these patients.

The authors' experiences from long-term group discussions with diabetic patients suggest that this group approach may produce better educational results than the classical vertical teaching. It enables the participants (doctors and patients) to devote equal attention both to the technical aspect of diabetes control and to the emotional aspects of the patient himself.

## RECOMMENDED LITERATURE

1. Anderson, C.M., Meisel, S.S. and Houpt, J.L. (1975): Training former patients as task-group leaders. *Int. J. Group Psychother.* 25, 32.
2. Barendregt, J.T. (1957): A psychological investigation of the effect of group psychotherapy in patients with bronchial asthma. *J. Psychosom. Res. 2*, 115.

3. Berger, I.L. (1978): Presidential Address: group psychotherapy today – ideologies and issues. *Int. J. Group Psychother. 28*, 307.
4. Berger, M.M. (1974): The impact of the therapist's personality on group process. *Am. J. Psychoanal., 34*, 213.
5. Cunningham, J., Strassberg, D. and Roback, H. (1978): Group psychotherapy for medical patients. *Compr. Psychiatry, 19*, 135.
6. Ford, C.V. and Long, K.D. (1977): Group psychotherapy of somatizing patients. *Psychother. Psychosom., 28*, 294.
7. Frank, J.D. (1975): Group psychotherapy research 25 years later. *Int. J. Group Psychother., 25*, 159.
8. Groen, J.J. and Pelser, H.E. (1960): Experiences with group psychotherapy in patients with bronchial asthma. *J. Psychosom. Res., 4*, 191.
9. Groen, J.J., Pelser, H.E., Stuyling de Lange, M.J. and Dix, P.G. (1979): Group discussions with diabetic patients and their families. *Pediatr. Adolescent Endocrinol., 7*, 164.
10. Groen, J.J. and Pelser, H.E. (1982): Newer concepts of teaching, learning and education and their application to the patient-doctor cooperation in the treatment of diabetes mellitus. *Pediatr. Adolescent Endocrinol., 10*, 168.
11. Pelser, H.E., Groen, J.J., Stuyling de Lange, M.J. and Dix, P.G. (1979): Experiences in group discussions with diabetic patients. *Psychother. Psychosom., 32*, 257.
12. McGee, T.E. (1974): The triadic approach to supervision in group psychotherapy. *Int. J. Group Psychother., 24*, 471.
13. MacLennan, B.W. (1975): The personalities of group leaders: implications for selection and training. *Int. J. Group Psychother., 25*, 177.
14. Reddy, W.B. and Lansky, L.M. (1974): The group psychotherapy literature: 1973. *Int. J. Group Psychother., 24*, 477.
15. Roberts, J.P. (1977): The problems of group psychotherapy for psychosomatic patients. *Psychother. Psychosom., 28*, 305.
16. Roman, M. and Porter, K. (1978): Combining experiential and didactic aspects in a new group therapy training approach. *Int. J. Group Psychother., 28*, 371.
17. Rosin, A.J. (1975): Group discussions: a therapeutic tool in a chronic diseases hospital. *Geriatrics, 30*, 45.
18. Sata, L.S. (1974): Group methods, the volunteer and the paraprofessional. *Int. J. Group Psychother., 24*, 400.
19. Sclare, A.B. and Crocket, J.A. (1957): Group psychotherapy in bronchial asthma. *J. Psychosom. Res., 2*, 157.
20. Skinner, B.F. (1968): *Technology of Teaching.* Appleton-Century-Crofts, New York.
21. Slavson, S.R. (1975): Current trends in group psychotherapy. *Int. J. Group Psychother., 25*, 131.
22. Stone, W.N. (1975): Dynamics of the recorder-observer in group psychotherapy. *Compr. Psychiatry, 16*, 49.
23. Vygotsky, L.V. (1978): *Mind in Society.* Harvard University Press, Cambridge.
24. Yalom, I.D. (1975): *Theory and Practice of Group Psychotherapy.* Basic Books, New York.

# 29.   ACTIVE LISTENING: How to make sure that what we heard was what the patient really meant

A. LACROIX AND J.-Ph. ASSAL

## EDITORIAL

*This paper is based on the assumption that a working dialog – an honest exchange of information based on demonstrating mutual respect – must exist between any health care professional and his patient to achieve maximum success in the management of a chronic disease. This requires physicians, nurses and dieticians to discern the various emotions behind patients' statements as well as the medical information in the message. To be able to achieve this level of sensitivity, the total individual patient must be considered in a scrupulous manner.*

*To create a real dialog with a patient, the medical professional must be aware of the effect produced by his or her words on the patient. Most medical care providers, who are often rushed as well as concerned about their patients, are unaware that their replies to the questions and statements of patients create feelings of anxiety, confusion and intimidation. These patient reactions then restrict the quality and quantity of information and true feelings which the patients want to share. This, in turn, decreases patients' possibilities of understanding and compliance. It is therefore crucial for the medical care provider to observe what type of reply he or she normally chooses in a given situation and what resulting emotional reaction it produces in the patient. (The editors.)*

## I.   THERE IS NO THERAPY WITHOUT DIALOG

Sooner or later every medical care provider discovers that, in addition to the cases and professional situations which can be solved by his scientific knowledge, there are problems for which he or she is not prepared. These problems include questions related not only to an illness, but also to the patient's attitude towards illness. This leads to the consideration of how the patient lives with illness; whether he or she is adjusted to it or rejects it. This approach, which can be termed 'global' as it requires consideration of the patient's emotional as well as physical being, is not only legitimate, but in fact indispensable in many situations. This is particularly true when the illness is chronic and irreversible with possible complications which may be very serious in the long or even in the short term.

Medical training is dominated by scientific, organic perspectives and hardly prepares the physician to face the personal interrelationships of doctor-patient and patient-illness. The doctor intends to treat, but the effects are rarely commensurate with the efforts exerted to persuade, caution, reassure, teach...

The doctor acts not only on the basis of his acquired knowledge, but also in the light of his own personality, character, values and the authority which he represents. The kind of relationship which results is unidirectional, with most of the information going from doctor to patient and little or no patient-initiated information returning to the doctor. This does not help the patient-doctor dialog. It is incumbent on the doctor to adopt an attitude that enables the patient to feel sufficiently accepted as a person to permit real doctor-patient and patient-doctor communication.

Messages from patients are not always clear. The doctor's attitude needs to encourage feelings of acceptance even when the patients' messages may be concealed in all sorts of statements which are difficult to understand; for patients, like all of us, have feelings which they do not express directly. Even when the doctor receives the message it is not enough for him merely to identify the problem. He or she must know how to react, what to say and how to say it. In other words, what the patient says must not only be understood by the doctor, but it is also necessary for the doctor to answer in a way that helps the dialog to continue and assists the patient in the expression of what he feels (his fears, his wishes ...).

'Active Listening' is a positive attitude adopted by the listener. It implies an effort by the listener (doctor) to decode and understand messages which are often poorly or unskillfully expressed by the speaker (patient). How frequently have we experienced the maddening question, 'By the way, doctor, what do you think ...' as the patient leaves the surgery or the consulting room? Such questions are often the result of how poorly doctors have previously listened to their patients.

## II. SPONTANEOUS REPLIES OR LACK OF COMMUNICATION: NOT BEING 'ON THE SAME WAVELENGTH'

Whether a medical professional is talking with a colleague or a patient, he answers in a way which is his own. It is to be expected that the individual's answer will depend upon the question asked, the problem presented, the timing or the person asking the question. Whether or not the doctor is sympathetic to the questioning patient or feels a risk – and with patients there is always an element of risk – affects the answer. However, independent of all these variables, all medical professionals have a personal style and this unconsciously reflects a whole range of ideas, principles, opinions and feelings towards the patient which collectively will influence the manner of the medical person's reply. All the elements which combine to produce the reply can be called total attitude.

Are there as many styles and as many attitudes as there are people? Studies and observations made in this field have shown that the attitudes of responders are not unlimited in number. While there are shades of meanings and while each person has his own style, there are 8 categories of responses which reflect 8 possible kinds of attitudes. These different attitudes are described below, with the examples from the responses of Matthew's father.

Matthew comes home from school on his bicycle and at lunch he says, 'Dad, all my friends have a motorcycle...' Matthew's father could then express different attitudes towards his son through 8 possible categories of responses:

| *ATTITUDES EXPRESSED* | *CATEGORIES OF RESPONSES* |
|---|---|
| 1. Judgment | 'At your age I didn't even have a bicycle. It is much healthier to cycle ...' |
| 2. Interpretation (analysis of imagined causes) | 'I bet you have already spoken to your mother ... and that she agrees' |
| 3. Support (emotional reassurance) | 'You know we all have lots of fleeting wishes – me too' |
| 4. Interrogation | (Father) 'Do tell me, does your friend, John, have a motorcycle?' (Matthew) 'Yes.' (Father) 'Emmanuelle does not have one, I know this. Do Sylvain and Patrick have one?' |
| 5. Rapid solution for immediate application | 'Well, for the time being you can use my old scooter which is in the garage ...' |
| 6. Information – teaching | 'You must know that the 47 muscles we have in each leg have some purpose. The trouble is that if we do not use them they waste rapidly. Do you remeber when you broke your leg ...' |
| 7. Avoidance | 'By the way, have you done your Latin homework for tomorrow?' |
| 8. Reformulation – comprehension (reformulation of the question) | 'If I understand you correctly, all your friends have a motorcycle ...' |

**Why is it important to know these different attitudes?**

In the first place it is important to understand that each of us spontaneously and unconsciously adopts only 2 or 3 of these attitudes. Some of us have the habit of simplifying, others of moralizing and others still of investigating. Depending on the situation, some of these attitudes may be frankly inappropriate.

Secondly, knowledge of these different attitudes should not only enable a judicious choice of reply, but should avoid the emotional blocks in listeners caused by the unconscious use of these attitudes. The following example comes from a situation specific to the care of diabetics. It is accompanied by comments describing the characteristics of the attitude of each reply and the effects produced by the interviewer.

The diabetic patient being considered had a fasting blood sugar that was constantly elevated, but with episodes of hypoglycemia in the late afternoons. It was recommended to the patient to take a second injection of insulin at bedtime and to lower the morning dose. The patient replied to the physician: *'I will not have a second injection. You lied to me by promising that I only had to take a single daily injection and I know that having 2 injections means that my diabetes is worse'*.

**Answers of the physician to the patient**

1. *Judgment*
'It is not by rebelling against your treatment that you will achieve better control of your diabetes'.
2. *Interpretation (analysis of imagined causes)*
'You have no confidence in what has been prescribed for you and you think that you have been misled'.
3. *Support (reassurance, simplification)*
'Do not get into such a state; it is not such a major point'.
4. *Interrogation*
'Tell me who has said that having 2 injections means the diabetes is more severe'.
5. *Rapid solution for immediate patient application*
'The most important thing is to deal with these attacks of hypoglycemia. You are to take 25 g of carbohydrate at 4 pm every day'.
6. *Information-teaching*
'If you are prescribed a second injection, this does not mean that your diabetes is worse. In your case it is wise to redistribute your insulin, with small doses in the morning and in the evening. Thus...'
7. *Avoidance*
'By the way, are you keeping an eye on your blood pressure? It was too high last time'.
8. *Reformulation-comprehension*

'You think that your doctor has not told you the truth and this makes you angry'.

Let us look in more detail at each attitude and the reactions which they produce in the partners, who, in the following situations, will be patients. Let us analyze the example of the diabetic with an elevated fasting blood sugar and constant hypoglycemia in the late afternoons.

*Response 1: Type of attitude – JUDGMENT*

'*I will not have a second injection. In the first place, the doctor lied to me by promising me a single daily injection and I know that having 2 injections means my diabetes is becoming more severe*'.

If the answer of the physician is: '*It is not by rebelling against your treatment that your diabetes will be better controlled*', the attitude expressed is nothing else than a moral *judgment* on the conduct and the feelings of the patient. In this case it is negative criticism, but on other occasions it may be positive, e.g.: 'Well done, I am proud of you. You are great'.

This *judgment* response is a paternalistic attitude which addresses itself to the patient's conscience (good or bad) or to the 'super ego' in psychoanalytic terms (see Chapter 26). This response places the patient in an inferior position. Blame, warnings or praise will lead to the infantilization of the patient and may cause:
- inhibition and/or even blocking of expressiveness
- deception
- aggressiveness
- anxiety
- rebelliousness and guilt

*Response 2: Type of attitude – INTERPRETATION (analysis of imagined causes)*

'*You have no confidence in what has been prescribed for you and you think that you have been misled*'.

Anyone who gives this response interprets the ideas expressed by stressing such and such point which he regards as essential. This creates the risk that the interpretation may deform or even misrepresent what the patient wanted to say.

Often this type of attitude is expressed by an explanation: 'I am going to tell you what is wrong in your case...' What appear to be good reasons for the listener's interpretation may change the explanation into an accusation. This type of interpretative intervention is delicate and subtle. It raises resistance which is difficult to manage, even by experienced psychotherapists. If, in addition, the interpretation is incorrect, no further dialog is possible.

Here, too, is the risk of remoteness from the patient who is surprised or shocked. Some patients will feel confused in their inability to understand the motives underlying their own personal reactions. In the interview they might show lack of interest, a lack of concern, or even obvious irritation.

*Response 3: Type of attitude – SUPPORT (emotional reassurance)*

'*Do not get into such a state, it is not such a major point*'. With this type of attitude the intensity of the feeling detected is reduced by minimizing the importance and the drama of the situation. In some cases this amounts to generalizing or over-simplifying. It sometimes can be labelled as a maternal attitude.

Generally this type of support induces extreme patient reactions at the 2 poles: dependence and submission or disappointment and rejection. It infers that any situation is simple and requires little or no need for attention.

*Response 4: Type of attitude – INTERROGATION*

'*Tell me who has said that 2 injections means that the diabetes is more severe?*' The doctor who gives this response is looking for more information on the facts or feelings of the patients. However, by insisting on this or that item, the doctor may run the risk of over-stressing the importance of one detail at the exclusion of the rest. Here the physician is regaining the initiative in the interview by using the style of history-taking in which questions are legitimate, but it must be understood that when specific and precise questions are asked, the answers may be the same.

A number of questions will be necessary during the interview. If the first one is too specific it may channel or even focalize the interview on a false channel. A closed question restricts the answer whereas an open question allows varied and numerous inputs. A stimulating question encourages the patient to speak: 'What do you mean ... (then) ... carry on...'

*Response 5: Type of attitude – RAPID SOLUTION (for immediate patient application)*

'*The most important thing is to deal with these attacks of hypoglycemia. You must take 25 g of carbohydrate at 4 pm every day*'. As an immediate response, the solution proposed may well rob the patient of any opportunity for personal problem solving. This type of attitude does not allow the patient to collaborate actively with the medical team. Such haste may bring the interview to an end and produce a passive patient.

Although the doctor is qualified to make decisions and to put forward solutions, it is not always necessary to do so with a sharp and authoritative approach. This again reinforces narrow dependence of the patient upon the medical team.

*Response 6: Type of attitude – INFORMATION-TEACHING*

'*If you are prescribed a second injection, this does not mean that your diabetes is becoming worse. In your case, it may simply be wise to redistribute your insulin with small doses in the morning and in the evening ... thus...*' Information and teaching are aspects of treatment. However, information stated is not always understood by the patient. The right moment must be chosen. When a patient shows feelings of hostility or fear, an information-teaching response may be perceived as 'teaching him a lesson' or 'putting him down', both of which intimidate and usually silence the patient.

*Response 7: Type of attitude – AVOIDANCE*

'*By the way, are you keeping an eye on your blood pressure? It was too high last time*'. This answer clearly sidesteps the question. It is popular among health care providers. It is to be hoped that it is rarely used in the therapeutic relationship. Strategies can be employed to divert the emphasis of the problem posed with another type of feature, such as a question on another subject, or a joke. However, if the question is systematically sidestepped or the subject changed, the problem is not tackled. The doctor may give the impression that what the patient says is of little interest or can be ignored. Faced with such a systematic attitude, the patient is left with 2 possibilities: either to accept the manipulation or to change doctors.

These 7 types of responses all fail to encourage communication with the patient and prevent real dialog with the doctor. The attitudes which underline these responses induce submissive or uncooperative patient patterns of behavior. Is there another attitude and a form of response which does not produce these effects?

*Response 8: Type of attitude – REFORMULATION–COMPREHENSION*

This response is none other than the active listening which guarantees real, true communication. Before considering this response, let us look again at what the patient said: '*I will not have a second injection in the evening because the doctor lied to me when he promised me a single daily injection. Also I know that having 2 injections means that the diabetes is becoming worse*'.

If this situation was represented in diagram form with the terms of communication defined, it would be as shown in Table 1.

If the patient's message is accepted literally, it could be perceived that the patient has understood nothing at all or that he is a difficult person to communicate with. Decoding is necessary if the feelings behind the words of the patient are to be understood. The immediate, spontaneous response does usually not permit decoding. It takes little time to decode, i.e. to analyze and identify the feelings hidden inside the message of the speaker's words (encoding).

*The crucial point is to know whether the listener (the medical personnel) has decoded the patient's message correctly.* Only by *reformulating* the patient's message in his presence is it possible to know if the listener correctly understood the speaker's intents. This is the aim of the eighth response in which the doctor says: 'If I understood you correctly, you think that the doctor has not told you the truth and this has made you angry. You also mentioned that the second injection is a sign that your diabetes is worse'.

After the listener has stated what he believes to be the speaker's points, the patient can then indicate whether this is what he really meant. The first reaction of the doctor should be a mirror reflection of the patient's message

Fig. 1 The effect of ENCODING and DECODING
on the inter-personal communication system

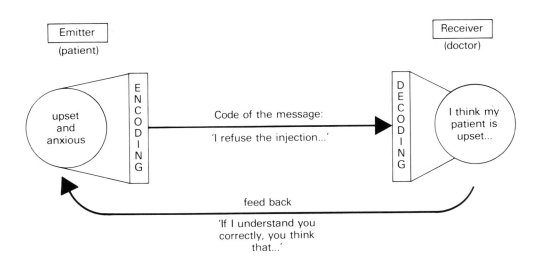

ENCODING: This is the personal and sometimes disguised language used by a person to express himself.
DECODING: This is the receiver's perception of the true, real meaning of the message spoken (often disguised) by the speaker (emitter).

which focuses upon what the patient really feels. There are 2 components in active listening: the first is to paraphrase (to put 'in other words') what has just been said without deforming it. The second is *to uncover the underlying feelings*.

One hears well only those persons whose ideas are welcome and whom one accepts without reservations. Therefore, to truly comprehend another person's words, one must be interested in the total individual. This includes his life style as well as his medical problems. This translates into using a 'global approach' with each patient. If such an approach, which creates an atmosphere of acceptance, manifests itself in the initial attention given to the patient, it must also be conveyed in the act of intervention.

The main tool in active listening is *reformulation*. It can reflect and clarify what has been said. The effects produced by a true and adequate reformulation have advantages for the 2 partners in the dialog. The patient, who has basically an emotional experience of his situation, is rarely in a position to formulate it objectively. The strength of his feelings blurs the message (encoding). The offered reformulation tells the patient that what he feels is recognized and accepted as being important. This will enable the patient to move from a momentary emotional perception to an idea reflection of his own situation.

The doctor or therapist, by taking into account the emotional state of the patient, is in a better position, at the right time, to mobilize the elements needed in the realization of a shared treatment plan. The cooperation gained by the patient's understanding is a stable basis for a better acceptance and application of recommendations and prescriptions. Active Listening may thus play a crucial role in securing the patient's motivation and compliance.

## III.   PRACTICAL EXAMPLES

The following examples, which are transcriptions of situations encountered in our Diabetic Unit, should help the reader to become familiar with the types of attitudes just described.

*Example 1*: Poorly controlled insulin dependent diabetic, age 39, diabetes began at the age of 24. Patient's statement from interview with dietician: 'I do not eat rice or starch because they contain bread equivalents. In fact, how much glucose is there in a bread equivalent?'

Possible responses of the dietician:
1.   'I can see that you have understood very little.' (Judgment)
2.   'It seems that you avoid starch and rice because you are afraid of eating too much glucose.' (Interpretation)
3.   'You get too worried about these equivalents. You must not think that starch is forbidden.' (Support)

4. 'Do you like rice and starch?' (Interrogation)
5. 'We must reinvestigate the whole problem of equivalents. Look at the sheet of equivalents and at your diet form.' (Rapid solution)
6. 'Simple! In one bread equivalent there are 25 g of glucose.' (Information-Teaching)
7. 'By the way, could I see your records of urine tests?' (Avoidance)
8. 'If I understand you correctly, you would like me to go over the question of carbohydrate equivalents again.' (Reformulation-Comprehension)

*Example 2*: Mrs. V., age 76. Diabetic peripheral neuropathy with almost total anesthesia of the foot. Hospitalized for 2 weeks, 6 months earlier with a perforating ulcer of the foot. Repeatedly advised on hygiene and care of the foot. Did not keep last appointment. Suddenly returned to the clinic and said to a nurse: 'My leg with the ulcer has been swollen for 3 weeks, but there is no pain. I cannot get on my shoe. Do you think I should get a larger size shoe?' Examination of the foot shows a suppurating perforating ulcer, a dirty foot, cellulitis and edema.

Possible replies of the nurse:
1. 'But you knew that you have to be careful with your feet.' (Judgment)
2. 'You must have neglected the care and hygiene of your feet.' (Interpretation)
3. 'Don't panic. We see a lot of this.' (Support)
4. 'What do you use as disinfectant?' (Interrogation)
5. 'I will deal with this at once. There is no time to lose.' (Rapid solution)
6. 'In your case, as your feet cannot feel pain, you must check each day that the skin is not red and that there are no wounds etc...' (Information-teaching)
7. 'I have the impression that you are not keeping a careful watch on your weight. You have gained weight since your last visit.' (Avoidance)
8. If I've understood you correctly, you think that a larger shoe will make you more comfortable and that the swelling will go away.' (Reformulation-Comprehension)

*Example 3*: Young, pregnant, insulin-dependent woman. Admitted to hospital in 34th week of pregnancy. Morning ketonuria with normal blood sugar and no hypoglycemia at night. In the clinic, before the doctor spoke, she said, 'I promise that I have not been cheating. I eat exactly what you have told me to eat, but I constantly have acetone, but no sugar, in my urine.'

Possible replies of the doctor:
1. 'You are in such a hurry to tell me this, that I think you are not telling me the truth.' (Judgment)
2. 'In your case you have not been taking enough carbohydrates.' (Interpretation)
3. 'Don't worry, there is no problem.' (Support)

4. 'Do you always keep down your meals or do you sometimes vomit your food?' (Interrogation)

5. 'It is a matter of diet. You must take 10 ounces of orange juice at 10 pm.' (Rapid solution)

6. 'Things are quite normal for your stage of pregnancy. Your baby is using more glucose and this requires compensation.' (Information-teaching)

7. 'Would you like a girl or a boy?' (Avoidance)

8. 'If I understand you correctly, you have said that although you have been doing as I prescribed, you have acetone but no glucose in your urine?' (Reformulation-Comprehension)

*Example 4*: Garage worker, overweight, heavy smoker. Patient announces to the physician, 'I have decided to have 10 days of intense physical exercise with a diet and massage in a Fitness-Club. It seems that I could lose 5 kg.'

Possible replies of physician:

1. 'It is obvious that if you had followed your diet better you would not be in this trouble.' (Judgment)

2. 'With the kind of life you lead the only way to lose weight is by an intensive cure.' (Interpretation)

3. 'What a good idea to want to lose 5 kg in weight.' (Support)

4. 'Is this what happens in this club? Is there any medical supervision?' (Interrogation)

5. 'There is no need to go to that club. We have everything here that is needed to solve the problem.' (Rapid solution)

6. 'The question of losing weight, which is your problem, depends on many factors. Of course, activity and diet come into it, but so do how and under what conditions you lose weight...' (Information-teaching)

7. 'By the way, do you know who is in the lead in the Paris-Dakar rally?' (Avoidance)

8. 'You mean you think you have found the most effective way to lose weight as far as you are concerned.' (Reformulation-Comprehension)

Attitudes develop spontaneously, mostly unconsciously. The fragments of interviews cited show us (sometimes as caricatures) the types of responses which reflect these attitudes.


## IV. TYPES OF ATTITUDES OBSERVED AMONG MEDICAL TEAM MEMBERS

Among the members of the medical team of our outpatient clinic, we have analyzed the types of attitudes developed spontaneously toward patients' statements. 20 doctors and a combination of 14 nurses and dieticians completed 4 questionnaires in which they selected 1 out of 7 categories of responses. They were asked to choose a response which they would have selected to use in reply to the statements of an imagined patient in a simulated situation. Each of the participants answered 4 questionnaires which represented 4 case studies. There was a total of 952 possible answers presented to each respondent.

Table 1  *Types of attitudes towards patients' statements observed by medical team members*

| Type of attitude | Percentages of 136 answers |
|---|---|
| * Information-teaching | 29% |
| * Rapid solution | 18% |
| * Reformulation-comprehension | 15% |
| * Interrogation | 12% |
| * Support | 12% |
| * Judgment | 9% |
| * Interpretation (causes imagined) | 5% |

Out of the total 136 recorded answers, the results expressed in decreasing order of frequency were as shown in Table 1.

As regards the attitude of Avoidance, not tested here, it is expressed fairly frequently by therapists working with seriously ill patients who ask questions about their state of health. For example, one of our patients with a nephrotic syndrome asked for information about his health; we observed one of our resident doctors saying: 'There are no problems with your eyes. Your blood sugar levels are excellent. I will see you again in 3 weeks'.


CONCLUSIONS

The therapeutic dialog, to be effective, requires a knowledge of various possible attitudes. It is not a question of wanting at all cost to acquire attitudes other than those which come naturally to the speaker, but to become aware of one's 'chronic' attitudes and learn to use them with more self-control.

To make the effort to use an approach which demonstrates understanding of a patient's spoken expression is based essentially upon the respect and the positive consideration of the other person. Thus one can really enter into true dialog with people who are different from oneself; understand them; and avoid judging or over-simplifying their statements. By listening to others better, medical professionals shall be able to accept, at least for a time, others' points of view and to restate them, regardless of their own judgment. Herein lies the core of the dynamics of successful treatment.

One of the main objections to the use of reformulation is that there may be a loss of natural spontaneity in a person's replies. It is not a trick, a device, but rather a genuine effort to understand others better. Each of us has to find his style between the 2 extremes: cold reformulation-repetition and effusive sentimentality.

## SUMMARY

8 categories of responses generally used by people are explained by the authors who advocate practicing one of these responses, the Comprehension-Reformulation response, based on the psychological works of E.H. Porter and Carl Rogers. This response allows a real therapeutic dialog to develop.

This article also presents a study in which the replies 34 physicians, nurses and dieticians gave to diabetic patients were recorded and analyzed to identify the most frequent types of replies. The reader is left with the necessary information to analyze his own responses in order to learn the emotional results of his own words on patients.

## SUGGESTED READING

1. Kinget, M. and Rogers, C. (1965): *Psychothérapies et Relations Humaines.* Second Edition. (Translated from Dutch.) Publications Universitaires, Louvain.
2. Porter, E.H. (1950): *Introduction to Therapeutic Counseling.* Houghton Miffling Co., Boston.
3. Rogers, C. (1960): *A Therapist's View of Personal Goals.* Pendle Hill, Wallingford, Pa.
4. Rogers, C. (1957): *Counseling and Psychotherapy: Newer Concepts in Practice.* Houghton Mifflin Co.
5. Rogers, C. (1961): *On Becoming a Person, a Therapist's View of Psychotherapy.* Houghton Mifflin Co.

# 30. MOTIVATION: A reciprocal engagement between doctor and patient

G. RUFFINO AND J.-Ph. ASSAL

## EDITORIAL

*Lack of motivation of the patient is one of the most frequent complaints of health care providers. This article describes various factors which might increase or slow the patient's motivation. The doctor/nurse/dietician play fundamental roles in this active process to move the patient towards the improvement of his or her treatment and, ultimately, towards a new sense of well-being. (The editors.)*

## MOTIVATION

The need to be motivated is not necessarily confined to the field of education. Everyone is propelled or pushed by someone or by something (external motivation), or is motivated by the goal he or she has personally set (internal motivation). What role should the doctor play in order to see that the diabetic patient has this 'push' to enable the treatment to be as effective as possible?

First of all the doctor describes the goal which is to be achieved; he or she then motivates the patient by giving reasons as to why an action is necessary. Even though for certain persons the need to be motivated is self-evident, there exist practical ways which permit techniques to be learned in order to promote and reinforce the motivation. These include the way in which objectives are presented to the patient and the manner in which one listens to the patient.

### What is motivation?

The words 'motivate' and 'motivation' find their origin in the Latin word 'movere', which signifies: 'move', 'agitate', 'set in motion', 'push', 'provoke' or 'bring forth'. The doctor who wants his patient to follow a course in order to first acquire knowledge and then to use this knowledge pragmatically, must provoke in him a sense of *curiosity* which will induce a desire to learn. This is indispensable for reaching efficiency in treatment and will, in turn, lead to a more balanced and active life for the patient.

To motivate someone, an explanation should first be given about the following question: 'What do I want the patient to do in order to reach my objectives?' This explanation will require, from the health care providers, pedagogical skills. In this approach the doctor becomes a teacher and, as a teacher, he or she will also be adviser and director. Through motivation, the doctor/teacher orients the behavior of the diabetic by providing the goals to be strived for together. In order for the motivation to make the patient *voluntarily* orient his or her behavior and activity, an objective (or objectives) must be proposed with the means of reaching it.

## Therapeutical objectives: the supports of motivation

Objectives, whether they be short, medium, or long-term, must be precise, concrete and evaluable. They must be adapted to each patient. The doctor/nurse/dietician as teacher must be assured that the way in which the motives are presented is precise. It is these motives which will persuade the patient/student to accept what has been prepared for him or her and to react accordingly. The power of motivation, when executing particular tasks, depends on the clear and precise vision of the given objectives both for the physician/nurse/dietician and the patient.

## Precise objectives in order to motivate the patient

To decide to attend a course for diabetics, the patient must understand clearly what the aim of the course is and what the results of his efforts will be. It is insufficient to say: 'You will learn about diabetes' or 'You will learn how to plan a diet'. It is necessary to tell the patient that he or she will learn something specific: for example, what the word 'alimentation' means in relation to what can or cannot be eaten and in what circumstances; that he or she no longer will have to refuse invitations to business luncheons or special dinners, which can often be copious.

## Concrete objectives

The diabetic must be convinced that in attending a course he or she will realize how to be capable of carrying out concrete and practical activities to maintain the best health possible. Concrete objectives could include learning to take care of the feet once a day in water heated to 35 degrees (95 degrees F); why it is necessary to wash well between the toes with the soap 'X' or 'Y'; how to dry the feet; never to use metal scissors or instruments with metal points to cut nails; or never to remove calluses with a razor blade. *One cannot motivate in an abstract manner, but must use real situations, giving attention to details which are sometimes considered boring and banal.* With such a concrete approach, the diabetic student will realize *why* it is necessary to learn, while actually in the process of learning.

**Evaluative objectives**

In order to see if the objective has been reached, an evaluation is mandatory. The patient should be able to evaluate if he or she has reached the objective and to measure the results. A diabetic who likes sports, for example, may not have the courage to engage in it. This person will be motivated to come to a course only if expecting to obtain tangible results leading to an improvement of his or her illness which will make participation in sports easier. To do this, the patient will need to learn techniques (adaption of insulin 'doses' and food) which will permit sports. The evaluation will require blood glucose measurements before and after sports activities (using a Home Blood Glucose Monitoring Kit, for example). The patient will thus be able to appreciate the results brought about by what he or she has learned.

**Necessity of global knowledge (medical and psycho-social) of the patient**

In the search to find ways to produce motivation, the doctor/teacher must take into account different factors about each diabetic: the patient's overall physical condition with the absence or presence of complications; the degree of acceptance of the illness and the character of the individual as well as his or her professional, social, affective and past life. The doctor must also consider to what extent the patient/student is able to understand and assimilate what is being taught. A clear understanding of the patient is fundamental in the dynamics of motivation.

Motivation, in order to be effective, must not surpass the actual abilities of the patient. The goals must not be exaggerated. The teacher must make sure that there is a balance between what is being asked of the patient and his or her capacity to meet these demands and to handle each new situation. The diabetic person has the right not to be motivated. The causes which motivate must be such that, in quantity and in quality, the patient can accept them and react voluntarily and naturally according to his or her needs.

Motivation addresses itself more to the 'ego' of the individual than to the 'super-ego'. These terms were used by Sigmund Freud to explain his structural theory of exploring the unconscious and conscious mind. According to Freud, the mind is divided into 2 parts: the 'id', which is the source of all instinctive drives and the 'ego', which regulates or mediates between the drives of the 'id' and society. The 'super-ego' is a section of the 'ego' which corresponds to one's conscience as created by the morals of the surrounding society. The total personality represents how well a person's 'id', 'ego' and 'super-ego' can act together [1].

To prescribe a diet following only the nutritional requirements of the disease without regard to the social and emotional aspects of the patient is to deal only with the 'super-ego' while ignoring the other two-thirds of the individual's personality. This one-sided approach is the major reason for teaching failures in all fields.

It is the 'ego' which is expressed by what the patient is able to do naturally. There is an optimal threshold at which the process of motivation is triggered. If the reasons that produce the motivation process are not sufficiently strong, the patient will think that what is being demanded is not worth the trouble and, therefore, will not react well or at all.

There may also be an absence of any positive reaction. In this situation, the patient will be passive if the conditions of the motivation are too demanding. To ask too much calls only upon the 'super-ego' of the individual. In such a situation the patient feels anxious and incapable of doing what has been demanded. Sometimes the fear of failure can also block motivation even though the patient could in reality perform the requirements. The doctor/nurse/dietician who becomes a teacher must guide and create the atmosphere for the patient/student to discover that there is nothing intimidating or superhuman about what is being asked of him or her.

The diabetic must simply remember in daily life that he or she must continue to act in the prescribed medical way with as natural a manner as possible. If it rains and you don't want to get wet, you must carry an umbrella, even if it is inconvenient. It might be a nuisance, but in such a precise situation one must submit to certain minor inconveniences. Thus, the insulin-dependent diabetic must know that snacks are necessary in certain situations, and must be willing to submit to the inconvenience of carrying the snacks when away from home. The level of motivation required for the effort in this situation is of the same magnitude as that of the effort in carrying an umbrella.

The level of motivation which produces the desired behavioral changes needs only to be enough to incite the patient to take action. A 'super-ego' motivation is not necessary, for it can create anxiety in the patient. Motivation which operates through the 'ego's' emotional instincts is the driving force which will make the person react naturally. The term 'emotion', from the Latin 'emovere', signifies 'to bring out, displace, or put away from'. True emotional motivation which comes from within the patient produces an independence of action, whereas the motivation of 'you should' (the 'super-ego'), enforced from outside the patient, creates dependence on others.

The doctor/teacher who wants to motivate patients has to offer precise motives which are concrete and evaluable. These motives must be formulated with consideration for the personality of the patient, his or her degree of acceptance of the disease, as well as the patient's capacity to face the implications of the treatment. The personal experience of actually teaching the patient is one of the most active, creative methods in which medical professionals can discover the process of motivating the patient.

## The patient who refuses to be motivated

If it is relatively easy to motivate most patients because they already have a desire to improve their condition, it becomes more difficult to motivate someone who does not care. The doctor/teacher must know that he or she will meet situations where the motivation is inhibited. This can be observed in 3 groups of situations:

1. *Absence of clinical signs*: this is the situation when the illness does not manifest any outward signs in a person who feels well. In a number of discussions with patients, it becomes apparent that medical professionals have not considered that there are often few outward signs of which the diabetic patient is aware. Examples are found in hyperglycemia without thirst, peripheral neuropathy with sensory loss in the legs, and background retinopathy.

   In situations with few clinical signs there is insufficient motivation both in the medical person treating the patient and in the patient himself. Such a patient might say: 'But I feel well. I do nothing in excess; my diabetes should be under control'; or 'I do not understand why I have such a serious foot infection. I never experience pain in my legs', or 'What is wrong with my eyes? I have good vision!' This type of patient has no intrinsic motivation which will convince him or her to follow a certain treatment course for his or her illness. This absence of outward signs is also found in other chronic illnesses where the adherence to a therapeutical program can be very disappointing. This is true for instance in hyperglycemia, arterial hypertension etc. Therefore, the success of motivating a patient can be somewhat dependent on the degree to which he or she is confined by the disease.

2. *Incomplete acceptance of the disease*: this situation is found in patients who have not yet accepted their disease as part of themselves. They might be in a phase of denial, revolt or 'bargaining'. (See Chapter 26.) This could be true of an insulin-dependent patient who is in a phase of revolt and personal manipulation, refusing to accept the various facets of the treatment, to take snacks or to follow the meal timetable imposed by the insulin treatment. Such a diabetic may refuse the program because he or she feels that the need for insulin is only temporary.

   How can one motivate those persons who are not coping? As a first step, the doctor will use his or her scientific competence to explain, like a teacher, the clinical condition to the patient. The description of the illness will help the patient to become more conscious of the situation even if the signs of the disease are absent. For the patient who refuses to recognize that he or she is ill, the medical explanation will permit getting this 'monster', which is how this type of patient often considers his or her illness, in better perspective.

3.   *State of depression*: the individual who is in a pathological state of depression with a loss of deep, existential interest will not be able to be motivated, either externally or internally. In this situation, the depression must be treated before the motivation can be considered.

## The motivation of the medical team

The patients will feel more motivated if they see that the doctor/nurse/dietician are motivated to help them. In order to convince someone else, it can help to be convinced oneself of the importance of a positive change in the other person. In certain professions, like salesmanship for instance, the conviction of the salesperson can be simulated. The situation is different in medicine where the only motivation of the physician/nurse/dietician is usually a real desire to improve the patient's health.

The ideal situation occurs, obviously, where a motivated doctor is teaching a motivated patient. The doctor/teacher who actively engages in the learning process with the 'bearer' of the illness is in a new situation compared to most doctors and patients. This situation can result in a relationship of mutual confidence, help and collaboration. The aim of this doctor/patient teamwork is to attain the independence of the diabetic patient and to achieve the most satisfying state of health possible.

## The motivation of the doctor/nurse/dietician

### 1.   *The role of the immediate therapeutic effect*

The medical team, in general, might not be motivated to teach the patient because they think that educating the patient is not an essential part of the treatment. Members of the team may argue that they consider it useless to teach because 'the patients will do what they think best for themselves', or '... the socio-cultural environment is so unfavorable that ...'

It is easier to motivate someone to take medication than to follow classes for better treatment of the illness. *Using specific medications like insulin, the patient and doctor know what benefit can be expected from this treatment.* The sooner the therapeutic effect is felt and observed, the more the doctor and the patient will have reciprocal confidence in each other and the medication. The more success is attained, the more they will be motivated by the ascendancy of the medication over the illness.

With the overweight diabetic the situation is not always as clear as with type I diabetics. The physician or the dietician is aware that weight loss may not always improve diabetes control. Faced with these uncertainties, it is not always easy to be motivated in order to motivate the patient to make an effort. Both patient and doctor must, however, have at least sufficient interest to try the therapy.

Can one motivate without oneself being motivated and personally convinced? It is quite possible. Not being motivated does not necessarily mean to be opposed to an idea. Just being interested in better health for the patient is sufficient. A non-motivated doctor/nurse/dietician can still motivate a patient if there is at least an interest in a minimum effectiveness of the treatment.

## 2.   *Improvised teaching during a consultation or a class with patients*

A physician can say: 'I prescribe my patient medicine; I give him advice; I propose directives and steps to follow'. These medical actions are in fact part of a teaching process. The name 'doctor', in Latin, means teacher. The opinion presently held by some is that a doctor should receive pedagogical training to improve his teaching approach to patients.

Is this opinion correct? Two remarks follow, for the reader's consideration, on the meaning of 'teaching': a) most teaching is composed of advice and directives; and b) each person who patiently transmits directives and advice on how the student should act is already teaching. This is what occurs often in a medical consultation.

What then, strictly speaking, is meant by 'education'? This form of transmitting a message has several possible structures which help the efficiency of transmitting the message. These structures can be learned and will help to prepare a more effective lecture or other teaching approach that will truly penetrate the patient's understanding.

A minimum of educational training provides added advantages, in quantity and in quality, over the spontaneous education given 'off the cuff' during a consultation. It permits a better utilization of the time allotted during the consultation. The advantages obtained are of as much benefit to the teacher as they are to the patient. Ultimately, all the patients will benefit.

The doctor who has learned how to teach the patient is more effective in less time. We observed this in training physicians to teach patients in our Diabetes Unit. When giving medical information and advice at the time of consultation, there is always some improvisation which means that the information given is not very precise. Short-term objectives are given which tend to deal only with immediate priorities. The patient who listens will, despite his willingness, only register the main points in the doctor's advice and directives: 'Your new medication is called ...'; 'You should take this pill after lunch, after supper ...'; '... don't forget your prescription'; '... the next appointment is ...'. In the outpatient consultation, the patient is really anxious when he or she is not able to assimilate everything. In the short consultation, doctor and patient concentrate their attention on what appears to be essential, or, in any case, what is judged to be most urgent.

The teaching of the patient, which takes place over a number of sessions, necessitates preparation, use of teaching methods and good organization, for nothing must be omitted. In mentally and physically preparing the lesson, the doctor/nurse/dietician acting as teachers have a better chance to foresee the possible objections and/or difficulties which the patient might have. The medical teacher might then be able to prepare replies, solutions and alternate modes of presenting information in advance.

The basic problem in giving a series of lessons is that it is necessary, on the one hand, for the physician/nurse/dietician to want to present the lessons and, on the other hand, for the patient to want to listen and comprehend. It is only during a *series* of lessons that the teacher will manage to provoke the patient's deep interior reactions. These reactions are sometimes long in revealing themselves, but are indispensable to bring forth the patient's desire to try. This desire will become the patient's motivation for action. Pedagogical methods, well-conceived and followed, can be a guide for stimulating motivation.

In awakening their own curiosity, interest and desire to improve the patient's health, the doctor/nurse/dietician, as teachers, motivate the patient. The motivation must use to the maximum the exterior and interior world of the patient (extrinsic and intrisic motivation). The demonstration of possible results to be achieved with the treatment will excite the diabetic's imagination and the patient will then become susceptible to the idea that 'maybe it's worth the trouble to make an effort'. This self-effort will provide the patient with the hope of better things to come.

In education, as in the simple doctor/patient consultation, it is essential to know the person or group that one is addressing. An old British saying is still valid: 'If you want to teach Jack anything, you must first know the subject matter, but you must also know Jack'.

CONCLUSIONS

Motivation is an abstract concept meaning activation of an individual toward a given task. This drive can be created through a dynamic process involving external and internal personal objectives. This dynamic process can be formed by short-term objectives leading to action.

A few points should be remembered:
1.   The motivation of the patient is activated by the doctor/nurse/dietician in the majority of cases.
2.   Motivation of the patient proceeds through a whole series of concrete, simple, daily actions which have to be planned in structured steps. The health care providers have a fundamental role in planning these actions with the patient. Using the technique of planning short-term objectives is a good way to enter the dynamic process of motivation. The precise, concrete and evaluable objectives for treatment should be designed to define clearly what has to be achieved by both the doctor/nurse/dietician and the patient.
3.   The process of creating and maintaining motivation is difficult. It goes normally through both positive and negative phases. Both doctors/nurses/dieticians and the patients have a tendency to become discouraged too

easily when difficulties arise. There are probably a number of valid reasons for a patient's lack of motivation. It is the task of the medical team to try to understand why patients have lost their motivation to follow the treatment by actively listening to them.

4.  Having a definition for the optimal level of motivation for a given patient is mandatory. There is no motivation if too little is asked of the student/patient. Asking too much of a patient can produce anxiety and even block the active process of motivation. The discouragement felt by the medical team and the patient when confronted by the absence or loss of motivation is frequently due to a concept of motivation that is too abstract, idealistic or perfectionistic.

5.  Patient motivation is also strongly dependent on the doctor/nurse/dietician and patient relationship in which the technique of careful listening to the patient plays a fundamental role (see Chapter 29).

## SUMMARY

Motivation is the key to success in all efforts to live with a chronic disease. Diabetes is a good example of a disease requiring constant motivation on a daily basis to monitor blood or urine glucose levels, keep records, take insulin injections, understand and follow a system of food exchanges, pay special attention to problems of blood circulation and foot care, etc. What role should the doctor/nurse/dietician play to help create the necessary drive within the diabetic individual so that the treatment can be as effective as possible? This article considers this question.

## REFERENCES

1.  Arlow, J.A. and Brenner, C. (1964): *Psychoanalytic Concepts and the Structural Theory*. International University Press, Inc., New York.

## SUGGESTED READING

1.  Aebli, H. (1951): *Didactique Psychologique*. Delachaux et Niesté, Paris.
2.  Brown, J.S. (1961): *The motivation of Behavior*. McGraw-Hill, New York.
3.  Cofer, C.N., and Appley, M.H. (1964): *Motivation: Theory and Research*. Viley, New York.
4.  Cohen, S.J. (1979): *New Directions in Patient Compliance*. Lexington, Toronto.
5.  Diel, P. (1966): *Psychologie de la Motivation*. Presses Universitaires de France, Paris.
6.  Fourcade, R. (1975): *Motivation et Pédagogie*. Editions Sociales Françaises (ESF).
7.  Fraisse, P. (1980): *La Motivation*. Presses Universitaires de France, Paris.

G. *Ruffino and J.-Ph. Assal*

8. Not, L. (1979): *Les Pédagogies de la Connaissance*. Privat, Toulouse, France.
9. Mager, R.F. (1968): *Developing Attitudes towards Learning*. Fearon, Palo Alto, California.
10. Mager, R.F. (1969): *Pour Éveiller le Désir d'Apprendre*. Ganthia-Villars, Paris.
11. Osterrieth, P.A. (1958): *La Motivation*. Symposium de l'Association de langue française, Presses Universitaires de France, Paris.

# 31.   COMPLIANCE: One aspect of the doctor-patient relationship. An overview

ANDRÉ HAYNAL AND PIERRE SCHULZ

## EDITORIAL

*No physician would say that all his patients consume precisely the prescribed amount of drugs or strictly follow dietary restrictions, since disobeying and having counterproductive behaviors are also part of human nature.*

*This paper on non-compliance underlines that considering the phenomenon as quantitatively negligible would be wrong, and this might be worth hearing once more. From the review of a few studies and on the basis of their personal convictions, the authors give us a check-list of what could be done to improve compliance. They say that the majority of these proposals cannot be carried out without many efforts from the physicians. When considering the patients, the authors state that '… common sense indicates that most of the strategies proposed (to improve compliance) are not detrimental to the patients'.*

*However, many of the proposals from the authors still have to go through a formal demonstration of their efficiency, and such studies will by no means be methodologically easy to carry out. (The editors.)*

Non-compliance with treatment is increasingly recognized as a major problem in the field of medicine. However, it is not a new problem related to the complexities of highly evolved and impersonal modern medical technology. Hippocrates had already recognized the phenomenon: 'The physician should be aware of the fact that patients often lie when they state that they have taken certain medicines' [1, 2]. The concept of compliance applies to behavior such as taking medications, following diets, making life style adjustments, following up on referrals and keeping appointments. This definition excludes from the concept of compliance related problems of health care, namely delay in seeking medical care, non-participation in community health care programs or self-neglect. Indeed compliance involves a preexisting patient-doctor relationship, i.e. a field of physician-patient interactions and instructions given in this setting which should be followed by adequate behavior in self-care.

Some critics have expressed uneasiness as to the concept of compliance, suggesting that the connotation of the verb 'to comply' implies necessarily some submissiveness on the part of the patients, and the idea of self-righteousness or an authoritarian wish for power on the part of the physicians. In this perspective strategies designed to improve compliance could be criticized on the basis of psychological or social, if not ethical, considerations. We feel that the term of non-compliance is legitimate when the study of the phenomenon remains on a descriptive level and does not involve a judgment of the patients based on moral considerations.

Not following medical advice creates a gap between the therapy prescribed and the treatment actually adhered to by the patients. That this gap is a significant explanation for the failure of numerous therapies appears to be a sensible statement. Medical work, with all the efforts on the part of patients and physicians and with the increasing cost of diagnostic procedures and treatment, might not fulfil its purpose and might become inefficient in a large percentage of cases: services are solicited and finally not accepted. However, the deleterious effects of non-compliance are limited to situations where diagnoses were correct; the therapy was clearly supposed to do more good than harm; neither the illness nor the therapy could be considered trivial and the treatment was carried out on the basis of informed consent [3]. We are convinced that in certain situations the refusal or the interruption of treatment can be safe and in some cases even beneficial to patients. We think every physician has such cases in mind from his clinical experience.

Table 1 gives a list of the frequency of non-compliance, evaluated in a few studies. In the literature, the range of values for non-compliance is even wider than reported in Table 1: from 0 to 93% of the patients were considered non-compliant. In the majority of studies, more than half of the patients were non-compliant. In the field of diabetes, Gabriele and Parabble, in a somewhat pioneering study [4], indicated that 61% of the children in a diabetes summer camp spontaneously reported that they did not follow their diet carefully. In a study of adult outpatients it was found that 50% made errors in insulin dosage and 77% did not sterilize the needles properly. Only one-third of the diabetics tested their urine correctly, and half of the patients were considered by the authors as using the results of urine tests in a way unsuited for a good control of diabetes. In the same study, about three-fourths of the patients followed the diet inadequately [5]. The above studies clearly indicate that non-compliance is a problem that applies to the majority of our patients.

The variation in the frequency of non-compliance is not only due to the many factors that influence compliance, but it is also explained by the criteria taken to assess the phenomenon. For example, should we define as compliant only those patients who regularly take 100% of their pills at the right moment in the day, or is a patient who takes two-thirds of the prescribed amount of drugs also considered a compliant patient? Various methods were used for the determination of non-compliance such as pill counting (comparison between the amount of drugs remaining and the amount that should remain if medications were taken according to prescriptions), determining plasma drug concentration or measuring urinary excretion of either the drug or metabolic by-products, interview of patients, registration of non-attendance to scheduled visits, observation of consequences of non-compliance [1, 6]. Unfortunately these methods are rarely used in clinical studies. Nemitz and Schelling complained that among 700 publications printed between 1969 and 1972 in 2 English medical journals, only 19% mentioned the use of the methods for the objective study of non-compliance [6b].

It is also important to insist that prediction of non-compliance is a difficult task for doctors. Results by Mushlin and Appel showed that interns and residents were right for approximately half of their evaluation of patients' compliance [7]. Similar results were obtained by Gilbert in a group of 10

Table 1  *Frequency of non-compliance*

| Type of patient studied | Number of subjects | Drugs | Non-compliant subjects (%) |
|---|---|---|---|
| General practice | 82 | Imipramine | 24 |
| | 48 | Antibiotics | 31 |
| | 58 | 'Long term'.e.g. digoxin, thyroxine | 34 |
| | 62 | Prophylactic iron (3 × daily) | 71 |
| | 24 | Once daily | 25 |
| Rheumatic centre | 78 | Phenylbutazone or placebo | 49 |
| Psychiatric OP | 125 | Chlorpromazine or imipramine | 48 |
| Tuberculous OP | 705 | Isoniazid | 34 |
| Tuberculous OP | 151 | Para-aminosalicylic acid | 50 |
| Tuberculous OP | 114 | Para-aminosalicylic acid | 31 |
| Tuberculous OP | 153 | Para-aminosalicylic acid | 49 |
| Pregnancy | 60 | Ferrous fumarate | 32 after 2 months |
| Tuberculous OP | 50 | Isoniazid | 30 |
| Neurology OP | 254 | Meprobamate or placebo | 46 |
| Children | 103 | Oral penicillin | 67 |
| Tuberculous OP | 26 | Isoniazid | 32 |
| Elderly, chronic sick, OP | 26 | Various | 61 |
| Elderly, chronic sick, OP | 178 | Various | 59 |
| Children | 107 | Oral penicillin | 19 after 5 days |
| | 352 | Oral penicillin | 44 after 9 days |
| Children | 587 | Various | 49 |
| Various at general clinic | 154 | Various regimes | 37 |
| Tuberculous OP | 98 | Isoniazid | 72 |

Adapted from a review by Stimson [42]. OP = out-patients.

family physicians: they were unable to predict compliance of their patients to oral digoxin, giving answers that were no better than those obtained by chance only. And this was even the case for patients who were known to the doctors for more than 5 years [8]. Norell concluded that the interview of patients was inaccurate in detecting non-compliance in a group of 73 patients treated for glaucoma [9]. However, both Enlund [10] and Haynes [11] found that interviewing patients, which is the simplest approach to assess adherence to treatment, was very useful in the case of hypertension, and correlated well with the prescription-filling patterns and pill-counting. Interviews of the patients can be complemented by collecting retrospective data on the behavior of the subjects and predicting future behavior from these data. Using the profile of weight gain between dialysis sessions, Agashua showed that this criteria could reliably classify patients into probable compliers or non-compliers to dietary restrictions [12].

Being able to predict non-compliance has obvious consequences on the management of individual patients. Some factors which have been recognized as useful for this purpose are listed in Table 2, based on a summary of the review by Haynes [13]. This author used stringent statistical criteria

Table 2   *Correlation between various factors and compliance*

| | Number of studies showing the association with compliance to be | | |
|---|---|---|---|
| | positive | negative | not significant |
| *Disease factors* | | | |
| diagnosis | 3 | 5 | 11 |
| severity | 0 | 4 | 7 |
| disability | 3 | 1 | 1 |
| duration | 0 | 0 | 10 |
| *Clinical setting factors* | | | |
| time between screening and appointment | | 3 | |
| waiting time before consultation | | 2 | |
| distance to clinic | 1 | | 4 |
| *Therapeutic regimen factors* | | | |
| alternative parenteral drug for the same disease | 6 | | |
| duration of therapy | | 13 | 3 |
| number of drugs or treatments | 1 | 11 | |
| frequency of dosing | | 2 | 3 |
| side effects | | 2 | 2 |

Adapted from a review by Haynes [13].

in his presentation of factors which showed a correlation with variations in compliance. Table 2 lists the number of studies in which the above association was present or absent at the 5% level of chance ($° < 0.05$).

## FACTORS THAT ARE ASSOCIATED WITH COMPLIANCE

In summarizing the different items discussed in the studies on compliance, we constructed the following 4 groups of factors listed in Table 3.

The factors of the first group, those related to the experience and subjective understanding of illness, are patient- and disease-related variables. They include the intellectual and emotional understanding of illness, the expectations, fears and hopes related to it (based on knowledge of similar cases), the intensity and the pattern of the symptoms (e.g. the character and duration of pain or impairment), the meaning of the disease to the individual (e.g. guilt, punishment or relief through secondary gains) and often the symbolic meaning and fears attached to the malfunctioning of particular systems (e.g. genital or psychiatric diseases). An example of the patient-related variables can be given for diabetic children. Some children falsely report that the urine test is negative and this can be a means for them to get attention, to engage in some desired activities, to be allowed more sweets or to avoid hunger or anger [14]. The somatic problems of a bad control of diabetes therefore does not always lead the child to the logical behavior of improved compliance. The factors of non-compliance that are related to the personalities of patients were not included in Table 2, except for the mention of a negative correlation between schizophrenia, paranoia or personality disorders and compliance. Denial, for example, which is not a mental illness but a defense mechanism, could influence compliance. Illness often activates latent personality traits and preexisting conflict which can lead to non-compliant behavior which was not predicted by the personality of the previously healthy individual. The particular form in which the disease is experienced (e.g. loss of control by obsessive individuals, intolerable limitations on dominant personalities) can lead to mental symptoms (e.g. paranoia) and influence the patients' collaboration.

Table 3   *Groups of factors that might influence compliance*

1.   Factors related to the experience and subjective understanding of illness

2.   Factors related to the doctor-patient relationship

3.   Factors related to the treatment

4.   Factors related to the environment of the patient

A. Haynal and P. Schulz

*The first group of factors is related to the experience and subjective under-standing of the illness.* It is easy to understand, and apparent in many studies, that patients with diseases with few or no symptoms at all, showed low compliance [15]. The diminishing compliance in case of anxiolytic medi-cation seen after improvement may be relevant to this subject: according to Lipman there was a 40% drop-out rate by the fourth week of treatment. Of those who remained in treatment, about 30% took less than the pre-scribed amount of medication [15]. Long duration of the illness with con-comitant doubts about appropriateness of the treatment or about the pos-sibilities of healing have their negative effects on both the patient-doctor relationship and compliance. Chronic diseases often create episodes of mental depression. Engel and Schmale spoke about 'giving up — given up' as having a bad prognosis for most physical illnesses [16]. These depressions are often related to the image the patient has of himself as an ill person and to his evaluation of whether life is still worth living. These crises occur-ring in the course of chronic diseases probably have a great and sometimes sudden influence on compliance. On the other hand we have to keep in mind that depression is a necessary part of human adaptation in face of a chronic illness: a 'mourning process' is needed to learn to cope with the disease. Previous habits and pleasures must be abandoned, new perspec-tives and limitations must be accepted. The stages of revolt and then of resignation are unavoidable steps. Being sick always generates some level of anxiety. At the 2 extremes of low or high levels of anxiety compliance diminishes. When anxiety is important the 'reminder' of being sick as-sociated with the taking of medication is avoided by 'forgetting' this obliga-tion [17]. In this context, one could also speak of reluctance to assume a 'sick-role'. With low levels of anxiety, it has been shown that the feeling of threat seems to be a determinant factor of compliance: the less the illness is perceived as severe, the less the likelihood is of compliant behavior [18, 19].

The *second group of factors is related to the doctor-patient relationship.* The presence of mutual trust is a condition for a good therapeutic alliance. The concept of trust may however have more of the qualities of an emotion than those of an intellectual judgment, hence the relative difficulty of assess-ing it by direct interviews or by questionnaires. On the cognitive level, patients may consider that they trust their doctors and they may continue to show up at appointments, although there sometimes appears a feeling of insecurity, 'things' being momentaneously 'no more as they were'. This kind of consideration makes us drift away from our customary, rationally based medical approach, where facts are conceived as variables which can be scrutinized in a fairly detached manner by observers. It becomes neces-sary to take into account our personal emotional clues in evaluating the quality of our relationships to patients and their environment. In our understanding of compliance we must include these and other psychological aspects, as they play a paramount role. In a careful examination of doctor-patient interactions, compliance was associated positively with the patient's expressing agreement with the physician, the patient's seeking the physician's opinions, and tension release during the therapeutic encounter. Non-compliance was associated with the physician's manifesting disagreement or even rejection [20]. In the patient-doctor relationship the belief of the doctor in the efficiency of the prescribed treatment enhances compliance [21]. Sometimes the patient has never had the intention of following any treatment, through fear of dependence or because of other irrational apprehensions. When this situation is recognized by doctors, the patient is often resistant to interventions aimed at improving compliance [22].

Conflicts with doctors, lack of adequate, understandable and acceptable explanations, the sense of irritating or confusing complexity and the feeling of not receiving the expected information all have negative effects on compliance. Ideally, a good doctor-patient relationship would improve compliance by creating a clinical setting favorable to the physical and psychological needs of patients. It would permit a relaxed atmosphere and the opportunity to give the necessary explanations concerning treatment and allow patients to inquire into other issues related to their fears about the disease and its treatment. It would diminish anxieties, feelings of guilt, overdemanding or self-destructive behavior. Moreover, the evaluation of compliance supposes a sufficiently good relationship with patients so that direct questions on compliance would receive adequate answers from patients.

The physician should strive to prevent patients from having a passive behavior towards their diseases and treatments. This is particularly important for chronic patients. Haynes [23] improved the drug-taking behavior of 38 non-compliant hypertensive patients by providing them with a device for self-measurement of blood pressure and asking them to take pills prior to a specified daily behavior and to record their pill-taking. Long-term compliance was also improved with these patients. For the chronic patients, some stimulation and reminder may be helpful, although perhaps not always efficient in the long run. Cummings [24] demonstrated that weekly telephone calls or behavioral contracting can improve the compliance of hemodialysis patients to dietary and fluid restrictions, with repercussions on serum potassium concentrations and weight gains between dialysis sessions. But these beneficial effects had disappeared 3 months after the intervention program, showing that the program was not sufficient to improve compliance on a long-term basis.

The *third group of factors is related to the treatment setting.* The fact that different drugs can be prescribed for the same disease enabled a few authors to compare compliance of patients having the same disorders but receiving various drug regimens. These studies led to conflicting reports. However, when different drugs are prescribed for different diseases, it appears that compliance is higher with drugs such as diuretics, insulin, oral hypoglycemic agents and cardiac drugs than is the case for tranquilizers or antacids. In

Table 4   *Strategies aiming at improving compliance*

| Recommendations | Potential efficacy at improving compliance | Costs to the health professionals | Costs to the patients | Deleterious effects on the patients | Difficulty to accomplish by health professionals |
|---|---|---|---|---|---|
| Verify the level of compliance of patient | high* | small to moderate | none | none | difficult |
| Classify patients as to their potential compliance | high* | small | none | none | very difficult |
| Simplify the drug regimen | moderate | none | none | none | easy |
| Educate the patients about sickness and treatment | moderate | moderate | small | ? | easy |
| Influence health beliefs of patients | high | moderate | small | ? | very difficult |
| Modify the clinical setting of the consultations | high | important | none | none | difficult |
| Give adequate descriptions of the practical modalities of treatment | moderate | small | none | none | easy |
| Improve the doctor-patient relationship | high | moderate | none | none | difficult |
| Influence attitudes of health professionals | moderate | small | none | none | difficult |

\* Detecting non-compliant subjects enables health professionals to center their efforts on a subgroup of the total population of patients.

most, but not all, studies side effects were considered to diminish compliance [25, 26]. It is established that the parenteral slow-release pharmaceutical formulations of antipsychotics or antibiotics have a big advantage in enhancing compliance. Paradoxically, one study showed that whether the treatment involves a single dose rather than multiple daily doses does not appear to enhance compliance [27]. However, patients are more likely to take 1 medication daily than 2 or 3 different drugs each day, and it remains a general rule that the higher the number of treatments prescribed to one patient, the lower his chance of adhering to the recommendations will be. The amount of behavioral changes required by the therapeutic regimen is directly related to non-compliance [28]: changes in eating, drinking or smoking habits or vocational changes are much more difficult to achieve than the less complex behavior of taking a drug [29, 30].

The *fourth group of factors is related to the environment of the patients*. It appears to be a well-established fact that having to wait for the consultation (either because a first appointment is given only in a few weeks or because the physician cannot see the patient rapidly after his arrival at the clinic) increases non-compliance. The lack of money can diminish adherence essentially for patients who have to pay themselves for their own health care [31-33]. Another factor linked with the environment of the patients is the family. Compliance is higher among patients with supporting families and is lower among those from unstable family units or living alone [34]. Family size by itself, however, does not appear to influence compliance [35].

The factors that we have assembled into the above 4 groups are all accounted for in the theory of the health belief model (HBM) [36]. Originally conceived for the field of preventive health care, the HBM served as a tool to study the probability of individuals to show adequate behavior (such as prophylactic dental care or immunizations) toward potential illnesses. The HBM was later used to assess sociological and behavioral determinants of compliance with medical treatments. The HBM states that the likelihood of action of a patient (i.e. to ask for treatment and follow recommendations) is determined by his perceived susceptibility to a disease, seriousness of the disease, advice from family, friends or the media, benefits from treatment and barriers to initiate help and treatment seeking. The HBM rightly underlines the role of patients' beliefs. For example, it implies that non-compliers believe themselves to be less threatened by illness than others such as hypochondriacs, who are good compliers. In a study by Becker the HBM was a useful predictive tool for the result of treatment of obese children [37]. In another study health beliefs related to arterial hypertension were however not predictive of compliance with treatment [38]. Overall, results showing positive correlations between components of the HBM and compliance outnumber those showing no significant correlations. Haynes [35] notices that 'while both prospective and retrospective studies support the predictive value of the model, the prospective studies generally show weaker relationships, suggesting that changes in compliance may precede, rather than follow alteration of the patient's health beliefs. Description of the formalization of the factors conditioning compliance leads to the question of the possibility to influence patients' HBM.

## EDUCATION AND OTHER STRATEGIES TO IMPROVE COMPLIANCE

It is distressing to note that health education does not always give the expected positive results: among 230 hypertensive steelworkers, those receiving health education and/or being able to see their doctors during work shifts did not adhere any better to the drug regimen. After 6 months, 50% of the men were considered non-compliant [39]. Tanner concluded that health education increased knowledge but not blood pressure control [40]. Educational counselling improved the re-attendance rate of patients at a sexually-transmitted-disease clinic; however, the re-attendance rate was also much influenced by the persistence of symptoms [41]. However, more elaborate forms of health education can have important consequences that are beneficial to patients. The educational approach to diabetic patients, on the psychological and socio-psychological levels, includes training in skills, transmission of information, occasions for mutual identification between persons having to live with the same chronic illness, group support and the opportunity to change from a passive sick role to an active one. We believe that all these events may be implemental to new doctor-patient, nurse-patient, dietician-patient and patient-patient relationships and may enhance compliance.

Education of patients is one of the many strategies aiming at improving the adherence of patients to their treatment. These strategies are summarized in Table 4, together with their potential benefits and their costs. For many of these recommendations, we only have preliminary or contradictory information on the efficiency of each strategy. However some of the recommendations imply very little cost to patients and physicians and common sense indicates that most of the strategies proposed are not detrimental to the patients.

## CONCLUSION

The probability that any given patient does not adhere to the prescribed treatment is high and difficult to assess. The determinants of non-compliance can be objective such as cost, waiting time or complexity of the drug regimen. Compliance is also one aspect of the patient-doctor relationship and as such is influenced by the subjective issues inherent to human interactions. In this sense one could speak of mutual compliance in that both patients and doctors work together in an alliance to find the best way out of an illness or to establish the best possible equilibrium between the constraint of treatment and the affective needs of patients.

The few studies we have summarized show that specific and quantifiable criteria are increasingly being used to quantify non-compliance and describe its causes. We will probably obtain a clearer image of all determinants of non-compliance in the coming years. At this date, it appears that some recommendations can already be made to improve the compliance of patients.

## SUMMARY

Non-compliance is a well known and frequent cause of failure of treatments. However its clinical recognition and its prediction are difficult tasks. We therefore reviewed studies in which non-compliance was quantified and in which factors leading to non-compliance were identified. The improvement of patients' compliance should be a goal for every physician. We list a few guidelines which are suggested to help achieve this goal. The issue of compliance should be considered within the framework of the interpersonal exchanges between patients and therapists.

### ACKNOWLEDGEMENTS

We thank Ms. R.C. Peduzzi and M. Struchen for their secretarial work.

## REFERENCES

1. Gordis, L. (1976): Methodologic issues in the measurement of patient compliance. In: Sackett, D.L., Haynes, R.B. (Eds.), *Compliance with Therapeutic Regimens*, p. 51. The Johns Hopkins University Press, Baltimore.
2. Lasagna, L. (1973): Fault and default (Editorial). *N. Engl. J. Med., 289,* 267.
3. Haynes, R.B. (1979): Introduction. In: Haynes, R.B., Taylor, D.W., Sackett, D.L. (Eds.), *Compliance in Health Care*, p. 1. The Johns Hopkins University Press, Baltimore.
4. Gabriele, A.J. and Parabble, A. (1948): Experience with 116 juvenile diabetic campers in a new summer camp for diabetic boys. *Am. J. Med. Sci., 218,* 161.
5. Watkins, J., Williams, F., Marler, D. et al. (1967): A study of diabetic patients at home. *Am. J. Public Health, 57,* 452.
6. Soutter, B.R. and Kennedy, M.C. (1974): Patient compliance assessment in drug trials: usage and measures. *Austr. N. Z. J. Med., 4,* 360.
6b. Nemitz, I. and Schelling, J.L. (1979): Un aspect particulier de la pharmacothérapie: la compliance. *Rev. Méd. Suisse Romande, 99,* 451.
7. Mushlin, A.I. and Appel, F.A. (1977): Diagnosing potential non-compliance. *Arch. Intern. Med., 137,* 318.
8. Gilbert, J.R., Evans, C.E., Haynes, R.B. and Tugwell, P. (1980): Predicting

compliance with a regimen of digoxin therapy in family practice. *CMA Journal, 123*, 119.

9. Norell, S.E. (1981): Accuracy of patient interviews and estimates by clinical staff in determining medication compliance. *Soc. Sci. Med., 15*, 57.
10. Enlund, H., Tuomilehto, J. and Turakka, H. (1981): Patient report validated against prescription records of measuring use and of compliance with antihypertensive drugs. *Acta Med. Scand., 209*, 271.
11. Haynes, R.B., Taylor, D.W., Sackett, D.L. et al. (1980): Can simple clinical measurements detect patient noncompliance? *Hypertension, 2*, 757.
12. Agashua, P.A., Lyle, R.C., Livesley, W.J. et al. (1981): Predicting dietary non-compliance of patients on intermittent heamodialysis. *J. Psychosom. Res., 25*, 289.
13. Haynes, R.B. (1979): Determinants of compliance: the disease and the mechanics of treatment. In: Haynes, R.B., Taylor, D.W., Sackett, D.L. (Eds.), *Compliance in Health Care*, 49. The Johns Hopkins University Press, Baltimore.
14. Semonds, J.F. (1979): Emotions and compliance in diabetic children. *Psychosomatics, 20*, 544.
15. Lipman, R.S. (1965): Neurotics who fail to take their drugs. *Br. J. Psychiatry, 111*, 1043.
16. Schmale, A.H. and Engel, G.L. (1967): The giving-up complex. *Arch. Gen. Psychiatry, 17*, 135.
17. Ley, P. and Spelman, M.S. (1965): Communication in an outpatient setting. *Br. J. Soc. Clin. Psychol., 4*, 115.
18. Davis, M.S. (1967): Predicting non-compliant behavior. *J. Health Soc. Behav., 8*, 265.
19. Gordis, L., Markowitz, M. and Lilienfeld, A.M. (1969): Why patients don't follow medical advice: a study of children on long-term antistreptococcal prophylaxis. *J. Pediatr., 75*, 957.
20. Davis, M.S. (1971): Variation in patient's compliance with doctor's orders: medical practice and doctor-patient interactions. *Psychiatry Med., 2*, 31.
21. Irwin, D.S., Weitzel, W.D. and Morgan, D.W. (1971): Phenothiazine intake and staff attitudes. *Am. J. Psychiatry, 127*, 1631.
22. Sackett, D.L. and Haynes, R.B. (Eds) (1976): *Compliance with Therapeutic Regimens*. The Johns Hopkins University Press, Baltimore.
23. Haynes, R.B., Sackett, D.L., Gibson, E.S. et al. (1976): Improvement of medication compliance in uncontrolled hypertension. *Lancet, 1*, 1265.
24. Cummings, K.M., Becker, M.H., Kirscht, J.P. and Levin, N.W. (1981): Intervention strategies to improve compliance with medical regimens by ambulatory haemodialysis patients. *J. Behav. Med., 4*, 111.
25. Caldwell, J.R., Cobb, S., Dowling, M.D. and De Jongh, D. (1970): The dropout problem in antihypertensive therapy. *J. Chronic Dis., 22*, 579.
26. Weintraub, M., Au, W.Y.W. and Lasagna, L. (1973): Compliance as a determinant of serum digoxin concentration. *J. Am. Med. Assoc., 224*, 481.
27. Taggart, A.J., Johnston, G.D. and McDevitt, D.G. (1981): Does the frequency of daily dosage influence compliance with digoxin therapy? *Br. J. Clin. Pharmacol., 1*, 31.
28. Donabedian, A. and Rosenfeld, L.S. (1964): Follow-up study of chronically ill patients discharged from hospitals. *J. Chronic Dis., 17*, 847.

29. Zisook, S. and Gammon, E. (1980-81): Medical noncompliance. *Int. J. Psychiatry Med., 10*, 291.
30. Davis, M. and Eichhorn, R.L. (1963): Compliance with medical regimens: a panel study. *J. Health Human Behav., 4*, 240.
31. Francis, V., Korsch, B.M. and Morris, M.J. (1969): Gaps in doctor-patient communication: patients' response to medical advice. *N. Engl. J. Med., 280*, 535.
32. Sackett, D.L. (1970): Does the periodic health examination affect health? *Sci. Forum, 15*, 9.
33. Antonovsky, A. and Kats, R. (1970): The model dental patient: an empirical study of preventive health behavior. *Soc. Sci. Med., 4*, 367.
34. Porter, A.M.W. (1969): Drug defaulting in a general practice. *Br. Med. J., 1*, 218.
35. Haynes, R.B. (1976): A critical review of the 'determinants' of patient compliance with therapeutic regimens. In: Sackett, D.L., Haynes, R.B. (Eds.), *Compliance with Therapeutic Regimens*, 26. The Johns Hopkins University Press, Baltimore.
36. Becker, M.H., Drachman, R.H. and Kirscht, J.P. (1972): Motivations as predictors of health behavior. *Health Serv. Rep., 87*, 852.
37. Becker, M.I., Maiman, L.A., Kirscht, J.P. et al. (1979): A test of the health belief model in obesity. In: Haynes, R.B., Taylor, D.W., Sackett, D.L. (Eds.), *Compliance in Health Care*, p. 81. The Johns Hopkins University Press, Baltimore.
38. Taylor, D.W. (1979): A test of the health belief model in hypertension. In: Haynes, R.B., Taylor, D.W., Sackett, D.L. (Eds.), *Compliance in Health Care*, p. 103. The Johns Hopkins University Press, Baltimore.
39. Sackett, D.L., Gibson, E.S., Taylor, D.W. et al. (1975): Randomised clinical trial of strategies for improving medication compliance in primary hypertension. *Lancet, 1*, 1205.
40. Tanner, G.A. and Noury, D.J. (1981): The effect of instruction on control of blood pressure in individuals with essential hypertension. *J. Advanced Nursing, 6*, 99.
41. Kruse Goodrich, K. (1981): Gonococcal infection: the effect of educational counselling on patient compliance. *Br. J. Vener. Dis., 57*, 137.
42. Stimson, G.V. (1974): Obeying doctor's orders: a view from the other side. *Soc. Sci. Med., 8*, 74.

# 32. What I have to say to a young diabetes specialist after 35 years of experience

JEAN PIRART

You are a young graduate. You know every step of the metabolic pathways, every enzyme involved in gluconeogenesis, every detail on the microtubules that lead the insulin granules out of the beta cell. And the more you know about that, the less you have had time to talk with patients. You know diabetes as good as your books and your teachers know it. But today you are starting with your medical practice and you have to take care of diabetics (not of diabetes).

Your teachers have been for you wonderful masters in physiology, pathology, biochemistry. They were not so good in clinical knowledge and still less reliable in matters related to the everyday problems of diabetic life. Do not put a blame on them: they could not see patients and listen at patients if they had to succeed in the academic career. They were more familiar with rats and photometers than with diabetic persons in daily life. In fact do not count too much on teachers nor on books. You have now to tackle the problems *on the field*.

Do not trust schemas and classifications too much. After all a patient has right to be himself (or herself) regardless of the pattern he (she) should fit in accordance to *your* theories.

Be ambitious and always try to give the best of yourself for the care of your patients, but remain realistic. Do not try to normalize all parameters. Keep in mind a list of priorities in decreasing order. For the elderly with mild diabetes, comfort and security come first. For the adolescent, normoglycemia should receive priority of course, but not at the expense of joy of living. For that obese hypertensive survivor from a secund infarct, cardiovascular problems and body weight should be first considered. For this obese with progressive retinopathy or for that pregnant, plump lady, normoglycemia, not slimming, should receive most attention.

The same holds true with education. To the family of that teenager remitting from acute diabetes and perfectly controlled with 5 units insulin, do not loose their (and your) time in explaining glucagon at length. Better explain how and when relapse will occur and give them the appropriate preparation to adapt at the end of the honeymoon.

Be *quickly* efficient in education: full knowledge on hypos – glucagon included – is essential from the 3rd or 4th week of insulin treatment in the diabetic who has no remission. But, be together patient and *slow*. If he does not cough and is not too lean, your young diabetic can wait some more weeks before having an X-ray of the chest. Ophthalmoscopy can also wait a little. Do not overburden a new diabetic (new for the patient or only new for you) with too many exams. They will divert the patient's attention from basic knowledge on the disease and the treatment, and give additional worries and constraints.

Adapt your strategy and your tactical manoeuvres to each case. Tailor also their education. Group education will seldom succeed. At best it can help after the most important explanations and recommendations have already been given during personal interviews.

When you talk, never look at your hospital record. Look at the patient. Watch him (her) carefully. As soon as you see that he (she) does no longer understand, stop. Come back to the preceding idea that has not been fully apprehended, repeat and explain at length perhaps with oversimplified sentences, perhaps in a childish way (aren't you a child yourself when facing your lawyer or your tax-collector?). Remember, your talk is intended to be understood, not to be admired.

Be patient with your patient. Do not request him to be too patient! A one-hour lesson is usually meaningless. Half an hour is more realistic and even so, vary the topics: a bit on diet, a bit on shots, a bit on urine testing and a bit on the weather today or on the job or on family affairs. The more recent the diabetes, the shorter the lessons. In fact, in the very first days the patient, and often the family in case of acute severe diabetes, are *not* receptive. Emotions prevail over rational attitudes. You should take that into account. In the very first interviews, it is usually not appropriate to dissert upon diabetes in the long run, upon the future of scientific research or upon the danger of overproduction of glucose by the liver even if you avoid the term gluconeogenesis. Be more matter of facts: explain how to handle the syringe or the test tube.

Do not be afraid of repeating several times the same idea in various manners and even in using exactly the same words.

Do not teach new data before what you already taught has been really assimilated (check it). You are not facing students in medicine. The teacher ought to transmit clearly the best of his knowledge, but what every student has really understood and remembered is not *his* problem. If your message to the diabetic has not been properly received (misunderstood, poorly applied ...) you have failed. Simply failed because there is no treatment without selfcare and there is no selfcare without accurate and more or less extensive knowledge.

Do not talk in a scholar way: 'high blood sugar' or 'low blood pressure' are as good as 'hyperglycemia' or 'hypotension'. Remind: speak to be understood, not to be admired.

Use graphs but draw them yourself with a pencil on a sheet of paper or with a chalk on a blackboard. Do not forget to explain what you put on the vertical axis and what on the horizontal one and show that ... 'it goes up' or 'it goes down' etc. ... Avoid putting actual figures except very simple ones, for instance the clock time or the figures for blood sugar if the listener is familiar with glycemic readings.

Keep in mind that most patients are not used to play with figures, lines, graphs and even simple abstract ideas or symbols. Do not consider them stupid and unable to understand what they ought to know for their treatment. After all, do you feel entirely at ease with the mathematical or the musical language? Remember *your* 'stupidity' when you started playing tennis or skiing or learning French, or while at the driving school. Is it so long ago?

Avoid figures, actual figures because scientific knowledge impresses but terrifies. Just say: smaller than... or faster than... or very long or very slow... or a bit weaker... Not everybody is immediately fit to play chess or bridge or to play with dose adjustment of insulin.

You are familiar with some expressions such as 'hyper', 'hypo', 'positive', 'negative'. The patient is not. Or he is familiar with the term to whom he gives exactly the opposite meaning: a negative commercial balance and a positive discussion between the trade-union and the employer are not perceived the same way as a negative or positive Acetest. When you explain how to test a urine with enzymatic paper or a drop of blood with a Dexstrostix, you say 'one minute'. After many years of scientific training you give the term 'one minute' a meaning that does not correspond to that of the lay people (by the way, are you sure that when you ask your patient to wait one more minute in the waiting room of your office, you still use the same time unit as that of your watch?).

Thus explain everything slowly, gently, completely. Take time to do it. Your patient is to repeat the same procedures his whole life. Hopefully they will be done correctly. This is worth taking some more minutes talking and demonstrating in details.

When a diabetic is new for you, he (she) may well have a long past with cumulated experiences shared by the patient and the doctor(s) before your intervention. If the insulin regimen or the diet seem a bit surprising, do not immediately consider your colleagues ignorant or crazy. Both patient and doctor may well have reached a certain regimen after a long way of trials and errors. Be cautious in taking any decision to change something that apparently is running well, however odd a treatment seems to be.

Listen to your patients. The key of a problem is more often found in their talk than in a laboratory test.

Listen to their questions. They are scarcely stupid or even irrelevant. Try to address these questions to practitioners, even to diabetes specialists. Their answers will more often be stupid than your patient's questions. Sometimes naive questions coming from lay people will open surprising windows on the diabetic universe. Anyway they afford good opportunities to check the patient's knowledge and understanding.

Do not escape any question: if not appropriate for the
the question aside and answer it in due time, some weeks

Be carefully aware of quack remedies, misconceptions an
pain in reading oddities and silly theories. Be prepared t
destroy a belief that can mislead your patient. Go ahead i
such matters. They are sometimes kept carefully hidden be
and the family feel that you will refuse discussing them,
them if they dare to speak of such things.

Ask gently what kind of books your patient has read ab
might be surprised. Take pain to demonstrate how false t
tion is. Do not simply say 'it is false' or 'don't worry
patient may believe in the book and … possibly in you, a
middle of the road manner of thinking or try an imposs
between you and the author, a doctor as you are, after

Do not reject the obese, the alcoholic, the cheater, th
the stubborn, the liar. Are you sure you are right to cas
be in their shoes … only for one day, for one hour.

Check everything with firm but friendly skepticism: I
snack been taken every mid-afternoon including the day
sugar in all pockets? In the pocket of *that* trousers? Is
Glucagon not expired? Are you really sure you got m
wine … or from mayonnaise? Is the diary reliable if all
filled in with one and the same pencil? If all the pa
spotless? Or if the dates of February go up to 29
discover the fake try to save the patient's face: 'Ev
tracted…'.

Know, at least roughly, the calorie and carbohyc
main foods. Joslin once said that otherwise you migh
confidence and esteem. And know somewhat on cooki
just to avoid to be ridiculous while prescribing a die

Some patients adore chattering. This is a way to e
lems. Do not play their game however tempting it cc
them a lecture on the topic they want, for instance i
science-fiction sensationalism. They are fashionable
encourage too long diversions along these lines, part
who still have much to learn. Come back to reality
you constipated? On which hour do you prick at
change the site of injection? Please, show your thi

I know you are a distinguished specialist but dc
down to the slightest details of the treatment. Be p
a slice of bread that size, hold your syringe tha
trembling as strong as this … When you explain hc
with glucagon, make the whole rehearsal in fro
parents. Moreover, given them an expired box in c
the procedure at home.

276

*Pirart*

Be cautious to avoid ambiguity. When you ask 'do you change the site your injections every day?', the answer 'yes' may refer to the fact that e right thigh is used the even days and the left thigh the odd days, but inspection you will discover that on either side only one square inch has en used for many years with a resulting fat pad of lipohypertrophy, red- ss and hypoesthesia. And when you ask 'hypos?' you have in mind: quent mild reactions are a good index of a thrive for normoglycemia; ereas your patient who answers 'OK' has in mind: *not one* hypo, a very nfortable diabetes indeed (with a blood sugar ranging from 150 to 300 /dl every day!). What is the meaning of 'at morning'? In your mind it y be the whole morning, say from 8 to 12 a.m. In the patient's mind, it ht well be on rising ...

nother misunderstanding is common. If you try to explain how to con- hyperglycemia at night, speak of the night sample of urine obtained in ling on rising. Do not say 'the morning sample'. See that the patient's y is kept properly with the column for the urine test performed on rising he *right* side, thus not the first column but rather the *last one*. Otherwise diabetic will not easily understand which insulin he (she) ought to ge. Explain slowly, repeatedly and still more slowly with great em- sis that the urine sample on rising at 7 a.m. does not inform about the ing day, but about the last night. It is determined, of course, by the in- of the *preceding* day (the preceding evening or the preceding morning se of a one-shot regimen).

ambitious, insisting, obstinate, incentive even in treating less gifted le, uneducated people, forgetful aged people, undisciplined children, nic neglectors etc... Be proud when you get a nice (and reliable) diary her with a $HbA_{1c}$ of 7% from an illiterated foreigner with total dia- . It is good. But remain realistic and do not insist on having a two-shots en of self-adjusted mixtures of 2 insulins each in persons who can y measure accurately a fixed unmixed dose of 40 units in their syringe. nuch sophistication harms.

simpler and shorter your instructions, the better they will be under- and applied.

betology is a wonderful job. But be fully conscious that there often a large gap between what should be done and what is actually ed. Pessimists claim that the patient will understand 50% of what ught and will apply correctly 25% during the first months of his es. What will remain of your initial message after 10 years will be nore disappointing (maybe 10% of the bulk of all information given). imists are wrong. Anyway they never should take care of diabetics. miologic studies or animal experiments are better jobs for them. best wishes,

A white-haired but still
enthousiast diabetologist.

# 33. Patient education – recent events in the United States

DONNELL D. ETZWILER

## EDITORIAL

*This article by Doctor Etzwiler illustrates the position of the United States as a pioneer in patient education. Even with full recognition at the level of the official public health authorities, patient education is not systematically recognized and financially covered by the health insurance systems.*

*Successes and difficulties experienced throughout Europe by diabetologists could be very close to those described in this chapter. In the long run, these difficulties should be overcome by the fundamental role played by patient education, the training and cooperation in the quality of the care of the patient and treatment of the disease. (The editors.)*

Patient education is not a new concept in health care. It undoubtedly began milleniums ago when people were told by the local witch doctor or medicine man to 'be careful'. The recent impetus in patient education began in the United States after World War II and diabetes has served as an excellent prototype, since the need for instructing these patients has been generally understood and readily accepted. Dr. Elliott P. Joslin, one of the earliest pioneers in this field, established his diabetes clinic in Boston in a house where patients were taught to manage their diabetes on a day-to-day basis. The importance of that patient education program was not appreciated by most and was emulated by few.

Tuberculosis was a popular model for patient teaching in the 1950's as evidenced by the reports by Jordan on Patient Education at Rutland Heights [1] and by Vavra and Rainbath's paper on Patient Attitudes at Firland Sanitarium [2]. This reawakened an interest, which quickly subsided with the development of isoniazide and streptomycin therapy.

Diabetes again assumed leadership in the field in 1956 when Beaser published the results of a questionnaire distributed among adult patients with diabetes [3]. This vividly demonstrated their lack of information regarding the disease and its management. In the late 50's, while attending pediatric endocrine clinics at the University of Minnesota, I became grossly aware that many young patients there were having difficulties with their diabetes, not because of the intrinsic nature of the illness, but rather from a lack of basic knowledge concerning its management. A multiple-choice questionnaire covering fundamental concepts of the disease was developed, and the

277

results of the study, 'What the Juvenile Diabetic Knows About His Disease' were published in 1962 [4]. This survey was conducted at a summer diabetes camp, and we were appalled at the children's lack of basic concepts about diabetes. We rationalized, however, that since the campers were between 9 and 16 years of age, perhaps their parents were knowledgeable and were assuming the bulk of responsibility for the control of the disease. It was decided to test the theory, and a similar knowledge assessment was conducted among the parents of these campers [5]. This limited study revealed that the parents also lacked a great deal of very fundamental information and stimulated us to extend the studies to all families whose children with the disease attended the public high schools in the Minneapolis-St. Paul area. Results of this study confirmed our initial findings among the camp population [6].

Having identified a serious lack of knowledge among the diabetic patients and their family members, it was decided to further delineate the problem by determining where the breakdown in patient education and communication was occurring in the health care system. It was generally acknowledged at that time in the United States that the bulk of information pertaining to diabetes management was taught primarily by nurses and dieticians. Consequently, 6 schools of nursing in the Minneapolis-St. Paul area were surveyed and questionnaires on diabetes administered to 289 graduating students. Since most of these nursing students were scheduled to take their licensure examinations within a few weeks, we thought their general understanding of the broad field of nursing might be at its highest. Here again, however, a tremendous deficit in basic concepts of diabetes was discovered [7].

97 members of the Minnesota Dietetic Association were also given the same multiple-choice diabetes questionnaire, and again a gross lack of diabetes knowledge was discovered. Is was then apparent that the health professionals who were considered to be primarily responsible for teaching patients were themselves lacking much of the basic information deemed necessary to be conveyed to patients. The survey was then extended to include physicians in their second or third year of post-graduate training at the Minneapolis General Hospital, and again the results revealed a poor understanding of diabetes and the basic concepts of day-to-day management.

Others were then becoming interested in the subject, and Ellis published an article 'Patient Education for Diabetics' in 1965 [8]. About the same time the U.S. Dept. of Public Health began their assessment of the subject. Using the National Health Survey of 1965 as a screening tool, Dr. Glen MacDonald and his staff determined that what had previously been found to be scattered 'local' deficits in patient education was actually nationwide [9]. He noted, for instance, that while 77% of all diabetics were placed on diets, only 10% had sufficient knowledge to choose the proper foods. Williams and Watkins further delineated the lack of knowledge and skills among patients, and the subject stimulated the interest of others [10-12].

Using direct observation, they noted that 3 out of every 5 diabetics were making significant errors in insulin measurement, including incorrect dosage when compared to their physician's prescriptions.

In 1975 the Report of the National Commission on Diabetes defined and substantiated the lack of knowledge of diabetes management among patients and health professionals [13-15]. Patient education was clearly addressed in the recommendations of the Commission in the guidelines for the establishment of Diabetes Research and Training Centers, but no other fiscal support was included in the Commission's recommendations or budget proposals. The hope to improve the delivery of health care to those with diabetes was totally over-ridden by those seeking its elusive immediate cure.

While the diabetes model was pioneering the concept of patient education and patient participation in the 60's, there was a simultaneous 'do it yourself' movement in the U.S. and an increasing concern for minority groups. Patients were viewed as one of the oppressed minority groups which was being dominated by aloof, uncommunicative and authoritative health professionals. 'Intimidated strangers in a land of white'. Historically, the time had arrived for patients to speak out and to demand recognition.

In 1973 a Patient's Bill of Rights was drafted, approved, and widely publicized by the House of Delegates of the American Hospital Association [16]. One of the Bill's purposes was to demonstrate that hospitals would recognize the rights of individuals who were hospitalized for treatment. Sections of the document referred to the patient's right to obtain specific information from physicians and other health professionals working in hospitals concerning their care, management and understanding of procedures and treatment. The American Hospital Association received a great deal of favorable publicity from this action and shortly thereafter assembled an Advisory Committee on Patient Education. It was the Committee's responsibility to formulate the Association's *Statement on the Roles and Responsibilities of Hospitals and Other Health Care Institutes in Personal and Community Health Education* [17]. By 1976 the AHA Joint Accreditation Manual included specific statements regarding the scope of patient education programs. According to the JCAH Manual ... 'The patient has the right to be informed as to the nature and the purpose of any technical procedure to be performed upon him as well as to know by whom such positions are being carried out ... and to receive from persons responsible for care adequate information concerning the nature and extent of his medical problems, planned course of treatment and prognosis. In addition, he has the right to expect adequate instruction and self-care in the interim between the visits to the hospital or to the physician' [18].

Having served as a member of the Advisory Committee of the American Hospital Association, I was impressed that a major component of the health care system had recognized 'patient education as an essential part of quality health care'. This encouraged me to bring the subject before other health professional groups and to urge them to issue similar statements. In 1975 a subcommittee was formed within the American Diabetes Association and a policy statement was published which declared that ... 'Patient education is an integral part of quality health care' [19]. Simultaneously, while a member of the American Group Practice Association's Committee on Patient Education, a similar policy statement was developed and declared by that group [20]. In 1975, we were also successful in persuading the Minnesota State Medical Association to approve a statement on patient education which was later forwarded to the Council of the American Medical Association and endorsed. The resolution confirming patient education as an integral part of quality health care was passed by the House of Delegates of the American Medical Association in June of 1976. Since then, other professional groups in the United States have issued similar statements.

While recognition and acceptance of patient education was occurring in the medical world, our legal system was simultaneously cognizant of the trend and the increasing responsibilities of health care institutions and professionals. This has resulted in litigation which quickly gained the attention of physicians and hospitals alike and has fostered the provision and the documentation of such services. This was emphasized particularly in the area of consent forms. Legal counsel to the California Hospital Association, Charles T. Forbes, has stated that hospitals per se are involved only indirectly in legal questions concerning informed consent; the primary responsibility is the physician's [21].

Others have proposed that clear and concise consent forms be developed and that office and hospital records include a description of the effort made to inform the patient concerning the nature and extent of the procedure, the risks and the consequences as well as the physician's interpretation of the patient's response [22].

Quality patient education requires planning, assessment, delivery, evaluation and documentation, all of which require professional time, time which must be reimbursed, but by whom? Patients themselves are frequently reluctant to pay, since most education in our nation is largely tax-based and education is generally considered a 'free' service. Even private schools and universities in the U.S. fail to charge tuitions which are self-sustaining and must resort to alumni support and periodic fund drives. In a country already acutely aware of staggering health care costs, it is difficult to add yet another costly service. The advocates of patient education have claimed that patients like it and that it will save money in the long run. Opponents say that any new service only adds to the total cost of care and are unwilling to commit millions to an effort which may not show any benefits for 10 or 20 years.

In 1976, a White Paper on Patient Education was issued by Walter McNerny, then President of the Blue Cross Association [23]. In this paper, health care institutions were encouraged to initiate and support patient education programs through existing payment mechanisms. While this concept was endorsed by leaders at the national level, few of the state or regional divisions of the company accepted those recommendations, and the effort had virtually no effect at the local levels where approval of payment occurs. Local groups were reluctant to pay for patient education which they felt was not a proven entity; not in sufficient demand by their insured policyholders to warrant an increased policy rate; and third-party payers had no real assurance of the services they were buying. Consequently, the lack of identified payment for patient education has been a major deterrent to the acceptance and integration of the service in our health care system.

Undoubtedly, one of the greatest deterrents to reimbursement has been the paucity of studies which have clearly demonstrated that patient education is valuable in actually cutting health care costs. Significant studies include one on cardiac patients who required fewer re-hospitalizations and another which demonstrated that patients who were taught prior to hospitalization about their surgery and its expected after-effects were able to be discharged earlier [24]. In the field of diabetes, the most influential study was published by Miller and Goldstein showing a savings in a single institution of over $3 million per year by instituting an active education and support program [25]. The major difficulty with the bulk of patient education evaluation literature is that it is subjective.

In 1965, we presented a paper on 'The Evaluation of Programmed Education Among Juvenile Diabetics and Their Families' in which 108 juveniles were evaluated according to their degree of diabetes control and their knowledge of the disease [26]. These patients were randomly selected from the community and were cared for by a variety of health care providers. Their knowledge of diabetes was initially assessed by questionnaires prior to their usage of an Auto-Tutor with an instructional program on diabetes, developed by the U.S. Public Health Service. Fasting blood glucose levels and 24-hour urine collections for quantitative glucose were obtained prior to the educational experience. The children were then permitted to use the Auto-Tutor which consisted of a single 2½ to 3 hour teaching experience. Following this session, retesting demonstrated a significant increment in knowledge of diabetes among all of the participants. 3 months later, when the participant's knowledge of diabetes was again assessed, it was found to have remained significantly elevated. Our primary concern, however, was to discern if there were any demonstrable differences in the fasting blood glucose levels or in the results of the 24-hour urines for quantitative glucose. These parameters were again evaluated 2 weeks and 3 months after the educational experience. No significant differences in either fasting blood glucose or 24-hour urine results were noted!

In the past few years we have subdivided the patient education process into acute, in-depth and continuing phases [27]. We believe that this is more effective in delivering information, sustaining knowledge, reviewing basic concepts, updating our patient population and stimulating compliance.

The results of our '67 paper were apparent to us at that time increasing patient knowledge alone does not necessarily influence patient behavior, improve disease management, or guarantee a positive outcome and dealt with patient cooperation and compliance. In 1973 we sponsored a conference on 'Education and Management of the Patient with Diabetes Mellitus' [27]. This conference and publication defined the responsibilities of diabetes care among health care professionals and patients, and encouraged the assignment of specific identifiable roles. This stimulated our interest in contracting with the patients. Our patient contracts have been simple written statements which clearly identify patient and physician responsibilities in specific areas of concern. It is obvious that at every office or clinic visit, contracts between patients and health care providers are made which constitute oral agreements or oral contracts. The health professional usually states what should be done, which medication should be taken, how often and when the patient should return. We chose to study patient contracting by identifying a single task and negotiating the specific terms of the contract with the patient [28]. Alternating the usual verbal contracting technique with written contracts, we evaluated the compliance of 100 juvenile diabetics seen consecutively at the St. Louis Park Medical Center. Although we sensed we had an excellent rapport with most of our patients, only 20% of the group complied with the oral contracts. Among those using written contracts, 64% of the patients complied with the stipulated terms. We found that contracting or delineating specific roles and responsibilities is important and does complement patient education by enhancing behavioral alterations. Thus, not only must we as health professionals teach patients about the nature of their disease and its management, but we must also address the concept of developing facets of the health care system which will support and encourage them to carry out their identified responsibilities. Marston's extensive review of the compliance literature in 1970 pointed out some of the factors contributing to patient cooperation or non-cooperation with medical regimes [29]. This literature has continued to grow and to verify that 'non-adherence is clearly one of the major problems and opportunities facing American medicine today' [30]. Zifferblatt's efforts to utilize behavioral analysis to improve drug compliance has been of limited success [31], as have Rosenstack's Health Relief Model [32], later modified by Becker [33, 34]. Thus, the definition of health education – the transference of knowledge which brings about a positive alteration in behavior – calls for teaching *and* ongoing efforts designed to enhance and sustain patient compliance.

The needs of patients are constantly changing. When the current model for the health care delivery system was developed in the U.S., the major causes of death and disability were infectious diseases. Here the physician was called to treat an acutely ill patient who immediately received whatever therapy was then available; a crisis was reached, and the patient either lived or died. The major causes of death and disability today, however, have changed and consist of chronic illness which cannot be cured but can be controlled over long periods of time. Treatment of these diseases frequently demands several daily tasks to be performed, usually by the patient in his/her home. As a result of changing health care needs, the patient has become a vital member of the health care team and not merely a recipient of care. The patient now constitutes a legitimate member of the provider team. Few professionals care to work with poorly informed or improperly trained colleagues; consequently, we all must have a commitment to patient teaching and make certain it is incorporated as an essential part of today's health care system. Quality health care can be achieved only with informed patients cooperating with knowledgeable and concerned health professionals.

## SUMMARY

During the last 50 years it has become increasingly evident in the United States that the education of the patient plays a crucial role in the successful management of his disease. Health care professionals have become more and more aware of the necessity of having a more *collaborative* relationship with their patients, as opposed to the hitherto one-sided relation in which the patient was simply the passive 'receiver' of treatment. A number of studies undertaken in the domain of diabetes confirmed the importance of the education of the diabetic. While the diabetes model was pioneering the concept of patient education, there was a simultaneous 'do-it-yourself' movement in other areas of medicine. An important step took place in 1976 when the House of Delegates of the American Medical Association passed a resolution confirming patient education as an integral part of quality health care. Since then other professional groups in the United States have issued similar statements. In the same year a White Paper on Patient Education was issued by the President of the Blue Cross Association, in which health care institutions were encouraged to support patient education programs through existing payment mechanisms. Despite these recommendations the response was poor; this was largely due to the paucity of studies on the subject, needed to prove the validity of patient education; the costs involved were considered too much of a burden on a health system already overstretched financially, and no insurance cover was integrated into this health system.

The commitment remains, however, that patient education is an essential part of health care, and that quality care can only be achieved by informed patients cooperating with knowledgeable and concerned health care providers.

## REFERENCES

1. Jordan, E.F. et al. (1950): *Patient Education at Rutland Heights, N.Y.* National Tuberculosis Association.
2. Vavra, C. and Rainbath, E.D. (1955): *A Study of Patient's Attitudes Towards Care at Firland Sanitarium.* University of Washington, Seattle.

3. Beaser, S.B. (1956): Teaching the diabetic patient. *Diabetes, 5*, 146.
4. Etzwiler, D.D. (1962): What the juvenile diabetic knows about his disease. *Pediatrics, 29*, 1.
5. Etzwiler, D.D. and Sines, L. (1962): Juvenile diabetes and its management: family, social and academic implications. *J. Am. Med. Assoc., 181*, 304.
6. Collier, P. and Etzwiler, D. (1971): Comparative study of diabetes knowledge among juvenile diabetics and their parents. *Diabetes, 20*, 1.
7. Etzwiler, D.D. (1967): Who's teaching the diabetic? *Diabetes, 16*, 111.
8. Ellis, E. (1965): Patient education for diabetics. *Health Educ. Work, 16*, 59.
9. McDonald, G.V. (1968): Diabetes supplement of the National Health Survey. *J. Am. Diet. Assoc., 52*, 118.
10. Williams, T.F., Anderson, E., Watkins, J.D. et al. (1967): Dietary errors made at home by patients with diabetes. *J. Am. Diet. Assoc., 51*, 19.
11. Watkins, J.D., Williams, T.F. et al. (1967): A study of diabetic patients at home. *Am. J. Public Health, 57*, 452.
12. Watkins, J.D. and Moss, F.T. (1967): Confusion in the management of diabetes. *Am. J. Nurs., 69*, 521.
13. *National Commission Report on Diabetes, Vol. II, Pts. 1-2*, 1975.
14. *National Commission Report on Diabetes, Vol. III, Pt. 5*, p. 129.
15. *National Commission Report on Diabetes, Vol. III, Pt. 3*, p. 41, 1976.
16. American Hospital Association (1975): *A Patient's Bill of Rights* (AHA Catalog 2415) Chicago, AHA.
17. American Hospital Association Policy Statement (1974): *The Role and Responsibilities of Hospitals and Other Health Care Institutions in Personal and Community Health Education.* AHA.
18. Joint Commission on Accreditation of Hospitals (1976): *Accreditation Manual for Hospitals.* Chicago, JCAH.
19. American Diabetes Association (1975): *Policy Statement on Third Party Payment – Report to the Board of Directors.*
20. American Group Practice Association (1974): *Policy Statement on Patient Education.*
21. Forbes, C.F. (1974): Medical legal forum. *Hosp. Forum, 17*, 4.
22. Horsley, J.E. and Lavin, J.H. (1977): An up-to-date guide to informed consent. *Med. Econ., 54*, 150.
23. Blue Cross Association (1974): *White Paper: Patient Health Education.*
24. Rosenberg, S.G. (1971): Patient education leads to better care for heart patients. *HSMHA Health Rep., 86.*
25. Miller, L.V., Goldstein, J. (1972): More efficient care of diabetic patients in a county-hospital setting. *N. Engl. J. Med., 286*, 1388.
26. Etzwiler, D.D. and Robb, J.R. (1972): Evaluation of programmed education among juvenile diabetics and their families. *Diabetes, 21*, 967.
27. Etzwiler, D.D., Hess, K. et al. (1973): *Education and Management of the Patient with Diabetes Mellitus.* Elkhart, Indiana, Ames Company.
28. Etzwiler, D.D. et al., in preparation.
29. Marston, M.V. (1970): Compliance with medical regimens: a review of the literature. *Nurs. Res., 19*, 312.
30. Stunkard, A.J. (1979): Adherence to treatment for diabetes. In: Hamburg BA, Lipsett L, Inoff GE, Drash, A (Eds.), *Behavior and Psycho-social Issues in Diabetes*, p. 129. U.S. Dept. of Health & Human Services.

31. Zifferblatt, S.M. (1975): Increasing patient compliance through the applied analysis of behavior. *Prev. Med., 4*, 173.
32. Rosenstack, I.M. (1966): Why people use health services. *Milbank Mem. Fund. Q, 44*, 94.
33. Becker, M.H. (1976): Sociobehavioral determinants of compliance. In: Sackett, DL, Baynes RB (Ed.), *Compliance with Therapeutic Regimens*, p. 40. The Johns Hopkins University Press, Baltimore.
34. Becker, M.H. and Maiman, L.A. (1975): Sociobehavioral determinants of compliance with health and medical care recommendations. *Med. Care, 13*, 10.

# 34.   The Grady Memorial Hospital diabetes unit ambulatory care program

JOHN K. DAVIDSON

## EDITORIAL

*Although no confirmatory data are available, the current medical belief is that patient education has a more effective impact on the educated middle and upper socio-economic classes. However, most of the patients in the care of Dr. Davidson's medical team emanate from the lower socio-economic class category. This paper, like the one published by Leona Miller in 1972, shows that patient education plays a fundamental role in the effectiveness of diabetes control, regardless of the patient's socio-economic status.*

*The efficiency of Dr. Davidson's diabetes center can also be attributed to its systematic management, which is not only concerned with the treatment of the various aspects of the patient's disease, but also lays emphasis on the importance of cohesive, interdisciplinary, medical teamwork.*

*It is only by evaluating the effectiveness of patient education that this form of therapy can be included in the complete armentarium for sound diabetes therapy. Evaluation (which in fact is the planned management of feedback) will allow new strategies to be adopted by the health-care providers. It is to be hoped that this evaluation will also lead to the development of a health-care system in which patient education can be transmitted and learned, as with any other therapy, rather than intuitively designed, as at present. (The editors.)*

## INTRODUCTION

Grady Memorial Hospital is the primary teaching hospital of the Emory University School of Medicine. It serves a medically-indigent, inner city population of about 350 000 people (82% black) who live in a 2-county area of metropolitan Atlanta. In 1982, about 12 950 (3.7%) of these individuals had diabetes mellitus (2.7% diagnosed, 1.0% undiagnosed). Of those with known diabetes, about 60.6% are black females, 22.6% black males, 11.3% white females, and 5.4% white males. The prevalence of diabetes in those under 20 years of age is about 0.1%, and the prevalence in those over 60 years of age is about 15%. 97% of those known to have diabetes were above their ideal body weight at the time of diagnosis. Females had, at time of diagnosis of diabetes, significantly more excess body weight than males. Body weight (as a percent of ideal body weight) was for black females 154%, for black males 116%, for white females 168% and for white males 116% [15].

## STRATEGY

Although patient education for those with diabetes in the United States was initiated at the Joslin Clinic in the early 20th century and several other private clinics had developed similar programs by 1950, no attempt to develop comparable programs for indigent patients was made until Runyan initiated the Memphis chronic disease program in 1964 [25, 26] and Miller initiated the diabetes program at Los Angeles County Hospital in 1968 [23, 24].

The decision to develop a medical care delivery system of high quality for patients with diabetes at Grady was made in 1968 [1, 4, 6]. By 1971, financial support had been mobilized (primarily from Medicare, Medicaid and the Georgia Regional Medical Program) that made it possible to change the strategy, structure and process of health care delivery from a *crisis-oriented* to a *prevention-oriented* approach (Table 1). In any given population of patients with diabetes, it is important to audit sequentially (preferably yearly) the effects of natural history, of intervention therapy and of professional-patient interactions on outcomes (Table 2).

At Grady prior to 1971, most available professional efffort was concentrated on treatment of acute complications (502 cases of severe diabetic ketoacidosis, i.e. carbon dioxide content of less than 10 mEq per liter, between 1 January 1969 and 31 December 1969) and chronic complications (172 lower extremity amputations between 1 January 1973 and 31 December 1973), leaving little time for comprehensive outpatient evaluation, education and follow-up care.

The strategy, structure and process of care changed significantly when the Diabetes Detection and Control Center (DDCC) opened on 11 January 1971 in 2000 square feet of space, and the *team approach* (physician, nurse, dietician, podiatrist) to patient evaluation, education and follow-up was started. Therapy with oral agents (sulfonylureas and phenformin) was discontinued [2, 5].

The *Diabetes Guidebook: Diet Section* [17], a color-coded picture manual designed for patients with limited reading ability, was published in November, 1971. Each patient is given a personal copy, which he is instructed to bring on return clinic visits. It has proven to be a valuable reference relative to what the patient has been taught concerning diet therapy, and it effectively coordinates the team's follow-up teaching efforts [3, 4, 7, 8].

Since 1973, insulin therapy has been reserved for those: (a) who are significantly hyperglycemic (fasting plasma glucose consistently $> 1.30$ G/L on appropriate diet and exercise therapy) when at or below ideal body weight (b) who acutely decompensate (diabetic ketoacidosis or hyperglycemic hyperosmolar state); and (c) who are pregnant (to protect the fetus). Since 1973 intensive diet therapy (including one-week total fasts, stringent hypocaloric diets and careful follow-up monitoring to encourage patients to attain and maintain ideal body weight) has been the cornerstone of diabetes therapy for those who are above ideal body weight [9, 11, 14, 15, 22].

## STRUCTURE (FACILITIES, PERSONNEL, EQUIPMENT, SUPPLIES)

Because space was not adequate between January 1971 and February 1975, follow-up care was provided in the Diabetes Clinic (DC), situated in an area of the hospital separated from the DDCC. On 10 March 1975, all

Table 1 *The objectives of a prevention-oriented approach to diabetes mellitus*

| Prevention-orientation | Objectives |
| --- | --- |
| 1. Primary prevention <br><br>(Applied to the general population, i.e. 240 million Americans) | To prevent the appearance of hyperglycemia throughout a lifetime by (1) avoiding or 'curing' excess body weight and (2) preventing viral-induced (?) and other beta-cell damage (research underway) |
| 2. Secondary prevention <br>(Applied when diabetes mellitus is diagnosed; an estimated 6.5 million Americans know they have diabetes, estimated 3.5 million have diabetes but do not know it) | To prevent the acute complications and to prevent or delay the appearance of the chronic complications of diabetes mellitus. These objectives may be accomplished by early detection of random glucosuria and hyperglycemia and by appropriate education, therapy (diet, exercise, insulin if needed) and follow-up to attain and maintain ideal body weight and normoglycemia or near-normoglycemia |
| 3. Tertiary prevention <br>(Applied when acute or chronic complications of diabetes mellitus are detected; an estimated 5 million Americans have, or will have, one or more of these complications) | To decrease mortality and morbidity resulting from acute and chronic complications of diabetes mellitus by prevention of, or by early detection and prompt and appropriate therapy of the complications |

Diabetes Unit activities (DDCC, DC, Podiatry Clinic, laboratory and other supporting services) were relocated and integrated within one area containing over 10 000 square feet of space.

Since 1976, the Diabetes Unit has provided comprehensive primary care for the majority of its patients [6, 13]. In 1982, the diabetes health care team consisted of 4 M.D. diabetologists, 16 nurse practitioners, 5 dieticians, a podiatrist, 3 laboratory technicians, a social worker and 15 supporting personnel (aides, clerks, secretaries, administrative assistants etc.). Each newly-diagnosed patient is seen promptly (within 24 hours if necessary) in the DDCC for team evaluation, education and therapy during a full-day visit. The same team members provide follow-up care in the DC on continuing basis.

The nurse practitioner is the primary contact professional to whom patients have access by telephone or by drop-in appointment (with physician supervision and dietician and podiatrist assistance). Each nurse provides follow-up care for a panel of about 500 active patients.

Table 2 *Auditing the effects of the natural history, of intervention therapy and of professional-patient interactions on outcomes*

| Professional's obligations to patients | Auditing outcomes |
|---|---|
| Give complete and accurate information; reference the natural history of diabetes mellitus and its complications and reference the benefits, risks and costs of available intervention therapeutic modalities | Audit by appropriate (yearly) sequential measurements of outcomes as affected by the natural history of the disease (compare to matched population of non-diabetic controls) and by the effects of intervention therapy (therapies) and adherence or non-adherence in a defined population of patients. |
| *Patients' obligations to themselves* Once patients become thoroughly knowledgable about diabetes and its natural history, their freedom of choice permits them to respond to professional recommendations in a self-determined way. This in turn determines whether a patient will adhere or not adhere to a prescribed routine, and for how long. It also may determine whether a patient will be rewarded by adherence, or penalized by non-adherence, to a prescribed routine | Ideally, all complications (diabetic ketoacidosis, hyperosmolar hyperglycemic state, retinopathy, nephropathy, arteriopathy and neuropathy) and associated problems should be audited. Practically, some problems (i.e. ketoacidosis and amputations) are easier to audit sequentially than others. In each program, the eventual aim should be to measure outcomes (mortality, morbidity) in terms of the natural history of diabetes as influenced by various types of available intervention therapy (benefits, risks, costs) |

## PROCESS (DETECTION, DIAGNOSIS, EVALUATION, EDUCATION AND THERAPY)

For detecting the unknown non-pregnant individual with diabetes mellitus (defined as a fasting plasma glucose > 1.40 G/L × 3, or a GTT sum of fasting plus 1, 2, and 3 hour post-one-hundred-gram-glucose-load plasma glucose levels > 8.00 G/L), a random urine glucose level > 0,25 G/L (Beckman glucose analyzer) [10] has a sensitivity of 100%, a specificity of 99.3% and a predictive value of 74%. In other words, 74% of those with a random urine glucose > 0.25 G/L will have diabetes mellitus on follow-up testing and 26% will have renal glucosuria [18].

When a diagnosis of diabetes is established in any inpatient, outpatient or satellite clinic division of the hospital, the patient is promptly referred for a full day of evaluation and education in the DDCC [12, 16]. During that day, a complete data base (subjective and objective) is collected on computer-compatible data sheets, and a complete problem list is constructed. Detailed information reference status of diabetes, its complications and therapy is recorded. Patient education is detailed, and patients responses to instructions are carefully noted. Indicated consultations, procedures and tests are scheduled. Urine testing and food measuring equipment and indicated prescriptions are supplied. The patient is assigned to the panels of 4 professionals (physician, nurse, dietician, podiatrist) who subsequently provide continuing primary care, and a return clinic appointment is given. During the day, the dietician instructs the patient on the diet prescribed by the physician, and prepares a copy of *Diabetes Guidebook: Diet Section* for the patient to use on a continuing basis. The patient is evaluated, educated and treated (if needed) by the podiatrist. Appropriate laboratory testing is done.

An electrocardiogram is routinely done on all new patients. If peripheral vascular disease is suspected, Doppler ultrasonography and plythesmography are done. If proteinuria is present, the patient is evaluated for nephropathy. If neuropathy is present, nerve conduction velocity measurements may be done.

After evaluation and education in the DDCC, a diligent effort is made to provide continuity of care for the patient. The nurse is the primary contact professional, and is available to the patient by phone or by drop-in visits to the diabetes clinic (DC) whenever the DC is open (Monday through Friday from 7:30 a.m.-4:30 p.m.). Physician, dietician and podiatry support are available at these times. If the patient misses an appointment, the nurse calls and/or sends the patient another appointment, and makes a maximal effort to keep the patient active in the prescribed treatment program.

## AUDITS OF OUTCOMES

By mid-1982, over 11 000 individuals had been evaluated, educated and treated in the DDCC and DC. About 1700 of these individuals died during the 11 year period (from the opening of the DDCC in January 1971 through December 1981).

In 1978, an audit showed that there were 24 993 visits and 8642 telephone calls to the Diabetes Unit [13]. This was a 6-fold increase in the number of visits to the Diabetes Clinic when compared to the number of visits to the clinic in 1967.

950 patients (73 per 1000 of those with diabetes) with a primary diagnosis of diabetes or one of its complications were hospitalized at Grady for 10 925 days in 1978 for a mean duration of 0.84 day per patient with diabetes (10 925 days for 12 950 patients) [19].

Decreases in preventable hospitalizations have been reported by Miller [23, 24] (from 5.6 hospital days per patient with diabetes in 1968 to 1.25 hospital days in 1973) and by Runyan [25, 26].

At Grady, there was a significant decrease in cases of severe diabetic ketoacidosis ($CO_2$ content $< 10$ mEq/l) and the hyperglycemic hyperosmolar state (serum osmolality $> 350$ mOsm/l) between 1969 and 1974 (from 38.8 episodes per 1000 patients in 1969 to 14.3 episodes per 1000 patients in 1974, and a further decline to 8.6 episodes per 1000 patients in 1978). There was a significant decline in total cases of diabetic ketoacidosis (severe, moderate, and mild) and the hyperglycemic hyperosmolar state between 1974 and 1978 (from 41.2 episodes per 1000 patients in 1974 (14.3 per 1000 were severe) to 20.6 episodes per 1000 patients in 1978 (8.6 per 1000 were severe) [19]. It is estimated that 1578 cases of diabetic ketoacidosis and of the hyperglycemic hyperosmolar state were prevented by the ambulatory care program between 1975 and 1981.

There was a significant decrease in lower extremity amputations after 1973 (from 13.3 amputations per 1000 patients in 1973 to 6.72 amputations per 1000 patients in 1980) [19]. It is estimated that 627 lower extremity amputations were prevented by the ambulatory care program between 1974 and 1981.

Audits to determine mortality rates in various demographic subgroups are underway, as are morbidity audits to determine the prevalence of retinopathy, blindness, nephropathy, renal failure, arteriopathy (coronary, peripheral, cerebral) and neuropathy.

In 1981, 81% of the patients were being treated with diet and exercise therapy alone, while 19% were being treated with diet, exercise and insulin. No oral agent therapy has been used since 1970.

Audits done in a cohort of 433 patients for whom oral agent therapy had been discontinued in 1970 and who were alive and active in the Grady Diabetes Clinic in 1979 showed that 311 (71.8%) were on diet and exercise therapy alone and 122 (28.2%) were on diet, exercise and insulin therapy [19].

In the diet and exercise group the average weight loss had been 20.3 pounds, with 87% having lost weight and 13% having gained weight over the 9 year follow-up period. The 1979 plasma glucose level was lower than the 1970 plasma glucose level (when patients were on oral agent therapy) in 151 (48.6%), unchanged in 58 (18.6%), and higher in 102 individuals (32.8%).

In the diet, exercise and insulin group, the average weight loss had been 11.3 pounds, with 72% having lost weight and 28% having gained weight over the 9 year follow-up period. The 1979 plasma glucose level was lower than the 1970 plasma glucose level (when patients were on oral agent therapy) in 67 (54.9%) and higher in 55 individuals (45.1%).

These audits confirm the fact that aggressive nutritional care (one week fasts, hypocaloric diets, intensive follow-up) [17, 20] will result in significant sustained weight loss in many of those who are overweight with a corresponding lowering of the plasma glucose level over a 9-year follow-up period.


## EVALUATION OF COSTS, BENEFITS AND RISKS OF ALTERNATIVE METHODS OF THERAPY FOR DIABETES

Demonstrable benefits of diabetes therapy should include: (a) weight loss in the obese, (b) return of sustained normoglycemia, (c) improved quality of life (fewer acute and chronic complications and hospitalizations) and (d) increased length of life. Benefits should be evaluated in terms of costs, i.e., resources expended and risks taken. When possible, monetary costs of structure and process (alternative methods of therapy) should be related to the monetary equivalents of benefits. One must guard against equating redundant (more) care and spending more money with quality. Frequently, quality declines as unnecessary care increases [21]. The cost of establishing and operating a monitoring apparatus (auditing and evaluating outcomes) should not only improve quality of care, it should be cost-effective. In other words, it should save more money than it costs over the long-term.

It now appears that a considerable amount of money is being wasted in health care delivery for those who are overweight and who have non-insulin dependent diabetes mellitus when oral agents or insulin therapy are substituted for appropriate weight loss as a result of aggressive nutritional education, treatment and follow-up. Also, drug therapy of obesity-induced diabetes is usually less effective and more risky than diet therapy [22].

No matter how careful and accurate the balance sheet of savings and expenditures is, a definitive judgment cannot be made regarding benefits vs. costs unless it is possible to measure the impact on the patient's health status. Because this has been so difficult, it is no wonder that an evaluation of the correlation between process and cost/benefits of medical care for patients with diabetes is just beginning [13]. The costs and benefits of alternate methods of therapy for diabetes should receive more attention in the future. Third-party payors are having an increasing impact on the way medicine is practiced, in that they usually determine which procedures are reimbursable and which procedures are not reimbursable. In the past, some decisions have been made on the basis of incomplete or misleading data. The prevention-oriented approach described in this communication has been supported from its inception by third-party payors. The prevention-oriented approach has provided better care for less money. As a result, third-party payors have saved money by decreasing markedly the use of resources that had been spent pre-1971 for hospitalizations that could have been prevented.

The total cost of operating the Grady Memorial Hospital Diabetes Unit Ambulatory Care Program for the last 9 years (January, 1973, through December, 1981) was approximately $6 300 000.00. It is estimated that the changes in strategy, structure and process of health care delivery initiated in 1971 prevented 627 amputations and 1578 cases of diabetic ketoacidosis during that 9 year period. Also, no oral agents and less insulin were used to control hyperglycemia because the expanded nutritional care program was successful in producing weight loss and lowering the plasma glucose in many of those with non-insulin dependent diabetes mellitus. The estimated savings from avoiding hospitalization for 627 amputations was $7 584 000 and for avoiding hospitalization for 1578 cases of diabetic ketoacidosis was $2 051 400. $549 835 was saved from not using oral hypoglycemic agents, and $55 190 was saved from using less insulin. Thus the estimated total cost avoidance from the 4 audited outcomes alone was $10 240 425. This means that the hospital spent $3 940 425 less than the total cost of the ambulatory care program ($6 300 000) by substituting the post-1971 prevention-oriented strategy for the pre-1971 crisis-oriented strategy in the treatment of diabetes mellitus. Also, the hospital recovered much of the $6 300 000 from third-party payors, especially Medicare and Medicaid.

## SUGGESTIONS FOR ORGANIZING AND OPERATING AN AMBULATORY CARE PROGRAM FOR PATIENTS WITH DIABETES

Much has been learned in the Grady program which can be transferred to other programs, i.e. 1) that the prevalence of ketoacidosis and amputations can be decreased markedly, 2) that aggressive diet therapy can result in significant sustained weight loss and frequently in normoglycemia in those with NIDDM, and 3) that oral agent and insulin therapy are relatively ineffective in the treatment of NIDDM. Other lessons about the natural history of IDDM and NIDDM and the effects of various intervention

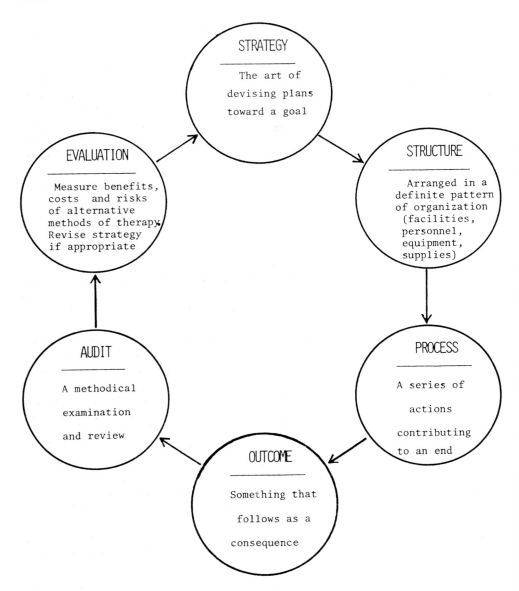

Fig. 1 Methods for developing, monitoring and evaluating a health care delivery system.

therapies will almost certainly be learned in the future. Meanwhile, how can contemporary knowledge be used to assist those who wish to organize and operate similar programs?

It seems appropriate to use a plan that conforms to the outline in Figure 1, proceeding from strategy to structure to process to outcome to audit to evaluation of costs, risks, and benefits of alternative methods of therapy, then back to strategy (and a revision of same if indicated) [13].

Structure (facilities, personnel, equipment, supplies) will vary depending on: 1) the size of the population with diabetes that is to be served, 2) the number in that population with IDDM and with NIDDM, 3) the ability of members of the population to pay for medical care (indigent or non-indigent?), 4) whether the provider is to supply primary, secondary and/or tertiary care and 5) whether the program is to develop in a public or private hospital, a public or private clinic, a group practice, or in a solo MD practitioner's office.

Using the team approach for evaluation, education and treatment (physician, nurse, dietician, podiatrist etc.), the Grady program has shown that the full-time physician can provide essentially all of the primary and secondary care and some of the tertiary care for about 1500 patients with diabetes if he has 1 registered dietician and 3 nurse practitioners working with him full-time.

The *Policy and Procedure Manual* of the Grady Memorial Hospital Diabetes Unit [12] and *Diabetes Guidebook: Diet Section* [17] contain considerable information on the organization and operation of an ambulatory care diabetes unit.

The National Diabetes Advisory Board published a report in 1980 [27] that it submitted to the U.S. Congress reference a national plan to reduce mortality and morbidity from diabetes in the 1980's. This report dealt with 5 problems: 1) foot complications and amputations, 2) diabetic ketoacidosis, 3) perinatal morbidity and mortality, 4) blindness and 5) nephropathy. It also dealt with health care financing, communications, professional education, health care planning and evaluation and health care systems that were needed to help reduce morbidity and mortality from these 5 problems.

Although serious impediments to the development of optimal programs were recognized (lack of provider and patient knowledge and lack of financial resources), the Board report gave an overview of the magnitude of the problems to which it addressed its deliberations. A lack of financial resources should not be used as an excuse for failure to expand provider and patient knowledge with resources that are currently available, since it is proven already from data provided in this and other communications that the prevention-oriented strategy described earlier is much more cost-effective than is the still commonly-used crisis-oriented strategy.

*J.K. Davidson*

## SUMMARY

The Grady Memorial Hospital Diabetes Unit Ambulatory Care Program has provided comprehensive evaluation, education, therapy, and follow-up care for more than 11.000 patients using the team approach (physician, nurse, dietician, podiatrist, laboratory technician, and supporting personnel) from January, 1971, through mid-1982. The prevalence of diabetic ketoacidosis and of amputations has been reduced markedly, and this has saved the hospital several million dollars. Aggressive diet therapy (including one-week fasts) has produced significant weight loss and has lowered the plasma glucose level in many of those with non-insulin dependent diabetes over a 9-year follow-up period.

## ACKNOWLEDGEMENT

This work was supported in part by the Georgia Department of Human Resources Diabetes Control Program Contract Number 4279300673 and by the Howell Diabetes Research Fund. The author expresses his gratitude to those who assisted him in data collection and in the analyses reported: James Johnson, Ilsa Mainzer, Rober Byers and Shirley Langella.

## REFERENCES

1. Davidson, J.K. (1971): In: Fajans, S.S., Sussman, K.E. (Ed.), *Diabetes mellitus: Diagnosis and Treatment, Vol 3*, p. 207. American Diabetes Association, New York.
2. Miller, M., Bennet, P.H., Davidson, J.K., Klimt, C.R. and Reid, D.D. (1972): *Panel on Diabetes. Epidemiologic Studies and Clinical Trials in Chronic Diseases.* Proceedings of a symposium held during the 11th meeting of the Pan American Health Organization Advisory Committee on Medical Research. Scientific Publication #257, 29.
3. Davidson, J.K. (1974): In: Conn, H.F. (Ed.), *Current Therapy*, p. 386. W.B. Saunders Co, Philadelphia.
4. Davidson, J.K. (1975): Educating diabetic patients about diet therapy. *Int. Diabetes Fed. Bull.*, *20*, 1.
5. Davidson, J.K. (1975): The FDA and hypoglycemic drugs. *J. Am. Med. Assoc.*, *232*, 853.
6. Davidson, J.K., Alogna, M.T., Goldsmith, M.P. and Riley, T. (1976): In: *Report of the National Commission on Diabetes to the Congress of the United States, Vol 3, Pt 5*, p. 227. D H E W Pub No (NIH) 76-1013.
7. Davidson, J.K. (1976): Diet therapy for diabetes mellitus. *Postgrad. Med.*, *59*, 115.
8. Goldsmith, M.P. and Davidson, J.K. (1977): Southern ethnic food preferences and exchange values for the diabetic diet. *J. Am. Diet. Assoc.*, *70*, 61.
9. Davidson, J.K. (1977): Plasma glucose lowering effect of caloric restriction in obesity-induced insulin-treated diabetes mellitus. (Presented at the annual ADA meeting in St. Louis, Missouri, June 1977). *Diabetes*, *26*, 355.

10. Davidson, J.K., Reuben, M., Sterberg, J.C. and Ryan, W.T. (1978): Diabetes screening using a quantitative urine glucose method. *Diabetes, 27,* 810.
11. Davidson, J.K. (1978): In: Melmon, K.L., Morrelli, H.F. (Eds.), *Clinical Pharmacology, 2nd Edn.,* p. 523. Macmillan, New York.
12. Davidson, J.K. and Delcher, H.K. (1979): *Policy and Procedure Manual.* Diabetes Unit, Grady Memorial Hospital, Atlanta, Georgia.
13. Davidson, J.K., Delcher, H.K. and Englund, A. (1979): Spin-off cost/benefits of expanded nutritional care. *J. Am. Diet. Assoc., 75,* 250.
14. Davidson, J.K. (1979): Diabetes mellitus and its treatment with diet, exercise, insulin and sulfonylureas. In: Wang, R.I.H., *Practical Drug Therapy,* p. 417. J.B. Lippincott, Philadelphia.
15. Davidson, J.K. (1980): Dietary control of diabetes in man. In: Tobin, R., Mehlman, M.A. (Eds.), *Advances in Modern Human Nutrition,* p. 138 Pathotox Publishers, Inc., Illinois.
16. Davidson, J.K., Alogna, M.T., Goldsmith, M.P. and Borden, J. (1981): Assessment of program effectiveness at Grady Memorial Hospital. In: Lawrence, P., Steiner, G. (Eds.), *Educating of the diabetic patient,* p. 329. New York, Springer Publishing Co.
17. Davidson, J.K. and Goldsmith, M.P. (1982): *Diabetes Guidebook: Diet Section, 3rd Edn.* Litho-Krome Co., Columbus, Georgia.
18. Davidson, J.K. (1983): Topic 167: Diabetes mellitus. In: Hurst, J.W. (Ed.), *Clinical practice of medicine.* Butterworth, Woburn, Mass. In press.
19. Davidson, J.K. (1983): The Grady Memorial Hospital experience. In: *Diabetes: The clinical perspective provided by epidemiology,* Ch. 13. Churchill Livingston, London, England. In press.
20. Davidson, J.K. (1983): Diet. In: Schnatz, J.D. (Ed.), *Diabetes Mellitus.* Addison Westley Publishing Co., Menlo Park, California.
21. Donabedian, A. (1978): *Needed Research in the Assessment and Monitoring of the Quality of Medical Care.* Off Sci Tech Information, Natl Ctr for Health Services, Research Report, 1978.
22. Knatterud, G.L., Klimt, C.R., Levin, M.E., Jacobson, M.E. and Goldner, M.G. (1978): Effects of hypoglycemic agents on the vascular complications in patients with adult-onset diabetes. 7. Mortality and selected non-fatal events with insulin treatment. *J. Am. Med. Assoc., 240,* 37.
23. Miller, L.V. and Goldstein, J. (1972): More efficient care of diabetic patients in a county-hospital setting. *N. Engl. J. Med., 285,* 1388.
24. Miller, L.V., Goldstein, J., Dumar, D. and Dye, L. (1981): In: Steiner, G., Lawrence, P.A. (Eds.), *Educating Diabetic Patients,* p. 349. Springer Publishing Co., New York.
25. Runyan, J.W. (1975): The Memphis chronic disease program. *J. Am. Med. Assoc., 231,* 264.
26. Runyan, J.W. (1980): Diabetes continuing care program. *Diabetes Care, 3,* 382.
27. US Department of Health and Human Services (1980): *A report of the National Diabetes Advisory Board. The Treatment and Control of Diabetes: A National Plan to Reduce Mortality and Morbidity.* Public Health Service, National Institutes of Health. NIH Publication No 81-2284.

# 35. Education of diabetic patients: Personal experience of a nurse

KERSTIN SPARRE

## EDITORIAL

*This paper by Kerstin Sparre shows the key-position held by the nurse in the health-system for diabetics. In order to meet the individual needs of the patient, there should exist in the medical team a unifying and coordinating presence; the nurse is ideally suited to play this role. (The editors.)*

The Diabetic Unit at the Karolinska Hospital is responsible for the health of an urban population of 143,100 persons, of whom 2,300 are known to be diabetic.

Generally speaking, all diabetics are checked primarily by their district doctor or private doctor. However, about 40% of them are regularly checked at the specialized unit at the hospital. These patients are mostly insulin-dependent, or in such a state of health that they need regular specialized attention.

Before 1968 no organized instruction existed for diabetics at the Karolinska Hospital. Doctors did not instruct regularly and dieticians were rarely called upon. In 1968 a medical team was formed consisting initially of a physician in charge, a nurse, a dietician and a chiropodist, all of whom had special educational training in diabetes care. An educational program for patients was then developed. In the beginning the difficulties were enormous, above all in the endeavour to get the doctors to recognize the advantages of this patient program. The impression given was that the nurse, the dietician and the chiropodist existed only to serve the doctor. As a rule the patient met the doctor first, and later one or two other members of the team. By that time the patient was already tired and not very motivated for instruction. The diabetic staff did not function well as a team but merely as 4 separate elements. Many times the patient felt that the instruction from the nurse or dietician was a 'punishment' for coming to see the doctor with poor metabolic control.

Gradually group teaching for the patients admitted to the hospital was arranged; at first a few times per week, later on every day, and finally twice a day. It has been difficult for the hospital staff to recognize the patients' real need for information and instruction and to realize the enormous need to support and understand their individual situations.

The instruction program has also been too theoretical and technical. At the hospital the patients had no real need to put into practice their new knowledge, living, as they did, in such artificially protected surroundings and being so well cared for. However, many problems confronted them at the time of their discharge from the hospital. It was also difficult to get the patients to come and attend the lessons while hospitalized.

The result of all this was that the patients only obtained a fragmentary knowledge of diabetes, and did not understand the whole picture of diabetes and its treatment.

## 'SCHOOL OF DIABETES'

To avoid these mistakes, in 1979 we reorganized the instruction program. The main emphasis is now placed upon a so-called 'School of Diabetes'. Patients with uncontrolled diabetes, but who do not need hospital care, are referred to the school. They have suffered the disease for either short or longer periods. These patients can be between 17 and 70 years of age. They are divided into 2 main groups: (a) younger and (b) older than 40 years. 5 patients, as near to each other in age as possible, are admitted as day patients to the hospital for a period of 1 week (Table 1). During this period they are taught in groups twice a day about diabetes theory, diet, control of the disease, insulin and injection techniques, what to do in case of hyper- or hypoglycemic states, as well as about sick-day rules. In addition, they are taught preventive foot-care. The disease is controlled through blood and urine glucose measurements 4 times a day, performed by the patients themselves in the presence of an instructor. With daily support of the team the patients analyze the results and are allowed to change the treatment themselves as necessary.

The patients have lunch and snacks together with some members of the team during which time special attention is given to teaching them practical diet habits, especially the exchange of carbohydrates.

A diabetic trained in teaching and psychology takes part in the program as well. Her task is to lead a discussion with the group on what it really means to have diabetes, and in the light of her own experiences she gives advice on how this knowledge can be adapted to everyday life.

The participants support each other tremendously and take pleasure when there are improvements in their blood glucose tests; we also observed that they expressed mutual sympathy when difficulties arose. Every day there is an opportunity to have individual consultations with members of the team, but the main interest is cooperation within the group. The social worker at the clinic takes part in the program, and when needed, gives supporting talks.

After the training period in our Diabetes School the patients check and actively adjust their treatment at home. This is achieved by a member of

Table 1  *Weekly program of the School of Diabetes*

| Time | Day 1 Monday | Day 2 Tuesday | Day 3 Wednesday | Day 4 Thursday | Day 5 Friday |
|---|---|---|---|---|---|
| 08.00 | Blood glucose testing, discussion of previous day's results. Modifying of treatment according to the results. Training for insulin-injections. | | | | |
| 09.00 | snacks | to be a diabetic | snacks | practice of foot care | snacks |
| | | | Urine testing | | |
| 10.15 | introduction what is diabetes | continued | diet 2 | foot care | diet 3 |
| | doctor | diabetic teacher | dietician | chiropodist | dietician |
| 11.00 | | | Lunch buffet | | |
| 12.00 | | | Individual consultation | | |
| 12.30 | diet 1 | blood glucose test. Test of urine glucose and ketones | insulin-treat-ment hypoglycemia | social ques-tions. Diabetic as-sociations | analysis of home-controls. Hyper-glycemia |
| | dietician | nurse | nurse | social worker | nurse |
| 13.15 | | | Blood glucose test | | |
| | | | Individual consultation | | |

the team being available to give advice when necessary. Afterwards the patients go back to the hospital or see their own doctor. No further follow-up is carried out in our centre.

The theoretical part of the course is open to patients admitted to the hospital. The diabetes team helps with individual advice to these patients together with the ward staff. The in-patients take as much of an active part in their treatment as possible and check their blood and urine glucose themselves.

## EVALUATION OF THE IMPACT OF THE 'SCHOOL OF DIABETES' ON THE REGULAR CARE OF THE PATIENT

We have recently finished a pilot study with the purpose of evaluating the school. The test included 40 patients attending the course. All were admitted to the Unit because of failure in their metabolic control and lack of diabetes knowledge. Before the course we tested aptitude and behavior regarding injection sites, snack intake, home control notebook and foot-care. Patients were tested on the same questions a fortnight and several months after finishing the course. The results of the test showed that:
* the knowledge of diabetes had increased considerably;
* skills improved, e.g. the patients chose adequate snacks, managed correctly their self-controls, injection techniques, and care of the feet;
* metabolic control improved;
* the patients were satisfied with the program – most of them appreciated the group dynamics because they were able to meet other diabetics and exchange useful knowledge. They also appreciated the time devoted to psychosocial problems and regretted that there was not more time allotted to these;
* they were positive about home blood glucose monitoring and adjusting the treatment accordingly.

4 and 8 months later, the knowledge, behavior and metabolic control were once again checked. The results then appeared to be different:
* knowledge acquired during the course had been retained;
* the positive effects on skills and behavior were only partly maintained: diet habits, injection techniques and foot-care seemed better than before the program; but the quality of self-monitoring and control dropped to the pre-course level;
* the same happened to metabolic control, which remained more or less the same as before the program.

8 to 12 months after the end of the school program, 8 patients who carried out home-monitoring and 8 patients who did not, or who did so only sporadically, were interviewed about their difficulties in managing the disease. Their answers suggested:
* that a stable family situation with its support is a prerequisite for adequate control of the disease;
* that it takes a long time and more than one week of a group program, to get a patient to assume responsibility for the control of his illness.

## THE DIABETIC CLINIC

The diabetic team usually has consulting hours 2 days per week. The doctor, the nurse and dietician work independently with their patients while the chiropodist and another nurse look after foot problems together. These members of the team are able to call on the assistance of the doctor if necessary. After the consulting hours the diabetic team meets and discusses the problems they have encountered. Once a month the whole team organizes an orthopedic consultation for patients with special foot problems. This consultation permits the members of the team to benefit from each other's experience and allows the patient to feel close to the health care providers.

## WOMEN'S CLINIC AND CHILDREN'S CLINIC

Pregnant diabetics are checked and treated at the women's clinic throughout their entire pregnancy. The diabetic team joins in, once a week, at the women's clinic and assists in treatment and training of the patients. After delivery, the women are checked once at the diabetic clinic.

The children's clinic has its own doctor and dietician while the same nurse attends both child and adult clinics. The children come to the clinic approximately every other month for a check-up where they see the doctor one time, and the nurse and dietician the next time. The advantage of this system is that parents and child meet the nurse and the dietician in a relaxed atmosphere and do not consider this visit as a 'punishment' for insufficient metabolic control. The doctor is always available for consultation.

## CONCLUSIONS

During recent years the diabetic team has worked together more than ever before. The work is jointly planned and developed. The basic training of diabetics will, in the future, be carried out by the diabetic school. To achieve more satisfying results we have to consider 2 points. First of all the follow-up, which should be carried out after attendance at the diabetic school, must be radically improved. We must look upon treatment as an essential part of the patient's daily way of life. It is necessary that the patient be assisted in coping with his diabetes by being encouraged to be realistic in order to help him progressively accept responsibility for the treatment of his illness. He should be helped to strive to attain a good balance between his own independence and dependence on the medical team. This approach requires more frequent check-ups than has hitherto been the case and should be started immediately after completion of the training program. The calls made on the doctor and nurse must take on another dimension in which medical requirements are met, while arriving, at the same time, at socio-psychological objectives.

The second point to be taken into consideration is that we have to improve pedagogical training and ultimately develop completely new methods in patient education. We must also be prepared to accept occasional failure, and the fact that the patient will sometimes reject what he or she has been taught.

## SUMMARY

This article attempts to focus attention on certain difficulties experienced in the treatment of diabetic patients, notably the problems involved in getting together a coordinated medical team and the problem of trying to obtain motivated physicians to teach patients. In order to attain the goals set for the efficacy and continuity of treatment, we have reorganized our service and have set up a 'school' for diabetics. This has permitted our team to work in closer contact, to the advantage of the diabetic patient. Some preliminary results of a study carried out in our centre have shown that knowledge and skill have improved and remained at the same level one year after the patients had attended the teaching centre: unfortunately, improvement in diabetes self-monitoring and control were not parallel to the improvement in knowledge and skill. This result suggests that further strategies should be formulated in order to ensure that the patient attains a state of health in which the effects of education on his diabetes are positive and long-lasting.

# 36. Discovery of the 'medical team' concept and the training of its members

TORBJORN GJEMDAL

## EDITORIAL

*In this article Dr. Gjemdal, at the request of the editors, describes his own painful developmental passage from treating no diabetic patients to finding himself responsible for all the diabetic patients in a 'large, regional hospital'. His growing interest in diabetic treatment finally expanded to educational activities about diabetes within a population of approximately 250,000. There will probably be readers of this article who can easily identify with Dr. Gjemdal's plight and find his progressive endeavors, findings and suggestions useful for application to their own situations. (The editors.)*

## BACKGROUND

In 1975 I worked in a large regional hospital in Norway as a hematologist mainly in internal medicine with blood diseases such as leukemia and other types of cancer. I was 1 of 5 senior physicians in our medical department, which also included a cardiologist, nephrologist, gastroenterologist, lung specialist, and a hematologist.

Suddenly something happened which was to alter the situation drastically. A 22-year old diabetic patient in her 7th month of pregnancy was admitted. When she arrived, the baby was dead. None of the doctors in the department had been treating her. Furthermore, no one had any interest in the treatment of diabetics, especially not pregnant diabetic patients.

It came as a great shock to the head physicians in our department that none of us had been treating this pregnant, diabetic patient. We agreed that one of us should be in charge of her treatment. The question was, who? Everyone had a great many responsibilities within their own specific field. None of us had the time, energy, or qualifications for the treatment of diabetic patients, who make up about 2% of the total population. I was elected for the job with only one opposing vote, my own.

My first reaction was to refuse to accept the situation. I did not want the responsibility for I had been educated and employed to treat blood disorders. I wanted to work with my specialty, not diabetes. This did not help my frame of mind.

My next reaction was anger and irritation when my colleagues referred all diabetic problems to me. A short period of depression followed. I did not want to treat diabetics, but, nevertheless, it was my responsibility.

Gradually, I became more realistic and began to accept the situation. However, it took 6 months for me to accept that I actually was permanently in charge of the treatment of diabetes. During these 6 months, I received no advice or help in facing the situation.

To increase my knowledge, I bought some books on diabetes which contained interesting topics, but practically nothing about the everyday treatment of diabetes. Perhaps I read the wrong books. I still had not read the terms 'diabetic team' or 'teaching nurse', but I had come across the word 'dietician', even if we did not have one at our hospital. The more I learned, the more interesting I found the subject. The final stage of my reaction to the problem began. There seemed to be some hope of improving the situation after all.

I was determined to make a serious attempt to improve the standard of treatment of diabetics in our district, in which 1 regional and 4 local hospitals served approximately 250,000 people. Perhaps if the other doctors and hospitals improved their treatment of diabetic patients, I might be able to concentrate on hematology again.

During 1976, several courses in the treatment of diabetes were arranged for local doctors. These were traditional and rather impersonal in structure, but attendance was very high. I also compiled a booklet on diabetic treatment, which was given to all district doctors.

I was pleased. The treatment of diabetes was to be improved and each doctor would take care of his own diabetic patients. I would no longer be 'responsible' for all diabetic problems and could return to my previous interest, hematology.

Then, what happened? More diabetic patients than ever were sent to me. My own suspicion was that what the doctors had remembered from the courses was: 'Diabetes ... Oh, Gjemdal knew something about that, didn't he?', and I was left with even more diabetic patients. Total failure! Two years had passed since I had been given the responsibility for the treatment of diabetes. I had tried to solve the problem on my own and the outcome had been one failure after another. However, this last failure was important for I finally understood that to succeed I needed help. Where could I find this help?

Norwegian hospitals, at that time, offered little or no organized treatments for diabetes, so I went on an educational trip to Steno Memorial Hospital in Copenhagen which specialized in diabetic treatments. My stay at the Steno Memorial Hospital totally changed my attitude towards diabetic patients and the treatment of the disease. I finally had had an opportunity to see a well-organized, diabetic program with specially trained nurses and a good outpatient department. Although I enjoyed talking with the doctors at the hospital, I derived most of my knowledge from the head nurse, the nurse for diabetics in the outpatient department, the dietician, and the chiropodist. It was a fantastic experience to participate in a well-organized team for diabetic treatment and to see cooperation of different members.

Soon I realized that in a large hospital one doctor alone is unable to handle the treatment of diabetes. The doctor can only work as part of a team. The same year, 1977, I took part in the symposium in Geneva on the education of diabetic patients. I realized that my problem was not unique, for others also found the treatment and education of diabetic patients problematic (see also 'Aims of the DESG', Chapter 2).

During the next 2 years our hospital employed a dietician. We established close cooperation with a local chiropodist and 3 of our nurses went on educational visits to 2 hospitals for diabetics in Copenhagen. However, it took 3 or 4 years for our hospital to get moving in the right direction. Why was that long period necessary?

I have since asked myself how the time could have been shortened so that we could have offered our diabetic patients proper treatment at a much earlier stage. I am sure that this problem is experienced by many of the doctors who have not been trained at a diabetic center. This frustrating problem I encountered is typical for a doctor who is working in a hospital without any background in treatments for diabetes. A doctor in this position who does not receive any help will be in danger of wasting as much time and energy in getting started as I did. The best help such a doctor could gain would be first-hand experience with a well-organized team trained in the treatments of diabetes. Only by seeing this him or herself, will the doctor understand the value of an experienced teaching nurse, dietician, and chiropodist working in close cooperation with the doctors. Therefore, I suggest that the Diabetes Education Study Group (DESG) should produce and maintain a current list of diabetic centers which would be open to educational visits from the people in the various medical disciplines concerned with diabetics. This list should be available to all hospitals in Europe.

Coming home after a study tour of a diabetic center can cause frustration. After seeing how a well-organized, adequately supplied diabetic team with good personnel can function, it is sad to return to an overfilled, busy, general hospital without a diabetic outpatient clinic or endocrinology unit.

Based on my own experience in this situation, I make the following suggestions in order of importance:

Employ a dietician and train a teaching nurse. The physician, dietician, and nurse must learn to work together. In the beginning they can meet the individual patient as a team. However, they must agree among themselves on the information to explain to the patients as well as their reasons for the choices to avoid confusion and misunderstandings for the patients. When routines are established, tasks can be divided among the members of the team.

After our diabetic team was established, various problems needed solving:
Training of medical personnel.
Instruction of earlier diagnosed diabetics.
Treatment and instruction of newly diagnosed diabetics.
Assumption of responsibility for treatment of diabetics with special problems.

## THE NORWEGIAN EXPERIENCE

These tasks were gradually accomplished by the following means:

### Training of medical personnel

Care of diabetics was concentrated on one ward in the medical department. The staff was given regular instructions on the subject of diabetes and its treatment and the same subject was often a theme during the twice weekly instructon sessions for physicians in the medical department.

A 2-day course on diabetes was arranged for general practitioners.

A 1½-day seminar on diabetes was held for nurses in children's centers and schools as well as for visiting nurses.

Diabetic teams were established at the 4 local hospitals in our district.

Instruction on diabetes has been given to 75 school teachers on 2 different occasions as part of in-service training.

A 25-page pamphlet on the treatment of diabetes was written and distributed to all doctors in our district. The second edition is now underway.

### Instruction of earlier diagnosed diabetics

We have held a series of short courses for various groups of diabetics: parents of diabetic children, teenagers, adults and older diabetics divided by insulin or non-insulin dependency. These short courses will be repeated at regular intervals. All newly diagnosed diabetics will also be included in this instruction.

We participate actively in the local diabetic patients' organization, both in the form of short lectures on various aspects of diabetes and its treatment and by conversation over a cup of coffee after the formal meeting. The latter gives patients themselves a better chance to communicate their particular concerns.

### Treatment of newly diagnosed diabetics

Newly diagnosed diabetics are instructed and treated individually by our diabetic team and, as much as possible, in an outpatient setting. Most of the older diabetics return to the care of their general practitioner, but the majority of insulin dependent diabetics continue under our care.

## Treatment of diabetics with special problems

It was not difficult to identify these patients. Some were referred by doctors outside the hospital and others approached members of the team directly.

## CONCLUSION

We have endeavored to increase knowledge about and interest in diabetes especially among medical personnel as well as patients and their families. The 'status' of diabetes has been improved by increased interest in the importance of well-coordinated treatment of diabetes. The individual patient seems to have benefited from our efforts.

## SUMMARY

This article is my personal account as a hematologist in the internal medicine department of a large, regional, general hospital in Norway. I was 'forced', by default, to be in charge of all diabetic patient treatment because the other 4 senior physicians voted me into the position against my will. This new, unwanted responsibility was followed by my attempts at self-education through reading; training local doctors to improve their treatment of diabetes; seeking concrete help by visiting a well-established, diabetic treatment program; and applying the information gained in my own hospital. This article expresses my doubts, frustrations, considerations, and results during and after 3 years of various levels of failures and success.

# 37.   A general practitioner's teaching therapy in a semi-rural Swiss area. A personal experience with diabetes

C. DANTHE

## EDITORIAL

*At the request of the editors, the author of this article presents his personal experience as a general practitioner who discoverd, in a semi-rural area of Switzerland, the need for a teaching therapy for diabetic patients. His increasing realization of the difficulties in reaching a clear understanding of how to plan and create such a medical teaching program followed. Too often medical papers only deal with final achievements. This paper, however, takes the reader through the various stages in planning and executing a practical, diabetic educational program.*

*The simultaneous presence of problems on 3 levels: (1) the true, organic health disturbance, (2) the weight of the psycho-social burden of the disease, and (3) the complexity of the educational aspects, makes a comprehensive, therapeutical approach to diabetes very difficult. The complexity of the total situation, without the needed exchange of ideas among doctors for possible solutions, often results in discouragements and failures of such teaching attempts.*

*The article of Dr. Danthe, as well as that of Dr. Gjemdal, is a remarkable illustration of the personal motivation, thoughts, doubts, and integration into action of physicians who seriously want to improve the medical control of a disease as well as the psycho-social well-being of the patient. These articles outline a one-man progressive development and application of a new medical dimension for active therapy.(The editors.)*

My medical office is situated in the mountainous Swiss area of the Jura at an altitude of 700 meters. The area is semi-rural and the nearest university is 40 km away. The population with which I work includes about 3,800 people who live in 2 villages which are situated approximately 5 km from each other. There are 3,000 people in one village and 800 in the other. Most of the inhabitants are workers, craftsmen, and small shopkeepers; a few are farmers. Few of these are either needy or belong to the aristocracy.

There were and still are 2 colleagues working full time in the area. Before my arrival in 1977 as general practitioner, my previous training had been in medicine, gynecology, psychiatry, surgery, and obstetrics. I was given a warm welcome both by my 2 colleagues and by the general population.

After a few months of practice, an important problem began to emerge. In the evening while going over the files of a series of diabetics, I was often struck by the gap that existed between the requirements for a well-conducted and efficient treatment and the actual results shown by high blood glucose values. The medical norms contrasted with the results I had before me. My patients may have been satisfied; I was not.

## IMPULSE

At that point I was faced with various areas of deep frustration from the comparison of my own ideas of what medical care in the area should be to the reality of what it actually was. Some of my most complexing concerns were as follows:
- being unable to explain the minimal scientific facts to guide effectively the patient in the management of diabetes;
- not having enough time to educate patients or not knowing if the time used was lost by incompetence;
- being faced with the impossibility of modifying behavior that might be detrimental to the health of certain patients;
- being unable to design or cook an attractive, varied diet which would appeal to patients as well as meet nutritional and dietary requirements;
- being ill-equipped to deal with the emotional circumstances which are the sources of so much overweight and uncontrolled diabetes.

The following example of one of my patients is an illustration of emotional problems leading to loss of diabetic control.

A 40 year old man takes up a managerial job in the area because of a job promotion. His family doctor refers him to me with the diagnosis of 'diabetes mellitus with a slight alcohol problem'. Instead of professional success for this man in the new job, there is failure. For the first time he is faced with his real personal problem which until then had been hidden: the inability to assert himself. He loses his diet control, steps up his alcohol intake and puts on 18 kilos in 6 months. His consequent loss of self-esteem brings a latent marital problem to the surface, exacerbated by the children being of an age to leave home. He loses the boss's confidence and is discredited in the firm's hierarchy. He progressively becomes an invalid.

This case illustrates the actual limits of the doctor's powers in a situation that is vital for his patient. There was frustration in the face of the patient's solitude as well as my own.

As a general practitioner I am faced with all the other diseases and problems, other than diabetes, of all my other patients. Even though we are in a semi-rural area, many of these patients suffer from psychosomatic problems which are expressed by functional disorders (palpitations, chest pains, stomach-ache, constipation, diarrhea, etc.). Other patients complain of sleep and anxiety problems, which gradually lead to the over-use of tranquilizers.

Over a period of several months I drew up a list of patients who would benefit from the self-relaxation technique called 'Schultz Autogenous Training'. Patients were questioned as to their willingness to attend an information seminar about this method of relaxation with the intention of forming groups to learn this technique.

I sent out invitations to the patients who showed interest in this relaxation course and then my wife and I re-read the literature about autogenous training. I had had 4 years' experience in this technique and in group therapy methods. Two groups were formed and the experiment proved a success. It improved not only the symptoms, but, as a by-product, provided personal serenity for both the patients and the therapist.

WHY NOT?

The positive experience of these relaxation groups suggested some connection between the pressing problems of chronic diseases in general and diabetes in particular. During a meeting on general medicine, I mentioned my intention to begin a group-teaching project for diabetics and was so much encouraged by a local diabetologist that it gave me the necessary impetus to put the project into practice.

The following professional experience significantly encouraged me to organize my first diabetic teaching team:

My practice took me to the bedside of a wealthy mother going through a nervous breakdown. For years she had been pursued by feelings of failure because of her diabetic son whom she over-protected and pampered. The psycho-sociological development of this young man had brought her into contact with the most qualified specialists in diabetes and mental illnesses. Her son, however, in spite of all professional help, continued to reject his condition and covered his mother with reproach. One day, the son died. He had been alone in a miserable one-room flat where he was discovered only 2 days afterwards. The water tap was still running ...

This tragic event was the deciding factor in my search towards a more rigorously structured approach to the education of diabetics.

Learning all that was possible, I visited several training centers for the out-patient care of diabetics. It became evident that the needs and problems of the diabetics at each center should be tabulated. I enlisted the help of

311

the district nurse, who is a nun specialized in home care, trained in group therapy methods, and very open to new ideas. She had a good understanding of the population from her personal observation of their living conditions and had made a list of those diabetics whom she thought would benefit from such a teaching method. I contacted, by letter, my colleagues who accepted the principle of this course for patients.

Having the moral support of my colleagues to launch a patient education program, I needed financial help. After the death of the young man whom I have just described, I was able to build up a deep relationship with his father, whose previous attitude had been somewhat distant. He introduced me to a private institution that gave me the necessary financial backing to set up a medical teaching unit in a social services building.

The district nurse and her substitute, together with the management committee of this institution, solicited financial participation in the project through the local press. Health league personalities were also interested and their local branch helped by donating teaching aids. I also informed the Samaritans League and the local Red Cross branch of the project. My primary aim was to encourage everybody to cooperate, while respecting their individual identities. Much to my surprise, everything seemed to work out right. To the call for help, there were 430 replies from the 3800 inhabitants.

Having financial support and professional approval, I now concentrated on organizing and planning a group established to work out various public health problems. The district nurse, her 2 assistant nurses and I continued our own brain-storming sessions. My laboratory assistant and my secretary pitched in to help. My wife has always backed me both with interest and understanding.

In my consultations with patients, I asked several diabetics the same question: 'If a group therapy class in diabetes was organized with practical exercises and discussions, would you be willing to take part?' Once again there was positive feedback. The next step was to write to my colleagues for a list of diabetics to whom they could recommend this type of instruction. A list of about 20 patients was drawn up from the 3 practices which would amply suffice for a first teaching and training programme.

## THE HYPOTHESIS OF A TECHNIQUE

The group of 20 diabetics on the list, advised by their own doctors and in answer to my invitation, would have to agree to a contract, accepted by themselves and the teacher/therapists, to attend and actively participate in a series of 12 sessions in 6 months. The patients would not stop seeing their personal doctors during this period. Routine visits to their doctors would be separate from the commitment to the group. Each patient's personal physician would receive a treatment report at the beginning and at the end of the course.

The 20 diabetics following this course would have to fast when coming to a morning meeting every 2 weeks for 6 months. They would be welcomed by a trained team (nurses aides, nurses, laboratory-assistant, secretary, and doctor). On arrival, their diabetes would be checked by a rapid quantative analysis method and weight measurement. Findings would be kept in a special group file. During breakfast together, there would be a 15 minute theory class to define the minimal cognitive and behavioral objectives of the treatment.

This brief session would be followed by practical exercises including various measurements, the manipulation of insulin, and meal planning. The method used would follow both the principles of active teaching and self-evaluation.

The group time would end with an open-discussion session about treatment and general problems relating to diabetes. In the course of the 12 sessions, each participant would keep a note book to record personal observations as well as a short duplicated summary of the teaching and group experience from the previous sessions.

## PLANNING OF THE COURSE

The study of the instructional methods used in other educational centers for diabetic patients in Amsterdam, Basel, Geneva, Lausanne, and Paris provided the models to establish my teaching program for patients. The following is an example of the content and the evaluation of the first lesson. The key words and basic knowledge which had to be provided to patients are as follows:

1. Where can sugar be found?
2. Sugar is equal to carbohydrates/glucose.
3. The sugar content of your diet is fundamental. The sugars, called carbohydrates, are transformed into glucose in the body.
4. The sugar concentration in the blood is also called the sugar level, or 'glycemia'.
5. An adult weighing 70 kilos has an average of 5 liters of blood. His 'glycemia' before eating in the morning is the equivalent of 1 lump of sugar in 5 liters of blood or 1 gr of sugar per liter, or 100 mg per 100 ml. This is the normal sugar level which we call 'normal glycemia'. It varies from one person to another between 70 mg/100 ml and 110 mg/100 ml.

*C. Danthe*

**Materials used for the course**

A list of foods, a card game representing different foods, 4 solutions of known glucose content and strips for semi-quantitative glucose determination.

**Evaluation of the course will include**

A. 1. What does the food we eat contain?
   2. What term is used to signify sugars?
   3. What are the essential elements for a diabetic's diet?
   4. The food containing carbohydrates is transformed into what in the blood?
   5. What is the term for the sugar content of the blood?
   6. How many mg of sugar per 100 ml of blood is a normal level of glucose in blood before eating in the morning?
B. *Testing food recognition*
   In an individually determined time limit, each person will sort cards representing different foods into the following groups according to the personal diet of that individual: (a) the foods he or she can use freely, (b) the foods to be measured, and (c) the foods only to be used in exactly measured quatities.
C. *Conducting practical glucose testing*
   Each participant will arrange from left to right the following solutions according to their glucose content: distilled water, 80 mg/100 ml, 180 mg/100 ml, and 250 mg/100 ml.
D. *Personal blood glucose levels* will be determined with the same testing technique and the result of the glucemia noted in the periodic check-up, either with the doctor or in the group, will be recorded in a special notebook.

THE PEGBOARD PUPPET

We designed a visual aid game to teach patients to understand physiological variations in blood glucose. The board or 'pegboard puppet' (Fig. 1) is divided into areas which represent the intestine, the circulatory system, the liver, the brain, muscles, and adipose tissue. The pegs represent glucose. The pancreas holds rings which represent insulin.

To play the game, the patient moves the glucose pegs from either the liver or the intestine. The glucose pegs can be easily moved through entrances to the brain without the need of the rings representing insulin. Or the contrary, the glucose pegs can be moved to the muscles or adipose tissue over barriers which can be crossed only when insulin rings released from the pancreas are placed on the glucose pegs. The purpose of this game

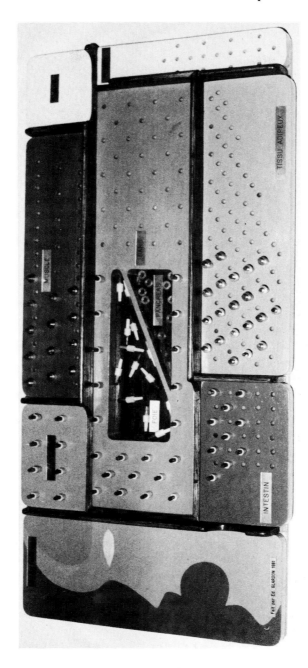

Fig. 1   The PEGBOARD PUPPET.

is to develop in the patient the understanding of the role of the pancreas and insulin as an agent to move glucose into muscles and adipose tissue.

Each patient receives a number of insulin rings according to his individual insulin dependency. As the puppet receives more food, the number of glucose pegs increases in the blood. The glucose pegs can flow freely to the brain until the brain section is filled, at which time the surplus pegs begin to fill the center or blood section. When the blood section is full of glucose pegs, the overflow 'spills' into a urine area because there is lack of insulin rings. Only by the use of the insulin rings can the patient move glucose from blood into muscle and adipose tissue.

The following is an example of the type of instructions that would be given to only 1 of the 4 or 5 patients playing 'The Puppet' during one session of the game: 'In this game you are the glucose (glycogen) pool in the liver. The section of the board directly in front of you represents the blood circulation. When the holes in this section become free, you fill them with your pegs which represent the glucose from the liver'.

Gradually each player restores the normal physiological balance of the puppet, only to have the doctor step in and upset this balance either by increasing or decreasing the values attributed to the pegs (the glucose) or the rings (the insulin) in one or another section of the puppet. Using the game and their own personal control notebook, each patient can have visual understanding of his or her various metabolic events and the effects of food and insulin. The positions in the puppet have to be managed by the diabetic himself according to his particular needs. The game has an experiental value and encourages the idea of personal diabetes in which each patient identifies the action in the puppet with his or her own system.

The emotional problems and difficulties in the treatments will be expressed and considered in a group discussion situation. The process of the acceptation of the illness and its treatment will be discussed with the therapists (see also Chapter 26).

## NEED FOR TRAINING THE MEDICAL TEAM

Such a complex teaching program could not be started without carefully trained collaborators. This has been done outside working hours in different training sessions.

## THE OPPOSITIONS

As soon as the project was known, opposition came from almost everywhere. First from the district nurse whose initial enthusiasm gave way to doubt because of the time required. However, this conflict produced a clarification of the status and role of each of the therapists.

Opposition came from the janitor of the building where the medical teaching unit was located. The dust and the noise from the transformation of the premises, coupled with the thought that people would occupy the previously rarely used rooms, represented change and extra work for her. Thoughtlessly, she spread pessimistic stories with decidedly negative results. Developing an acute backache problem, she came to me for a consultation, which also gave us the opportunity to discuss the problems generated by the teaching centre.

The insurance companies showed no interest in making the treatment elegible for insurance benefits. Their typical reply to payment inquiries was that 'Patient Education' was not mentioned anywhere in the administrative regulations concerning medical treatment.

I even became aware of conflict within myself. To take on the risk, to set the ball rolling, cannot be done lightly without some moments of great self-doubt. If I abandoned this project to go back to my old medical routine, would it not be tantamount to allowing the diabetes to overcome both myself and the diabetic?

## CONCLUSIONS

As a general practitioner, the difficulties experienced in treating diabetics have forced me to develop and combine educational and medical principles to ensure patients an understanding of their own treatment. Concrete learning experiences along with group dynamics helped me to reach the multi-dimensional aspects of the disease. These methods enabled me to discover a new dimension and interest in the treatment of diabetes as well as in other fields of my general practice, even though the difficulties were and are still great.

## POST SCRIPTUM

The above mentioned program for patient education has been completed. The first training session for diabetics has given positive results. Ten patients, aged 24 to 80, and 2 of their spouses, participated in the group sessions which were held twice monthly during 6 months. Half of the group was insulin-dependent. During this period we were able to achieve a weight loss of about 3 to 4 kg for the patients who had to lose weight. Except for 1 patient, HbA1C fell by about 25% at the end of the course when compared with the values obtained at the beginning of the training programme. These values as well as weight loss remained stable or even improved 5 months after the end of the course. Medical visits could be held at greater intervals; it was much easier for the physician to discuss diabetic problems with the patients thanks to their clearer understanding of the disease. Less time had to be spent on management of diabetic problems during the medical visit. The impression of these patients has been definitively favorable towards this type of training approach which gave less information in a given period and where repetition was part of its methodological approach.

For my medical team this experience was also well accepted and I could observe that the attitude of my collaborators towards diabetes was radically modified after these group sessions.

## SUMMARY

This article describes my personal experience in diabetic patients' education. I am a general practitioner working in a semi-rural area of the French-speaking part of Switzerland. Two other physicians and I share the medical care of the 4,000 inhabitants.

The methods used for patient education in my ambulatory clinic are group dynamics as well as active learning techniques. One concrete example of how theory is translated into practice is by asking patients to interact with a 'peg-board puppet'. The design of this program and its application gradually led me to discover a more active, interesting, and integrated way of treating patients.

## SUGGESTED READING

1. Luthe, E.W. and Schultz, J.H. (1969/1973): *Autogenic Methods*. Grune & Stratton. M8.272-232-240-288-368-441 (6 Vol.).
2. Gfeller, R. and Assal, J.-Ph. (1979): Le vécu du malade diabétique. In: *Folia psychopractica*, Hoffmann-La Roche.
3. Gfeller, R. and Assal, J.-Ph. (1979): Une expérience pilote en diabétologie clinique et en psychologie médicale: l'unité de traitement et d'enseignement pour diabétiques de l'hôpital cantonal de Genève. *Méd. Hyg.*, *37*, 2966.
4. Kubler-Ross, E. (1969): *On Death and Dying*. Mac Millan, New York.
5. Ruchti-Grabowska, M.-J. (1979): Psychothérapie dans le traitement des diabétiques. *Méd. Hyg.*, *37*, 1421.
6. Curchod, B. (1979): Remarques sur la pédagogie du diabétique. *Rev. Med. Suisse Romade*, *99*, 415.
7. Berger, W. and Staffelbach, O. (1980): Bale. Thérapie de groupe des diabétiques. Une aide dans le traitement et la maîtrise du diabète sucré. *Méd. Hyg.*, *38*, 3442.

# 38.  The emancipated diabetic patient

I. MÜHLHAUSER, A. KUNZ AND W. GRANINGER

## EDITORIAL

*This last paper represents not only the hopes of the editors, but also those of doctors, nurses, dieticians, psychologists, social workers, etc., as well as the hopes of the millions of diabetics themselves. The many meanings of the term 'emancipated' include 'mature', 'independent', 'autonomous' and 'responsible'. This term thus represents the general objective for which health-care providers and patients strive: a better quality of life.*

*The goals implicit in the word 'emancipated' cannot be attained without short-term objectives, which often are rather tedious (such as daily blood and urine controls, injections, dietary adherence, etc.). In a real adult-to-adult relationship between doctor and patient, the patient's emancipation can only occur if the health-care provider is himself a mature, responsible and autonomous person who accepts losing part of his classical medical identity. Medical efficiency in treating chronic diseases goes hand in hand with the abandon of the traditional attitude of health-care providers, in favor of one promoting a dialogue with, and encouraging the independence of patients. Improvement in the quality of the diabetic's life is not the result of better metabolic control alone: it also requires increased understanding of diabetes as well as a better psychological acceptation of the disaese. Attainment of these goals is a real challenge for the medical team. (The editors.)*

## PROLOG

*Tipo de medico educador [1]*

- humilde y compasivo, vea a los demas como iguales
- esta dispuesto a enseñar y a aprender de los que lo rodean, compartiendo sus conocimientos y sus responsabilidades
- esta dispuesto a trabajar con la gente, a ayudarlos a mirar al futuro y asi frenar la enfermedad antes que comience
- determine prioridades al canalizar los rescursos disponibles, humanos y non humanos, de mañera que rindan el mayor beneficio al mayor numero de personas
- esta dispuesto a trabajar por honorarios mas justos, cuya recompensa no resida en ganacias monetarias sino en la alegria de preocuparse por y de compartir con otra gente.

319

The eventual aim of diabetes education must be to give the diabetic patient the means of living as normal a life as possible, despite his chronic disease. A patient who does not know how to monitor his blood glucose level and, if necessary, to adapt his insulin dosage in time in order to maintain normoglycemia, will never be able to attain this goal.

In any case, a diabetic must be a trained diabetic; that is, one who is prepared to take over the responsibility for monitoring and treating his condition himself. Therefore the basic aim of diabetes education must at the very least be the effective training of the diabetic patient in every day management.

However, since it is extremely difficult to bring successfully under control a disease which entails so many restrictions in so many areas of life, it is not enough merely to master the immediate every day necessities. More than that, it presupposes a mode of thought and behavior in the patient, which will also enable him to cope efficiently with problems which do not occur every day. The highest aim of diabetes education is helping the patient to develop in this direction. We would like to characterize this type of diabetic as 'emancipated'*. Generally speaking, as a human being this ideal patient will also have developed a critical, self-confident and responsible attitude towards society. The following article is an attempt to describe him in terms of his relationship to his doctors and social institutions.

## RELATION TO THE DIABETES TRAINING CENTRE

What the emancipated patient surely expects from his diabetes training centre is advice in situations he is not able to cope with by himself. For example, he might come to his diabetes training centre having realized that, in spite of doing his best, he is having no success in keeping his glucose levels within the desired range. On many other occasions he will come merely for extra information, for instance about new sorts of food or drugs or new principles of therapy he might have heard of.

It might thus occur that a patient reads an article in a newspaper with the headline 'Acarbose instead of Insulin' (as reported in 'Bild am Sonntag', 25th September, 1981). Having developed a critical point of view towards this type of unresponsible reporting, he will try to obtain information about the proven effects of it before deciding whether or not to test it.

Sometimes a diabetic patient will also expect immediate around-the-clock advice and help from his training centre. Such situations could be acute or severe problems related to his disease, for example unsureness when faced with the necessity of altering his insulin dosage to an unusual extent.

Undoubtedly, the emancipated patient expects to be treated by his train-

*The word 'emancipated' must serve as a translation for the German 'mündig', an expression with a rather wide meaning, also standing for mature, independent, autonomous and responsible.

ing centre not as a 'petitioner', but as a partner on an equal footing. He therefore expects that the people responsible for his training at the centre will abdicate the traditionally dominant role played by the doctor in the conventional doctor-patient relationship.

In spite of all these justified demands, the emancipated diabetic does not remain in a passive 'consumer' attitude towards his training centre. He should rather be prepared himself to bear a large part of the social responsibility independently. This starts with the emancipated patient's relaying his own experiences, observations and suggestions to the training centre. In doing so, he will be aiding the centre to collect information which it could otherwise only obtain with difficulty and over a long period of time. This would not only concern matters such as metabolic control or further training of patients, but also, for example, observations on changes in the attitudes of various institutions (health insurance institutions, employment offices, the media) towards diabetics.

A diabetic patient expects as a matter of course to be able to rely on his training centre acting responsibly; this means above all that the doctors at the centre should not work for their own, purely personal career-oriented goals, especially with regard to research. They should be aware of their responsibility to use their knowledge and ability, as well as public and institutional means, primarily for the good of the patient, thereby meeting their public and social obligations.

The emancipated patient will, however, be fully aware of the fact that this situation will be more readily achieved if the patients themselves participate actively in the work at their training centre. To give a concrete example: in training centres which perform clinical studies on diabetes, for instance university hospitals, patients will demand the right to take part in deciding which clinical trials should be performed, depending on the evaluation of their practical relevance. The diabetic will of course insist on being thoroughly informed about the results of these studies, as well as about the consequences these results might have for him and his peers. To achieve this, the diabetic might aim at taking part in ethical committees, or, if none exist, they might found a patients' representation committee at their training centre.

## RELATION TO THE GENERAL PRACTITIONER

In the patient's relation to the general practitioner, we have to differentiate between 2 eventualities. In the first case, the diabetic meets a general practitioner who is not specialized in diabetes and is not used to taking care of trained diabetics, but who is the only doctor available in the area.

The emancipated patient is aware of this and accepts that not every general practitioner will also be a diabetologist, but he will try to be acknowledged by his doctor as a trained and emancipated diabetic with all the consequences that this fact might imply: for example, he will insist on obtaining the prescriptions which are necessary for the self-management of his condition; furthermore he will make sure that his doctor will not insist on hospitalization when it is simply a case of failure in management leading to a severe hypoglycemic reaction; if his doctor recommends hospitalization merely to improve diabetes control or taking a *Kur* at a diabetes rehabilitation centre every few years, an emancipated diabetic would reject these recommendations and try to convince his doctor that these are neither adequate nor useful methods for achieving or maintaining good metabolic control. On the other hand, the emancipated diabetic patient who realizes that, in spite of trying his best, he cannot sufficiently succeed in keeping his blood glucose levels within the desired range, will make sure that his doctor refers him to a more competent institution, for example, a diabetologist or a diabetes centre.

In the second case, the diabetic finds a general practitioner who is specialized in diabetes, or he visits a specialized outpatient unit. Here the relation of the diabetic to his doctor or outpatient unit would be comparable to his relation to a diabetic training centre.

In either case, the emancipated diabetic reminds his doctor of, and if necessary insists on, the regularly needed check-ups on blood pressure, blood lipids, kidney function, ECG, eyes, etc., about which he has been taught at the diabetes training course.

His relationship to his general practitioner will be determined by the degree of his emancipation, for whatever reason he is consulting him. He regards his doctor not as an oracle, but as a source of competent information, on the basis of which he can make informed decisions. For example, an educated patient will know of all the possible methods of birth control and how to use them. She/he will know the possible side-effects of different contraceptive methods and will know which methods are preferable for her/him, especially in relation to his/her condition. However, while taking this knowledge into account, the emancipated diabetic woman might temporarily consider choosing a contraceptive method less suitable for her condition, if it were more convenient for her personal situation. The diabetic woman will be aware of the difficulties which she could have to face in trying to obtain the contraceptive method of her choice as one aspect of a problem frequently encountered by women in general. Thus, if a diabetic woman fails to obtain the necessary prescription for the contraceptive method of her choice from her doctor or gynecologist, she will consult other doctors. If a woman decides to take the pill for some time, she will make sure that her doctor regularly monitors her blood pressure, blood lipids, parameters of liver function etc.

Since an educated diabetic has been informed about the mode of diabetes inheritance and the possible risks of diabetic pregnancy for both mother and child, she will, bearing all those factors in mind, be prepared to take over responsibility for deciding whether to become pregnant or not. The emancipated diabetic woman will therefore forgo having a child if her doctor believes that the resultant risk would seriously endanger her health. Should she, however, not find his arguments sufficiently convincing, she will consult another doctor for a second opinion as well. In this case she will be quite aware that neither her doctor nor anybody else has the right to advise her against becoming pregnant merely because of the possibility of transmitting the disease to future generations. The emancipated diabetic woman will thus of course reject sterilization or abortion if it has been recommended only on these grounds.

A diabetic woman who intends to become pregnant makes sure that her doctor refers her in good time to an adequate centre which is able to treat her appropriately before, during and after pregnancy. In the case of there being no diabetes centre specialized in the pregnancy and delivery of diabetic women, the pregnant diabetic will insist on close cooperation between her diabetes doctor, her obstetrician and the pediatrician.

## RELATION TO UNFAMILIAR HOSPITALS AND DOCTORS

Should the emancipated diabetic have to be hospitalized because of another, additional illness, for example for an operation, or in the case of an infectious disease, he will make sure that he can continue to manage his diabetes himself during his stay in hospital, i.e., he does not necessarily have to relinquish this reponsibility. If a hospitalization is already foreseen, an emancipated patient will contact the hospital in due time, in order to discuss with the doctors and nurses his conception of how the diabetes treatment should be organized.

The emancipated diabetic will expect and if necessary insist on having facilities to monitor his metabolism himself, or if the necessary monitoring is done for him, that he is given the results in time, should he for reasons of health be unable to perform the required tests himself. He will also expect and again insist that his dietary needs will be taken into account when the meals are planned, and that he can at least take part in fixing the level of his insulin dosage every day. He will also expect to be informed if he is given medicaments or therapy which could have effects on his metabolic balance [2, 3]. Should he be unable to achieve one or another of these aims for reasons of hospital administration and believes his metabolic balance thereby to be endangered, the emancipated diabetic will seek to realize these aims by contacting his training centre or perhaps by getting his relatives or friends to intervene. If an operation, narcosis or long-term restriction of his mental faculties or physical mobility can be planned in good time beforehand, the emancipated diabetic will find out who will be regulating his metabolism during this time and how this regulation will be performed. In certain specific situations, for instance long, difficult operations, or the delivery of a diabetic woman, the emancipated diabetic will insist on a diabetologist's being called in. On the other hand, it is surely a mark of emancipation when the educated diabetic is prepared to make compromises where the requirements of hospital organization are concerned. The limits of the diabetic's readiness to compromise, whether it concerns the times of meals, the exchange of carbohydrate groups or methods of monitoring the metabolism, should be set where his metabolic balance would otherwise deteriorate.

When the treatment for the illness which made hospitalization necessary in the first place is terminated and the doctors concerned keep the patient in hospital merely because the regulation of his diabetes is not yet optimal, the emancipated diabetic will discharge himself, if necessary against the advice of the doctors concerned.


OBTAINING INFORMATION

The emancipated diabetic patient knows where and how to obtain material which will help him to increase his knowledge of his disease. However, he will also be aware of the importance of knowing where certain information comes from, and that even specialist literature must be reviewed critically, since it is not always innocent of commercial interest, nor is it necessarily uninfluenced by the authors' personal goals.

The emancipated patient will also make sure that he has access to any literature on diabetes that could possibly be of interest to him, whether it be publications from pharmaceutical firms, scientific journals or other sources. He will definitely not accept the idea that there is any sort of 'literature for the privileged few' that could be withheld from him on the grounds of its presumed unintelligibility for him.


ATTITUDE TO NEW THERAPEUTIC PRINCIPLES AND PARAMEDICAL THERAPIES

Should the emancipated patient hear of new forms of therapy or of new therapeutic aids, he will know where he can obtain exact and objective information on them. Once he has obtained it, he will be able to evaluate the advantages and disadvantages of a new therapy (such as the insulin pump treatment in its present form) in relation to his personal situation. He knows that as long as good metabolic control is maintained, he may try out any of these remedies either to adopt it if it helps him or to reject it if it does not.

Furthermore, the emancipated patient evaluates advertisements for foods claiming to have beneficial effects on his metabolism, or he will at least consult different people on this subject. He knows that his condition does not indicate the use of special 'diabetic food', but nevertheless, should he want to eat such food, he does so under regular metabolic self-monitoring. The same is also valid for drugs, of which is frequently maintained in the media that they improve metabolic control and reduce the insulin requirement, or even replace it altogether.

The emancipated patient will also have a critical attitude towards forms of therapy which have not yet found acceptance in orthodox medicine. Should he decide to try out these methods of treatment, he will do so under strict monitoring of his blood glucose. In addition, the emancipated diabetic has learned to evaluate advice concerning problems of health which have not yet been generally resolved, for example, the possibly beneficial effects of regular exercise on prolonging life, especially concerning regular exercise as a part of his diabetes therapy.

## SOCIO-ECONOMIC PROBLEMS

The emancipated diabetic patient is aware, firstly, of the difficulty of achieving and maintaining metabolic balance under certain work conditions, and secondly, that there are also jobs where, if he were to practice them, he would be endangering not only himself but others as well. He will not consider himself eligible for such jobs.

The situation will be totally different, however, if a diabetic is forced to assume that, although he could perform a job perfectly well, he would not be given the position if the employer knew that he was a diabetic. In this case, the diabetic has no alternative but to conceal his condition. Thus, he is effectively deprived of the opportunity to act as an emancipated individual right from the beginning.

If a person should become diabetic while employed in a job unsuitable for diabetics, he would as an emancipated patient use every opportunity for job retraining.

The emancipated diabetic patient accepts that because of his illness, he is sometimes not capable of functioning as efficiently or bearing as great a degree of stress as someone who is non-diabetic, and that in certain circumstances he must reckon with special assistance and support from the world around him. On the other hand he will make sure that he does not exploit society unduly. That goes not only for claiming the legally provided advantages which a registered disability brings with it, but also for claiming sick leave and paid visits to health resorts. It is, however, a mark of emancipation when a diabetic claims the assistance that he needs and is entitled to, for example, the financing of self-monitoring materials through his health insurance. Moreover, the emancipated diabetic acts not as a petitioner, but as a partner on equal terms when dealing with institutions such as social insurance, the employment office, etc.

## SELF-HELP GROUPS

The emancipated diabetic patient will have heard of the existence and objectives of self-help groups or diabetic lay organizations. He will decide to participate in such a group if, by doing so, he sees a possibility of effectively solving his own problems and those of others. The emancipated diabetic will also see in a self-help group the opportunity of safeguarding his interests concerning the health and social security system.

The emancipated diabetic will also evaluate self-help groups under another criterion: as a rule, he will often enough have experienced the limits of the opportunities he has as an individual to achieve or maintain emancipation in relation to his illness or his position as a patient. He will thus see the essential significance of a self-help group as lying in the function such a group could have within general social structures. Such groups could for example bring the public's attention to the difficulties a diabetic has to reckon with when looking for work, and to the fact that there is often discrimination against a minority which is in any case at a bad disadvantage. In addition, self-help groups could bring pressure to bear on medical boards if there were no doctor available in the area who possessed sufficient knowledge about the care of educated diabetics.

## EPILOG

As mentioned in the introduction, one should consider that for any patient there is a degree of emancipation as a human being in general and in addition a specific process of emancipation with regard to his being a diabetic.

For those individuals who have not yet attained their highest subjectively possible degree of emancipation, appropriate diabetes teaching programs help them to emancipate themselves both as human beings and as diabetic patients. For those patients who have already reached this objective in general and not just as a diabetic, they should be instrumental in helping them to preserve this rate of mind and mode of behavior in relation to their illness and their situation as a patient.

Optimal training therefore presupposes that the diabetes teacher is himself sufficiently emancipated to be fully aware of these interactions. A teacher who is not aware of this will at best give the diabetic the knowledge which is the basic requirement for him to be in a position to emancipate himself as a diabetic patient. On the other hand, any good diabetes teacher will also be aiding the diabetic patient in his efforts to come to terms to the greatest possible degree of emancipation with the difficulties arising from his illness.

In conclusion, the less emancipated the patient, the more emancipated the teacher must be. However, the more emancipated the patient is, the less emancipated the teacher may be without doing any harm to the patient. This seems to us to be a valid principle for any system of information and education.

## ACKNOWLEDGEMENTS

The authors wish to express their deep gratitude to Ms. Sophie Kidd B.A. (Hons) for her expert help in translating this manuscript. Furthermore, we would like to thank all our patients who participated in discussions leading to the formulation of this review.

## REFERENCES

1. Morley, D., *Prioridades en la Salud Infantil.* Editorial Pax Mexico.
2. Travis, L.B., Hürter, P. (1980): *Einführungskurs für Kinder und Jugendliche mit Diabetes Mellitus.* Gerhards & Co Verlag OHG, Frankfurt.
3. Rusting, R. (1981): In the hospital. *Diabetes Forecast, 34,* 18.

# Author index